T0205855

# Nutrition for Brain Health and Cognitive Performance

. . . . . . . . . . . . . . . . . . . . . . .

# NUTRITION FOR BRAIN HEALTH AND COGNITIVE PERFORMANCE

Edited by

**TALITHA BEST**
School of Human Health and Social Science
Central Queensland University
Australia

**LOUISE DYE**
School of Psychology
University of Leeds
United Kingdom

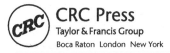

CRC Press
Taylor & Francis Group
Boca Raton London New York

CRC Press is an imprint of the
Taylor & Francis Group, an **informa** business

CRC Press
Taylor & Francis Group
6000 Broken Sound Parkway NW, Suite 300
Boca Raton, FL 33487-2742

First issued in paperback 2021

© 2015 by Taylor & Francis Group, LLC
CRC Press is an imprint of Taylor & Francis Group, an Informa business

No claim to original U.S. Government works

Version Date: 20150430

ISBN 13: 978-1-03-209857-9 (pbk)
ISBN 13: 978-1-4665-7002-3 (hbk)

**Visit the Taylor & Francis Web site at
http://www.taylorandfrancis.com**

**and the CRC Press Web site at
http://www.crcpress.com**

Publisher's Note
The publisher has gone to great lengths to ensure the quality of this reprint but points out that some imperfections in the original copies may be apparent.

*Dedicated to my dad, Robert Dye, who died before I could show it to him and who I miss everyday*

**Louise Dye**

*Dedicated to my family who inspire me with their commitment to share their lives with others*

**Talitha Best**

# Contents

## SECTION I    Big Picture: Nutrition for Brain Health

## SECTION II    Process and Methods for Measuring Brain Function and Cognition

# SECTION III   The Story So Far: Foods and Nutrition for Performance across the Lifespan

# SECTION IV   Technology and Brain Function

# Preface

This book critically reviews the evidence surrounding the impact of dietary patterns and nutrition on brain function and cognitive performance and the mechanisms which underpin this. The increase in public awareness of the role diet can play in brain function has been accompanied by a significant development of products, dietary supplements, functional foods, nutraceuticals, food programs and submissions of dossiers for health claims and public health recommendations for maintaining brain function. The area of nutrition–cognition research is an emerging interdisciplinary field of work that examines the impact of food, nutrients and diet on everyday aspects of cognitive performance and brain function. It is our hope that this book serves its purpose: to make available a detailed and innovative scientific summary of nutrition–cognition research to provide valuable information regarding nutritional and lifestyle choices for cognitive health.

We have purposefully sought to balance rigorous scientific information and analysis, with information for readers who are 'non-experts'. We have sought out contributions from internationally recognised scholars alongside the next generation of researchers to provide accessible, up-to-date reviews that consider the impact of dietary patterns, nutritional components, methods of assessment and technology and the underpinning physiological processes to support brain health and performance. This book is appropriate for health professionals, researchers, teachers, educators, health service providers, food and nutraceutical industry personnel, nutritionists, dietitians, psychologists and psychiatrists, public health workers and the general public. We trust it will serve as a valuable resource for your research, teaching and client support.

We offer our appreciation and thanks to the authors of each chapter for their thoughtful and skillful contributions. Their time, expertise and willingness to support this project to equip others with up-to-date information in this broad, multi-disciplinary field of cognition and nutrition is greatly valued.

Look out for the recommendations and summary boxes throughout the book that provide a summary of the key points to take away from the chapters that we hope support you in your life-long learning.

May your food choice promote a cognitively healthy life.

**Talitha Best**
**Louise Dye**

# Editors

**Talitha Best** is a researcher, practicing psychologist and lecturer with a passion for solution-oriented thinking and process innovation. Dr. Best addresses critical innovation related to translation of research into workable solutions for researchers, practitioners and industry in the areas of nutrition, food systems and products, brain function and cognitive performance.

Dr. Best received her PhD in clinical psychology and nutrition–cognition research from Flinders University, Adelaide, South Australia, and completed a joint post-doctoral position at the Nutritional Physiology Research Centre at University of South Australia (UniSA), Adelaide, and the Centre for Human Psychopharmacology, Swinburne University, Melbourne. Her research and clinical interests focus on the effects of nutrition to improve mood and neurocognitive function. Her research has explored the role of non-starch polysaccharides in everyday cognitive abilities and the well-being of middle-aged adults in order to understand the potential mechanisms by which dietary polysaccharides may have beneficial effects across the lifespan. In addition, Dr. Best's research focuses on processes of knowledge transfer between the research and industry sectors to promote innovation in food and nutrition research and development.

She has taught advanced statistics and research methods and psychological assessment at the undergraduate, master's and postgraduate levels, and currently teaches 'psychological assessment methods' at the honours level. With experience in clinical and research supervision, Dr. Best supervises undergraduate and postgraduate students across multidisciplinary settings within the food, nutrition, health and agriculture nexus at Central Queensland University, Bundaberg, Australia.

Talitha frequently speaks, writes, reviews, edits and lectures across multidisciplinary settings and contributes to national and international not-for-profit organisations committed to supporting health through community development in food, agriculture and education.

**Louise Dye** is professor of nutrition and behaviour in the Human Appetite Research Unit at the Institute of Psychological Sciences, University of Leeds, Leeds, United Kingdom. She received her BSc in human psychology from the University of Aston in Birmingham and her PhD in psychopharmacology from the University of Leeds. She has held Medical Research Council and Royal Society post-doctoral fellowships in the United Kingdom and Europe, including a Marie Curie professorial fellowship in Jena, Germany. Professor Dye is a chartered health psychologist and member of the British Psychological Society. She is associate editor of *Nutritional Neuroscience* and the *European Journal of Nutrition* and a member of the editorial board of *Human Psychopharmacology*. Currently, Professor Dye sits on four expert groups for the International Life Sciences Institute (ILSI). These are Postprandial Carbohydrate Metabolism, Benefits of Satiety, Measuring Subjective Mental Performance and Mood and BioMarkers for Cognitive Function. She has supervised more than 20 doctoral students and currently has seven doctoral students under her supervision, many in collaboration with industry or National Health Service partners.

For more than 20 years, her research has examined functional foods for cognitive performance and well-being across the lifespan. She has conducted numerous studies of the effects of foods and food components on glycaemic response, cognitive function and appetite control. In the last decade, she examined stress, obesity and cognitive function and the effects of breakfast interventions on cognitive performance and appetite control in children, adolescents and younger and older adults. Her research has been funded by ESRC, TSB, MRC, BBSRC and many food companies with whom she has formed strategic partnerships and led Knowledge Transfer Partnerships. Her recent research involves the effects of food components on digestive function and the impact of metabolic diseases such as cystic fibrosis and phenylketonuria on cognitive function. Louise has taught biological psychology and advanced statistics and research methods at the undergraduate, master's and postgraduate levels. Currently, Louise teaches a course called "Food and Health" on the MSc Psychological Approaches to Health at the University of Leeds and contributes to the Health Food Innovation Management Masters at Maastricht University, Maastricht, the Netherlands, and to an undergraduate module on "Nutrition and Behaviour" on the BSc psychology programme at the University of Leeds, alongside supervising undergraduate and postgraduate research in these areas.

# Contributors

**Samrah Ahmed**
Nuffield Department of Clinical
  Neurosciences
University of Oxford
Oxford, United Kingdom

**Valentina A. Andreeva**
Sorbonne-Paris-Cité
UMR University of Paris XIII
Paris, France

**Talitha Best**
School of Human, Health and Social
  Sciences-Psychology
Central Queensland University
Bundaberg, Queensland,
  Australia

**Kate L. Brookie**
Department of Psychology
University of Otago
Dunedin, New Zealand

**David Alan Camfield**
School of Psychology
Illawarra Health and Medical Research
  Institute
University of Wollongong
Wollongong, New South Wales,
  Australia

**Tamlin S. Conner**
Department of Psychology
University of Otago
Dunedin, New Zealand

**Celeste A. De Jager**
Division of Geriatric Medicine
Department of Medicine
University of Cape Town
Cape Town, South Africa

**Louise Dye**
School of Psychology
University of Leeds
Leeds, United Kingdom

**Jayde A.M. Flett**
Department of Psychology
University of Otago
Dunedin, New Zealand

**Rebecca J. Kean**
School of Psychology and Clinical
  Language Sciences
University of Reading
Reading, United Kingdom

**Emmanuelle Kesse-Guyot**
Sorbonne-Paris-Cité
UMR University of Paris XIII
Paris, France

**Daniel J. Lamport**
School of Psychology and Clinical
  Language Sciences
University of Reading
Reading, United Kingdom

**Robert K. McNamara**
Department of Psychiatry and
  Behavioral Neuroscience
University of Cincinnati College of
  Medicine
Cincinnati, Ohio

**Jose M. Ordovas**
Department of Nutrition and Genetics
Jean Mayer United States
    Department of Agriculture
    Human Nutrition Research
    Center on Aging
Tufts University
Boston, Massachusetts

**Lauren Owen**
School of Psychology
Keele University
Keele, United Kingdom

**Matthew Pase**
Centre for Human Psychopharmacology
Swinburne University of Technology
Hawthorn, Victoria, Australia

**Andrew Pipingas**
Centre for Human Psychopharmacology
Swinburne University of Technology
Hawthorn, Victoria, Australia

**Maria A. Polak**
Department of Psychology
University of Otago
Dunedin, New Zealand

**Aimee C. Richardson**
Department of Psychology
University of Otago
Dunedin, New Zealand

**Bernadette Robertson**
Department of Psychology
Lancaster University
Lancaster, United Kingdom

**Andrew Scholey**
Centre for Human Psychopharmacology
Swinburne University of Technology
Hawthorn, Victoria, Australia

**Con Stough**
Centre for Human Psychopharmacology
Swinburne University of Technology
Hawthorn, Victoria, Australia

**Sandra I. Sünram-Lea**
Department of Psychology
Lancaster University
Lancaster, United Kingdom

**Wei-Peng Teo**
Faculty of Health
School of Exercise and Nutrition
    Sciences
Deakin University
Melbourne, Victoria, Australia

**Christina J. Valentine**
Division of Neonatology
Perinatal Institute
Cincinnati Children's Hospital Medical
    Center
Cincinnati, Ohio

# Section I

**Big Picture: Nutrition for Brain Health**

# 1 Good News Story
## *Nutrition for Brain Health*

### *Talitha Best and Louise Dye*

## CONTENTS

## SUMMARY

The idea that nutrition can influence our health is not new. Most are aware of the significant impact food choices can play in health conditions such as obesity, type 2 diabetes and cardiovascular function and the importance of nutrition for physical and psychological well-being. Importantly, nutrition for brain function and cognitive performance is a rapidly increasing area of interest for scientists, industry and the general public. As a modifiable lifestyle choice, diet and nutrition are important contributors to brain health across the lifespan. In the chapters that follow, exciting, innovative research regarding the role of nutrition and diet in brain health is discussed. This chapter discusses a broad, good news story for *brain health*, innovative changes in nutrition–cognition research and provides suggestions for how to utilise the material presented in this book.

## 1.1  GOOD NEWS: PROMOTING BRAIN HEALTH

Developments from the fields of neuroscience, nutritional neuroscience and neurology provide converging evidence that the structure and function of the brain changes as a result of nutritional status (Lieberman et al., 2005). These changes and adaptations are called neuroplasticity, whilst neurogenesis refers to the creation of new neurons. These two properties of the brain underpin a good news story about how and why brain health can be supported with appropriate nutrition.

3

This good news helps to buffer some of the fear around the increasing prevalence rates of cognitive decline and neurodegenerative disease, such as dementia, the incidence rates for which range from 1.5% in over 65-year-olds to almost 25% in over 85-year-olds in western Europe with similar rates in North America (Alzheimer's Disease International, 2008). Worldwide, there are 4.6 million new cases annually. Dementia is estimated to affect over 65 million adults in countries with low and middle incomes by 2030 (Prince et al., 2013) which have far fewer resources to deal with its social and economic consequences. The prospect of *losing one's mind* and the ability to engage and remember interactions in the world due to declining brain health is frightening on an individual level, as it impacts at the core of how we define our identity and meaning in the world (Fjell et al., 2014). It is perhaps no surprise that across the world, there is a dramatic demand for pharmaceuticals, food products, nutraceuticals and technologies to support brain health from early childhood to allow optimal development into late adulthood to prevent or slow the progression of age-related cognitive decline.

Like any other organ in the body, the health of our brain relies on food and nutrients. The human brain requires a large proportion of the energy that is consumed because of high energy demands made by neuronal tissue. Twenty to twenty-five percent of our resting metabolic rate is utilised by the brain (Leonard et al., 2007). This energy is essential to maintain function (e.g. fundamental functions such as synaptic transmission and complex functions such as behaviour, cognitive performance and well-being) and structure (tissue connectivity and density of neuronal networks). Nutritional compounds are involved in the complex interactions and activity of the brain, from neurogenesis in the infant brain through to adulthood (Uauy & Dangour, 2008) to metabolic pathways, such as glucose regulation and inflammation involved in brain ageing and neurological disorders (Cutler et al., 2004). Nutrients also help maintain specific structures in the brain, such as the hippocampus which is directly associated with learning, memory and mood (Deng et al., 2010). Changes in dietary patterns and nutritional status, such as increased vitamin B, have been shown to impact the function and structure of the hippocampus in terms of size, activity and production of neurotransmitters related to cognitive performance (Deng et al., 2010; Monti et al., 2014; Stangl & Thuret, 2009; Stranahan et al., 2008).

The performance of the brain in terms of overall neural activity and cognitive ability, however, sits within a complex network of interactions. There are many external and internal influences such as changes in emotional states (Compton, 2003), social attachment (Young et al., 2001) and physical activity (Lista & Sorrentino, 2010) that can exert a direct effect on the neuronal circuits of the brain (Adolphs, 2003; Davidson & McEwen, 2012). For example, emotional states such as stress and low self-esteem have been associated with smaller hippocampi (McEwen et al., 2012) and disrupted neuronal function within the hippocampus and medial prefrontal cortex (McEwen & Gianaros, 2011). In addition, certain activities, such as prayer and meditation, can alter brain function in terms of neurochemical changes within the norepinephrine, dopaminergic and serotonergic receptor systems (Hölzel et al., 2011; Newberg & Iversen, 2003) and improve attention and executive function (Lutz et al., 2008).

Therefore, brain health can be influenced by a range of diverse external conditions, beyond the scope of this book. Although these are important, and there are networks of interactions that support brain health, we focus here on nutrition as one modifiable lifestyle factor that influences brain function. The focus of this book is to consider nutrition and how it might be studied, evidenced and ultimately applied in practical and public health settings to improve, maintain and promote brain health and cognitive function.

## 1.2 BRAIN, FOOD AND BEHAVIOUR

In the chapters that follow, we discuss dietary patterns, specific nutrients that may confer benefit for cognitive performance following both acute and habitual consumptions, with reference to how diet and nutrition may offer protection against cognitive impairment as we age. The diet contains hundreds of naturally occurring components that could impact a number of physiological and neurological mechanisms that underpin everyday cognitive functions. Dietary components can affect any one, or a series, of the processes that regulate hormone and neurotransmitter pathways, synaptic activity and connections between cells, membrane fluidity and signal-transduction pathways and neurogenesis (Gomez-Pinilla, 2008; Gomez-Pinilla & Tyagi, 2013).

Throughout the following chapters, the impact of dietary patterns (Chapter 2), micronutrients such as vitamins and minerals (Chapter 8) and omega-3 fatty acids (Chapter 7), as well as dietary constituents such as polyphenols and glucose (Chapters 6 and 10) and nutraceuticals and herbal remedies such as ginseng and green tea (Chapter 9) on cognitive function and mood, are discussed. Importantly, the potential impact of dietary interventions on cognition may be mediated by effects of these interventions on gene expression, as discussed by Ordovas in Chapter 3. In addition, technological advancements in techniques that could be used to capture nutrition effects on cognition and brain function are developing our knowledge of the effects of diet on brain health; see Chapters 11 and 12.

There is a pressing need to *round-out* the discussion and awareness of the relationship between nutrition and brain health. Due to the *brain diets* and *nutrients to help your brain* campaigns appearing in public awareness and media and drawing strong interest, the field of nutrition and cognition has a requirement to provide methods and evidence-based recommendations to government agencies, industry and consumers to support the substantiation of cognitive performance and mood claims for foods and food products.

The global demand for foods that are marketed for, or perceived to have, a significant health or performance benefit is growing exponentially. Innovative food products are continually launched and the market is estimated to be growing at a rate of 8%–14% per year, with an estimated value of US$477 billion by 2015 (Nutrition Business Journal, 2013). Less than a decade ago, estimates for complementary nutritional supplement and product consumption were $8.5 billion a year in United States and $4.05 billion in Australia (Xue et al., 2007).

Specifically, the consumption of brain/mental/cognitive supplements was reported to be around US$631 million in 2013, with an uptake of *cognitive-related* health products estimated to be a $2 billion industry (Nutrition Business Journal, 2013; Watson, 2013). As industry searches for new ingredients for product development, the value chain of information and knowledge about health claims will be important for long-term, beneficial impact for public health. In particular, claims which relate to the improvement of particular aspects of cognition and mood such as memory, alertness, mental energy, stress, depression and anxiety as functional outcomes will need critical appraisal via rigorous methodology. In order to provide recommendations for health claims related to nutrition, sound methodology and process innovation are needed in research questions, design and analysis.

## 1.3 BROAD METHODS AND INNOVATION IN NUTRITION–COGNITION RESEARCH

It is important that coherent and appropriate research methods are used to determine the quantity and quality of nutrition across the lifespan that may assist cognitive abilities (Kuczmarski et al., 2014). For example, higher intake of whole food dietary patterns has been associated with lowered risk of cognitive deficit compared to processed food dietary patterns (Kuczmarski et al., 2014). This finding was still significant after factors such as demographic characteristics (gender, age and marital status), comorbidities (diabetes, hypertension, coronary heart disease and mental health) and physical and behavioural factors (BMI, energy intake, smoking and physical activity) were controlled for. However, clear evidence on the association between dietary patterns and cognition is often diverse and may be related to methodological differences.

Throughout this book, a number of methods and critical factors for interpretation of nutrition–cognition research outcomes, such as cognitive and mood test selection, sources of nutrients and acute and chronic testing environments, are discussed. Thus, this book offers ideas to address the emerging opportunities to develop critical effectiveness in the design and conduct of nutrition–cognition trials that may increase the efficiency of recruitment, retention, testing and data management and potential data sharing that promotes the quality of the outcome (Ioannidis et al., 2014).

Nutrition–cognition research outcomes hold an intrinsic market value for investigators, sponsors, regulators and industry, as well as the community. Collection of data through mobile devices and Internet-based assessment and measurement tools, together with technologies for stimulation and imaging of the brain, is ushering the field into an increasingly competitive information environment (Berger & Doban, 2014). Innovation in tools and methods for collecting real-time data about everyday function could direct research outcomes into an entirely new, information value chain. This value chain of information is a competitive space underpinned by *big data* about health and health outcomes (Raghupathi & Raghupathi, 2014). The changing regulatory and economic environment may be a tremendous catalyst for competitive innovation and novelty in research and health care. It is exciting to consider where the next generation of research in this field will lead.

## 1.4   NEXT PART OF THE GOOD NEWS STORY: HOW TO USE THIS BOOK

The changing landscape for nutrition, food systems and sustainability, as well as food products and personalised nutrition, poses a unique challenge and opportunity for research into nutrition for brain health. The twenty-first century challenge has been called the *nutrition transition* or *nutrition paradox*, in which obesity coexists with malnutrition and vitamin deficiencies (Kearney, 2010). As practitioners, scientists and consumers, it is important to consider the types of psychosocial and economic influences on consumer behaviour underpinning the demand for and use of nutritional products. The interface between product health claims, generation of knowledge and information for public health provides great scope for nutrition and cognition research and nutritional neuroscience to interact with both industry and consumers. The role of industry is recognised by government and non-government organisations as critical to address under-nutrition and improve nutrition-related health outcomes (Luijten et al., 2012; Yach et al., 2010). Thus, it is important for research into effects of nutritional products, ingredients and formulations on brain function to consider and balance the input and goals of the manufacturers, developers, industry and marketeers of products and ingredients with those of the consumers and public health organisations.

The challenge ahead in the twenty-first century for the field of nutrition and behaviour is not only to address gaps between research, industry and the consumer but also to think about application and interpretation of the research findings. Research examples throughout this book highlight methodology (types of extract, tests, populations and cohort characteristics, such as age and level of ability) and offer a critical appraisal of the evidence about the impact of whole diets, nutrients, techniques and methods likely to confer benefit for brain function and structure across the lifespan.

### 1.4.1   FOR INDUSTRY

Use this book to support your research and development (R&D) agenda which might include the pursuit of health claims or the development of new products/modification of existing formulations. This book might suggest the methodologies and considerations required to develop the evidence base for claims of nutritional effects on brain health. In addition, use this resource as a guide from a range of highly regarded experts about the level of evidence available to you currently to develop and disseminate rigorous, high-quality information for your consumers.

### 1.4.2   FOR HEALTH-CARE PROFESSIONALS, RESEARCHERS, TEACHERS, EDUCATORS AND INTERESTED PUBLIC

Use this book to guide you in your understanding and appreciation of the role of nutrition to support psychological (cognitive function and mood) health and brain health. We hope that the explanations of the mechanisms and critical appraisal of the quality of the evidence will give you an awareness of issues that will enable you to make critical evaluations of key topics and methodological issues in the field.

Furthermore, we trust that this will enhance your knowledge and enable you to reduce confusion and assist your students and clients to appreciate the importance of nutrition for supporting brain health.

## 1.5  CONCLUSION

The subtle effects of food on the brain and behaviour mean that it is a complicated task to organise and distinguish those nutritional components and dietary patterns that are related to or likely to confer benefit for brain health. The promising effects of diet on brain plasticity and neurogenesis, together with the findings from human studies, reinforce the important translational concept that diet and nutrition can modulate brain health and function (Murphy et al., 2014).

This book presents the state-of-the-art scientific evidence, challenges and potential applications within this exciting field. By providing insight into the methodological considerations of research in this area, it is our hope that readers in the community, students, researchers and industry R&D use the information, techniques and insights of the book to support application of this research. In addition, it is our intention that this book be used to promote and extend the research, teach the process of research in this area and promote a collaborative understanding of the field between industry and academia.

More broadly however, we hope that this book is accessible to non-specialist readers and so can also be utilised by those in the community with keen interest in understanding this research to learn more about nutrients and dietary patterns which may confer cognitive protection or benefit. Use the summary boxes provided within each chapter that offer, from the authors' perspective, quick reference points to the key material and are a guide to the main issues and recommendations of the research in this area.

---

**TOP 4 SUMMARY POINTS FROM THIS CHAPTER**

- Brain health can be impacted by a range of external factors, such as exercise, meditation, social interaction and imagination that can influence/alter the function and structure of the brain.
- Nutritional intake and dietary patterns are critical for brain health across the lifespan. Certain dietary patterns and intake of particular nutrients are associated with both improved function and reduced risk of cognitive decline.
- Key methodological considerations in this field include appropriate methodology, research question and processes, type of intervention and design and sample selection especially the target group of the intervention.
- Innovation in research design, tools and methods is likely to support the transition of research outcome of this field into the twenty-first century information value chain which drives consumer and industry outcomes.

## REFERENCES

Adolphs, R. (2003). Cognitive neuroscience of human social behaviour. *Nature Reviews Neuroscience, 4*(3), 165–178.

Alzheimer's Disease International. (2008). *The prevalence of dementia worldwide.* London, U.K.: Alzheimer's Disease International.

Berger, M. L., & Doban, V. (2014). Big data, advanced analytics and the future of comparative effectiveness research. *Future Medicine, 3*(2), 167–176.

Compton, R. J. (2003). The interface between emotion and attention: A review of evidence from psychology and neuroscience. *Behavioral and Cognitive Neuroscience Reviews, 2*(2), 115–129.

Cutler, R., Kelly, J., Storie, K., Pedersen, W., Tammara, A., Hatanpaa, K., … Mattson, M. (2004). Involvement of oxidative stress-induced abnormalities in ceramide and cholesterol metabolism in brain aging and Alzheimer's disease. *Proceedings of the National Academy of Sciences of the United States of America, 101*(7), 2070–2075.

Davidson, R. J., & McEwen, B. S. (2012). Social influences on neuroplasticity: Stress and interventions to promote well-being. *Nature Neuroscience, 15*(5), 689–695.

Deng, W., Aimone, J. B., & Gage, F. H. (2010). New neurons and new memories: How does adult hippocampal neurogenesis affect learning and memory? *Nature Reviews Neuroscience, 11*(5), 339–350.

Fjell, A. M., McEvoy, L., Holland, D., Dale, A. M., & Walhovd, K. B. (2014). What is normal in normal aging? Effects of aging, amyloid and Alzheimer's disease on the cerebral cortex and the hippocampus. *Progress in Neurobiology, 117*(0), 20–40.

Gomez-Pinilla, F. (2008). Brain foods: The effects of nutrients on brain function. *Nature Reviews Neuroscience, 9*(7), 568–578.

Gomez-Pinilla, F., & Tyagi, E. (2013). Diet and cognition: Interplay between cell metabolism and neuronal plasticity. *Current Opinion in Clinical Nutrition & Metabolic Care, 16*(6), 726–733.

Hölzel, B. K., Carmody, J., Vangel, M., Congleton, C., Yerramsetti, S. M., Gard, T., & Lazar, S. W. (2011). Mindfulness practice leads to increases in regional brain gray matter density. *Psychiatry Research: Neuroimaging, 191*(1), 36–43.

Ioannidis, J. P. A., Greenland, S., Hlatky, M. A., Khoury, M. J., Macleod, M. R., Moher, D., … Tibshirani, R. (2014). Increasing value and reducing waste in research design, conduct, and analysis. *The Lancet, 383*(9912), 166–175.

Journal, N. B. (2013). The Highest Common Denominator. *Nutrition Business Journal, 18,* 1–9.

Kearney, J. (2010). Food consumption trends and drivers. *Philosophical Transactions of the Royal Society B:Biological Sciences, 365,* 2793–2807.

Kuczmarski, M. F., Allegro, D., & Stave, E. (2014). The Association of Healthful Diets and Cognitive Function: A Review. *Journal of Nutrition in Gerontology and Geriatrics, 33*(2), 69–90.

Leonard, W. R., Snodgrass, J. J., & Robertson, M. L. (2007). Effects of Brain Evolution on Human Nutrition and Metabolism. *Annual Review of Nutrition, 27*(1), 311–327.

Lieberman, H. R., Kanarek, R. B., & Prasad, C. (Eds.). (2005). *Nutritional neuroscience.* Boca Raton, FL: CRC Press, Taylor & Francis Group.

Lista, I., & Sorrentino, G. (2010). Biological mechanisms of physical activity in preventing cognitive decline. *Cellular and Molecular Neurobiology, 30*(4), 493–503.

Luijten, P. R., Dongen, G. A. M. S. v., Moonen, C., Storm, G., & Crommelin, D. J. A. (2012). Public-private partnerships in translational medicine: Concepts and practical examples. *Journal of Controlled Release, 161,* 416–421.

Lutz, A., Slagter, H. A., Dunne, J. D., & Davidson, R. J. (2008). Attention regulation and monitoring in meditation. *Trends in Cognitive Sciences, 12*(4), 163–169.

McEwen, B. S., Eiland, L., Hunter, R. G., & Miller, M. M. (2012). Stress and anxiety: Structural plasticity and epigenetic regulation as a consequence of stress. *Neuropharmacology, 62*(1), 3–12.

McEwen, B. S., & Gianaros, P. J. (2011). Stress- and allostasis-induced brain plasticity. *Annual Review of Medicine, 62*(1), 431–445.

Monti, J. M., Baym, C. L., & Cohen, N. J. (2014). Identifying and characterizing the effects of nutrition on hippocampal memory. *Advances in Nutrition: An International Review Journal, 5*(3), 337S–343S.

Murphy, T., Dias, G. P., & Thuret, S. (2014). Effects of diet on brain plasticity in animal and human studies: Mind the gap. *Neural Plasticity, 2014*, 32.

Newberg, A. B., & Iversen, J. (2003). The neural basis of the complex mental task of meditation: Neurotransmitter and neurochemical considerations. *Medical Hypotheses, 61*(2), 282–291.

Prince, M., Bryce, R., Albanese, E., Wimo, A., Ribeiro, W., & Ferri, C. P. (2013). The global prevalence of dementia: A systematic review and metaanalysis. *Alzheimer's Dement, 9*(1), 63–75.e62.

Raghupathi, W., & Raghupathi, V. (2014). Big data analytics in healthcare: Promise and potential. *Health Information Science and Systems, 2*(3), 2–10.

Stangl, D., & Thuret, S. (2009). Impact of diet on adult hippocampal neurogenesis. *Genes & Nutrition, 4*(4), 271–282.

Stranahan, A. M., Norman, E. D., Lee, K., Cutler, R. G., Telljohann, R. S., Egan, J. M., & Mattson, M. P. (2008). Diet-induced insulin resistance impairs hippocampal synaptic plasticity and cognition in middle-aged rats. *Hippocampus, 18*(11), 1085–1088.

Uauy, R., & Dangour, A. (2008). Nutrition in brain development and aging: Role of essential fatty acids. *Nutrition Reviews, 64*(s2), s24–s33.

Watson, K. (2013). Cognitive health ingredients drive category growth. *Natural Products Insider, June 25*.

Xue, C., Zhang, A., Lin, V., Costa, C. d., & Story, D. (2007). Complementary and alternative medicine use in Australia: A national population-based survey. *The Journal of Alternative and Complementary Medicine, 13*(6), 643–650.

Yach, D., Khan, M., Bradley, D., Hargrove, R., Kehoe, S., & Mensah, G. (2010). The role and challenges of the food industry in addressing chronic disease. *Globalization and Health, 6*(10), 1–8.

Young, L. J., Lim, M. M., Gingrich, B., & Insel, T. R. (2001). Cellular Mechanisms of Social Attachment. *Hormones and Behavior, 40*(2), 133–138.

# 2 Nutrition and Cognition in the Context of Ageing
## Role of Dietary Patterns

*Valentina A. Andreeva and
Emmanuelle Kesse-Guyot*

## CONTENTS

## SUMMARY

The worldwide increase in life expectancy portends serious consequences in all areas of life. As physical and mental health status generally deteriorates with advancing age, researchers forecast an unprecedented rise in disability and health-care costs, concomitant with marked declines in the quality of life of the elderly. Hence, the role of various modifiable lifestyle factors, such as healthy diets and engagement in physical activity (PA), has been evoked as paramount prevention strategies. Nutrition-based strategies – especially those focused on overall dietary patterns (DPs) which account for the marked synergies and interactions among nutrients in the food matrix – merit particular attention as primary prevention options regarding cognitive ageing and impairment. This chapter explores the current evidence that suggests a Mediterranean-type diet rich in fruit and vegetables (FVs), plant-derived products and seafood, with relatively low alcohol intake and low intakes of meat, saturated fatty acids and added sugar, could have important benefits for brain health. Beginning early in life, individuals can help reduce their risk of physical and mental impairment in the course of ageing by following a well-balanced, nutritious dietary regimen, maintaining a healthy weight and being physically active.

## 2.1 WORLDWIDE POPULATION AGEING AND ITS IMPLICATIONS FOR HEALTH CARE

Advances in medical science and technology, notable social and economic improvements and the demographic transition from high to low levels of fertility and mortality, initially observed in developed regions and gradually spreading to less developed regions of the world, have led to an unprecedented increase in life expectancy and population ageing (Korczyc et al., 2013; United Nations, 2002). In most developed countries, the age of 65 years or older has been accepted as a definition for elderly or older persons, whereas the age of 60 years has been used to mark the beginning of old age in less developed countries in Africa (World Health Organization, 2014). Whereas in the 1950s, the proportion of older persons worldwide was approximately 8%, at the beginning of the twenty-first century, it was approximately 10% (i.e. 600 million people), and by the year 2050, it is expected to reach 20% (i.e. 2 billion people). The annual increase of 2% of the elderly population is higher than the overall population growth rate, with individuals aged 80 years and over representing the fastest-growing segment (i.e. annual increase of 3.8%). Despite demographic heterogeneity across different world regions, female life expectancy is generally higher than that for males. In the United States, for example, by the year 2050, there will be more than 48 million women and about 40 million men aged 65 and over (Figure 2.1).

    The worldwide population ageing portends serious consequences in all areas of life, including decreasing labour force participation owing to retirement and increasing demand for health care, special housing and changing family composition (Korczyc et al., 2013; United Nations, 2002). As physical and mental health status

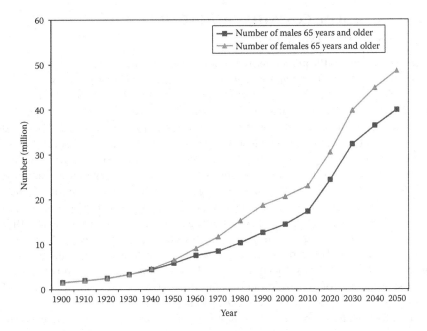

**FIGURE 2.1** The U.S. population 65 and over by sex: 1900–2050. (From Projections of the population by age and sex for the United States: 2010 to 2050 (NP2008-T12), Population Division, U.S. Census Bureau; Release date: August 14, 2008; Data for 1900–2000 from Census 2000 Special Reports, Washington, DC, Series CENSR-4, Demographic Trends in the 20th Century, 2002.)

generally deteriorates with increasing age, demand for long-term care is likely to grow (United Nations, 2002). In addition, given the impact of population ageing along with that of the obesity epidemic, the increasing cardiovascular disease (CVD) morbidity and declining CVD mortality (partly due to improvements in treatment), researchers forecast an unprecedented rise in disability and health-care costs, concomitant with marked declines in the quality of life of the elderly (Pandya et al., 2013). A recent report by the American Academy of Neurology Workforce Task Force also predicted a marked future shortfall of neurologists provoked, in part, by ageing of the population and by increased health-care utilization rates of neurologic services (Freeman et al., 2013).

In Europe, one-third of the population is expected to be aged 60 and over by the year 2050 (Korczyc et al., 2013). The rapidly declining share of the working-age segment of the population concomitant with an increasing demand for long-term care services and the rising costs for supporting an expanding elderly population are seen as major challenges throughout the region, with especially serious repercussions for Bulgaria, Croatia, the Czech Republic, Estonia, Latvia, Lithuania, Hungary, Poland, Romania, Slovenia and the Slovak Republic (Korczyc et al., 2013). In turn, alarming social security data from Germany suggest that by the year 2030, employed individuals will be working to sustain twice as many retired elderly as they did in the early 1990s (Borsch-Supan, 1992).

## 2.2   COGNITION, COGNITIVE AGEING AND COGNITIVE IMPAIRMENT

Cognition comprises the numerous and complex mental processes involved in acquiring knowledge, learning, attention, memory, intelligence and consciousness (Harada et al., 2013; Lezak et al., 2012). These processes are dependent on the transmission of electrical and chemical signals between neurons (nerve cells). With age, the rate at which neurons receive and transmit such signals declines which leads to declines in learning, recall and multitasking skills (Institute for the Study of Ageing, 2005). Importantly, there is marked variation in the age-related rates of decline across the various cognitive abilities, with some abilities, such as those related to vocabulary, knowledge and social cognition possibly improving with age (i.e. crystallized intelligence), while others, such as working memory, reaction time and processing speed (i.e. fluid intelligence), typically show salient age-related decline (Depp et al., 2012; Lezak et al., 2012). Despite substantial heterogeneity among individuals, normal ageing generally leads to a reduction in the volume of different brain structures (e.g. caudate nucleus of the basal ganglia, cerebellum, hippocampus, prefrontal areas), decreasing number of synapses and decreased integrity of white matter tracts, all leading to potential cognitive deficits (Depp et al., 2012).

Cognitive decline represents a continuum of subjective and objective symptoms, ranging from normal (healthy) cognitive ageing through subjective memory complaints, mild cognitive impairment (MCI) and preclinical dementia and ending with Alzheimer's disease (AD) (American Psychiatric Association, 2013). Reviews of the scientific evidence suggest that the prevalence of memory complaints – defined as everyday memory problems – varies between 25% and 50% in the general elderly population. Older age, female sex and low education have been linked to an increased risk of memory complaints which are regarded as a risk factor for cognitive impairment and dementia in community-dwelling elderly (Jonker et al., 2000).

MCI represents a heterogeneous cluster of symptoms, which might not always be detected (Shankle et al., 2005). Despite the lack of a precise definition, MCI pertains to some cognitive impairment (in recall, judgment, etc.) that does not affect instrumental activities of daily living (shopping, housekeeping) (Shankle et al., 2005). Its overall prevalence varies widely across different populations of elderly, ranging from 3% (Ritchie et al., 2001) to 46% (Drexler et al., 2013). In fact, much of the variation can be attributed to the diagnostic criteria used, for which there is currently no consensus (Drexler et al., 2013). Generally, MCI increases the risk of dementia (Brodaty et al., 2013), which consists of marked and irreversible cognitive decline from a previous level of functioning. Dementia is characterized by progressive deterioration in different cognitive domains (attention, concentration, memory, executive function) that is severe enough to interfere with daily life (American Psychiatric Association, 2013). In epidemiological studies, cognitive decline is typically assessed via neuropsychological tests measuring global cognition, such as the mini-mental state examination (MMSE) (Folstein et al., 1975) or its modified version (Teng & Chui, 1987), administered at least twice over a period of several years.

Each individual cognitive domain (language, memory, visuospatial ability, information processing speed, attention, executive functioning) can be evaluated by specific neuropsychological tools (Reichman et al., 2010); see also Chapter 4. Generally, impairment in episodic (autobiographical) memory and impairment in executive functioning are considered as principal markers of dementia (Lezak et al., 2012). Magnetic resonance imaging (MRI) has shown that episodic memory loss is associated with hippocampal deterioration (due to lipid peroxidation, loss of neuronal integrity, oxidative stress, etc.), primarily involving the left hemisphere (Thomann et al., 2012); see Chapter 12. Other cognitive domains (abstract reasoning, conceptual formation) also become progressively impaired in the preclinical phase of AD (Amieva et al., 2008; Jacobs et al., 1995).

AD is the most common cause of dementia among the elderly, accounting for up to 70% of all dementia cases (Querfurth & LaFerla, 2010). It is a complex multifactorial disease characterized by two principal neuropathological features: increased extracellular amyloid plaque deposits in the brain and presence of intracellular neurofibrillary tangles (Querfurth & LaFerla, 2010). Such lesions gradually result in neurodegeneration, associated with increased inflammation and oxidative stress (Querfurth & LaFerla, 2010). Neuroimaging studies have reported that the AD process is initiated many years before the manifestation of cognitive impairment (Masdeu et al., 2012). In turn, epidemiological studies have shown that abnormally low performance in different cognitive domains (e.g. semantic memory and concept formation) can be seen a decade or more before the clinical diagnosis of AD, underscoring the existence of a very long and progressive prodromal phase of AD, with successive emergence of cognitive deficits, depressive symptoms and functional impairment (Amieva et al., 2005, 2008). Finally, vascular dementia is the second most common cause of dementia in the elderly and is defined as loss of cognitive function resulting from ischemic, hypoperfusive or haemorrhagic brain lesions due to CVD (Roman, 2003).

## 2.3   MENTAL HEALTH PROMOTION: MODIFIABLE FACTORS WITH A FOCUS ON NUTRITION

The increasing life expectancy across the world necessitates urgent public health action aimed at preserving the physical and mental health status and autonomy of the elderly via optimal control of chronic diseases and a focus on the various dimensions of quality of life (physical, psychological, social) (Woo, 2011). In fact, cognitive impairment and AD have a profound negative impact on health and quality of life not only of patients but also of their caregivers. Given the current lack of a cure for dementia, prioritizing prevention is critical. The role of various modifiable lifestyle factors, such as healthy diets, prevention of nutritional deficiencies, engagement in PA and social interaction, has been proposed as paramount prevention strategies (Hughes & Ganguli, 2009; Solfrizzi et al., 2008).

Nutrition-based strategies – focused on individual nutrients or on overall DPs – merit particular attention as prevention options regarding cognitive ageing and cognitive decline, with potentially far-reaching public health impact (Alles et al., 2012;

Otaegui-Arrazola et al., 2014). These strategies stem from research on the preventive role of nutrition in different age-related chronic diseases. Specific nutrients and dietary components that have received substantial attention in prevention research, albeit with marked heterogeneity among the findings, include B vitamins (see Chapter 8), antioxidants (vitamin C, vitamin E, flavonoids and their principal food vectors – FVs), omega-3 fatty acids (see Chapter 7), vitamin D, fish, (green) tea, caffeine and caloric restriction (Daviglus et al., 2011; Gillette-Guyonnet et al., 2013; Joseph et al., 2009). Conversely, certain dietary components, such as saturated fatty acids, have been linked with increased risk of cognitive impairment and AD (Gillette-Guyonnet et al., 2013).

## 2.4  DIETARY ASSESSMENT METHODS

In order to study individuals' eating habits and dietary intake, a number of research tools have been developed (Table 2.1). They can be broadly grouped into *real-time* tools, where data are recorded at (or close to) the time of eating, and retrospective tools, where data collection pertains to past (or habitual) intake. The 24 h dietary record (providing detailed information on all foods and beverages consumed during a 24 h period) is an example of the former type of dietary assessment, whereas diet histories (providing information on habitual dietary intake over a relatively long period of time) and food frequency questionnaires (FFQs) are examples of the latter type (Thompson & Byers, 1994; Willett, 1998).

FFQ can be self-administered or interviewer administered and constitute the most common dietary assessment tools used in epidemiological research. They are intended for the collection of information on the type of food and beverage consumed (selected from a predefined list) and the frequency of consumption. FFQs differ in the number of food/beverage items included, the measures of frequency (servings), weight (grams, litres) (Thompson & Byers, 1994), the description of portion sizes (i.e. using photographs or predefined standard portions), the period of time covered (past week, past month, etc.) and the presence of additional questions regarding food preparation methods and dietary supplement use (Thompson & Byers, 1994; Willett, 1998). Validation studies often compare FFQ against another dietary assessment method (e.g. 24 h recalls) or a biomarker of nutritional status (Willett, 1998; Gibson, 2005).

The development of innovative tools allows the collection of dietary intake via information and communication technologies: videotaped dietary assessment (Ortiz-Andrellucchi et al., 2009), computerized FFQ and 24 h recalls (with built-in audio and video aids), personal digital assistants, digital photography and smart cards/phones (Ngo et al., 2009). Such tools have the potential to improve dietary assessment quality and decrease researcher and respondent burden (Ngo et al., 2009). Finally, gathered information on food and beverage consumption can be used to extract data on nutrient intake via food composition tables (Willett, 1998). However, the exact nutrient content of each type of food might be difficult to calculate, as food composition varies by environmental conditions, geographical location, food production and preparation methods (Gibson, 2005; Otaegui-Arrazola et al., 2014).

**TABLE 2.1**

**Comparison of Common Dietary Assessment Tools**

| Dietary Assessment Tool | Strengths | Limitations |
| --- | --- | --- |
| *Retrospective assessment* | | |
| FFQ | Easy self-administration | Lack of precision in estimating exact quantities consumed |
| | Assessment of habitual consumption/ intake patterns | Possible over- and/or under-reporting |
| | Relatively cost and time efficient | Differences in portion size description across FFQ |
| | Does not impact eating habits | Inconsistent number of items across FFQ |
| | Can be administered to very large study samples | Heterogeneity in time period covered (past week, past month) across FFQ – difficult to complete when longer time periods assessed |
| | A number of validated FFQ available | |
| | Streamlined data format | |
| Diet history | Assessment of habitual dietary intake over a long period of time | Possible misreporting/ under-reporting |
| | Information on food intake by meal | Might lack precision in estimating exact quantities consumed |
| | Structured interview with prompts | Might be burdensome and time-consuming for investigator and for respondent |
| | Does not impact eating habits | Lack information on current dietary habits/potential dietary modifications |
| | Stability of dietary intake data | Might not be suitable for very large study samples |
| | Data available on rarely consumed foods | Cost-efficiency might be low |
| *Real-time assessment* | | |
| 24 h dietary record/recall | Detailed information on all foods and beverages consumed during a 24 h period | Might impact dietary habits if day of assessment is known in advance |
| | Precise assessment of quantities consumed | Might be burdensome and time-consuming for respondent |
| | Assessment of current (actual) eating behaviour | Lack information on past dietary habits |

*(Continued)*

**TABLE 2.1** (*Continued*)

**Comparison of Common Dietary Assessment Tools**

| Dietary Assessment Tool | Strengths | Limitations |
| --- | --- | --- |
| | Possibility to assess rarely consumed food items when multiple 24 h records are administered | Possible under-reporting |
| | Method appropriate for most study populations | Cost-efficiency might be low |
| | | Time-consuming data entry |
| Food diary (food record) | Detailed information on all foods and beverages consumed (usually) during a 7-day period | Heterogeneity in data format |
| | Assessment of current (actual) eating behaviour | Method not optimal for large study samples |
| | Precise assessment of quantities consumed | Might impact dietary habits |
| | Can serve as a weight-loss aid | Lack information on past dietary habits |
| | Method better adapted for small study samples | Investigator and respondent burden |
| | | Time-consuming data entry |

It should be kept in mind that research data gathered in nutritional epidemiology might be subject to several kinds of bias due primarily to the fact that individual consumption/intake data are self-reported (Willett, 1998). In particular, the issues of recall bias, prevarication bias, measurement error linked to the estimation of portion sizes and under-reporting, among others, have been extensively discussed (Gibson, 2005; Willett, 1998).

## 2.5 DPs: DEFINITION, IMPORTANCE AND A PRIORI AND A POSTERIORI INDICES

Food constituents are not independent but are in fact interrelated in complex ways, showing synergistic, additive and antagonistic effects which, in turn, support the idea of dietary variety and the importance of consuming nutrient-rich foods (Jacobs, Jr. et al., 2009). The combination of naturally occurring food components is the food matrix which has a differential, arguably greater influence on the human biological systems and on health overall than the influence exerted by the individual components (Jacobs, Jr. et al., 2009). Generally, DPs fall into two principal categories (see Table 2.2): (1) hypothesis driven, *a priori* indices or scores taking into account the role of nutrition in disease prevention, and (2) data driven, exploratory *a posteriori* factors and clusters (Gu & Scarmeas, 2011; Hu, 2002; Kant, 2010). Recently, a third category which is a hybrid of the hypothesis-driven and data-driven methods has been used for the evaluation of DP reflecting intake

**TABLE 2.2**

**Comparison of *A Priori* and *A Posteriori* DPs**

| Characteristics (Including Strengths and Limitations) | *A Priori* DPs | *A Posteriori* DPs |
|---|:---:|:---:|
| Theory (guideline) based | X | |
| Hypothesis driven | X | |
| Data (sample) driven | | X |
| Characterize overall (total) diet | X | X |
| Diet quality index or score | X | |
| Generalizable (high external validity) | X | |
| Multiple components included in score | X | |
| Account for entire quantity of intake | | X |
| Latent factors reflecting correlations among diet variables | | X |
| Nutrient or food group clusters (mutually exclusive) | | X |
| Exploratory in nature | | X |
| Allow for synergy among dietary/nutrient components | | X |
| Describing eating habits/dietary behaviour | | X |
| Subjective decisions about food groups | X | X |
| Subjective decisions about scoring | X | X |
| Can be studied in relation with health outcomes | X | X |

of specific nutrients or biomarker concentrations with hypothesized associations with predefined health outcomes (Gu & Scarmeas, 2011; Hoffmann et al., 2004; Kant, 2010).

### 2.5.1 A PRIORI DPS

The *a priori* approach is based on the investigation of diet quality via dietary intake variables (quantified and summed up) considered important for various health outcomes (Waijers et al., 2007). There are diet quality indices based on nutrients (e.g. micronutrients, dietary fat, total energy), indices based on food or food groups (i.e. FV, dairy products, etc.), as well as indices based on nutrients and foods (Kant, 1996; Waijers et al., 2007). More than 20 different *a priori* DPs have been created, largely belonging to two main categories: (1) indices based on official nutrition guidelines (recommendations) and (2) indices or scores based on specific dietary styles (Gu & Scarmeas, 2011; Hu, 2002; Roman-Vinas et al., 2009). Examples of the former category include the Healthy Eating Index (HEI) (Kennedy et al., 1995), Dietary Approaches to Stop Hypertension (DASH) (Appel et al., 1997), diet quality index (Patterson et al., 1994), healthy diet indicator (Huijbregts et al., 1997), Programme National Nutrition Santé Guideline Score (PNNS-GS) (Estaquio et al., 2009) and the Canadian HEI (Shatenstein et al., 2012). An example of the latter category is the Mediterranean diet (MeDi) (Trichopoulou et al., 2003).

The *a priori* approach entails the assignment of sub-scores for each of the predefined food or nutrient groups and the calculation of a graded score or index using predefined cut-offs (or sample median values) and reflects the degree to which an individual's diet conforms to dietary recommendations or to predefined health-conducive DP (Alles et al., 2012; Gu & Scarmeas, 2011). The inclusion of specific nutrients or foods in *a priori* indices is largely determined by their presence (or absence) in the particular guidelines or reference source utilized in defining the score, according to the researcher's judgment, and the available data. The principal strength of *a priori* measures is their generalizability (external validity) and applicability across different samples (thus permitting comparisons across studies), even though dietary recommendations might have greater pertinence for certain populations and be less applicable to others (Roman-Vinas et al., 2009). However, *a priori* indices also entail some limitations, as outlined at the end of this chapter.

### 2.5.2 MEDITERRANEAN DIET

The olive-growing Mediterranean region comprises about 20 different countries where prevailing DPs share some important, health-conducive features. Apart from the salient presence of olive oil in the largely plant-based MeDi, the following nine desirable characteristics of this *a priori* DP have been identified (Trichopoulou et al., 2003): (1) high ratio of monounsaturated to saturated fatty acids (mainly olive oil); (2) high consumption of fruit; (3) high consumption of vegetables; (4) high consumption of legumes and nuts; (5) high consumption of non-refined cereals, including bread; (6) moderate consumption of milk and dairy products; (7) moderate ethanol consumption (mainly red wine); (8) low consumption of red meat, meat products and poultry; and (9) high consumption of fish. This DP is known as health conducive due to its protective impact regarding chronic conditions such as CVD, cancer, AD, hypertension, obesity and mortality (Perez-Lopez et al., 2009; Trichopoulou et al., 2003).

The classic Mediterranean diet score (MDS) takes into account the nine components listed earlier (Trichopoulou et al., 2003). For FV, legumes, cereals, the ratio of monounsaturated to saturated fatty acids, fish and mild-to-moderate alcohol intake (i.e. beneficial components), individuals whose calorie-adjusted amount of intake in grams is below the sex-specific median are given 0 points, while those whose intake falls above the sex-specific median are given 1 point for each component. For meat and dairy products (i.e. detrimental components), individuals whose calorie-adjusted amount of intake is below the sex-specific median are given 1 point, while those whose intake is above the sex-specific median are given 0 points. Next, MDS is computed by adding the scores on the individual components. Its value ranges from 0 to 9, with a higher score representing closer adherence to MeDi (Trichopoulou et al., 2003). Yet another approach for assessing MeDi adherence is to give a score according to recommended frequency of intake defined by the MeDi pyramid (Willett et al., 1995). A revised MDS has also been developed in order to account for consumption of refined grains and sweetened beverages (Issa et al., 2011). Finally, a Mediterranean-style DP score was developed for the U.S. population (Rumawas et al., 2009). Using the Framingham Offspring Cohort, the authors assessed the intakes of 13 food groups in the MeDi pyramid, with each food group scored from 0 to 10 based on the degree of adherence to the recommendations. Exceeding the recommendations results in a lower score proportional to the degree of overconsumption, resulting in a bell-shaped score distribution. The food group scores are summed, standardized and weighted by the proportion of total energy consumed from MeDi foods (Rumawas et al., 2009).

### 2.5.3 OTHER A PRIORI INDICES

The DP known as DASH was first promoted in the late 1990s by the U.S. National Heart, Lung, and Blood Institute (Appel et al., 1997). This DP supports increased consumption of FV, whole grains, nuts, fat-free or low-fat dairy products, fish and poultry, while discouraging consumption of red meat, sweets and sugar-containing beverages. The DASH index is thus high in protein, fibre, magnesium, potassium and calcium and low in sodium, cholesterol and saturated and total fat (Appel et al., 1997).

In turn, the HEI, developed by the U.S. Department of Agriculture using the Dietary Guidelines for Americans and the Food Guide Pyramid, is a diet quality index which accounts for 10 components (each scored from 0 to 10): 5 food groups (FVs, grains, dairy and meats), 4 nutrients (cholesterol, fats, saturated fat, sodium) and 1 measure of dietary variety (Kennedy et al., 1995). This DP was initially designed for monitoring dietary intake trends and for informing nutrition promotion activities (Kennedy et al., 1995). A revised HEI (alternate HEI) additionally takes into account cereals, fibre, protein sources, the ratio of polyunsaturated fatty acids to saturated fatty acids, moderate alcohol consumption and dietary supplement use (McCullough et al., 2002).

In France, the National Nutrition and Health Program (PNNS, Program National Nutrition Santé) was implemented in 2001 with the aim of improving the health status of the general population via nutrition-focused prevention (Hercberg et al., 2008). An *a priori*, 13-component PNNS-GS has been developed to assess adherence to these national guidelines. This score takes into account the consumption of FV, starches, whole grains, dairy products, meat, eggs, fish and seafood, beverages, sweets and desserts, fat and salt. The score also includes *bonus* points (> 1) for engagement in PA and for increased consumption of FV, as well as *penalties* (with points being subtracted from the total score) for the intake of salt and sweetened products. An additional *penalty* for overconsumption is applied when the total energy intake is higher than the estimated energy expenditure (Estaquio et al., 2009).

### 2.5.4 A POSTERIORI DPS

A posteriori DPs are data and population specific and are derived via multidimensional techniques such as principal component analysis, factor analysis or cluster analysis. In general, this approach allows the reduction of data collected via FFQ, 24 h dietary recalls or diet records into smaller sets of variables that constitute a DP (Hu, 2002; Roman-Vinas et al., 2009). Input variables can include specific nutrients, foods, food groups or a combination of the three, with food groups being the most common, given the fact that they represent total dietary intake and capture the interaction/synergy among nutrients (Hu, 2002).

Principal component analysis is the most frequently used technique in this context. It produces linear combinations (representing DP) of the measured variables along with factor loadings reflecting the relative weight or importance of each dietary variable to the respective DP. Next, principal component analysis provides a score reflecting the degree to which an individual's diet conforms to the DP (Gu & Scarmeas, 2011; Hu, 2002). This statistical approach also entails important subjective decisions regarding variable selection, food groupings and number of DP retained (Moeller et al., 2007). In turn, factor analysis is useful when transforming many original dietary variables which are intercorrelated into fewer uncorrelated (orthogonal) factors (Hu, 2002; Newby & Tucker, 2004). The derived factors represent DPs which are named according to the input variable with the highest factor loading (e.g. vegetables) or according to a quantitative description (e.g. low fibre). A review of the literature in this domain reported that the number of extracted factors ranged from 2 to 25 and the percent variance explained ranged from 15% to 93% (Newby & Tucker, 2004).

Over four decades ago, researchers began applying cluster analysis for the development of classification schemes for categorizing individuals into groups with similar dietary intake patterns and diet quality (i.e. light eaters, heavy eaters, salty food consumers, etc.) (Akin et al., 1986). In cluster analysis, the individual-level data are grouped into mutually exclusive clusters (anywhere from 2 to 8, as previously reported) of DP with each individual being assigned a cluster-specific indicator (Gu & Scarmeas, 2011; Newby & Tucker, 2004). Thus, there is dietary homogeneity among individuals belonging to the same cluster (Gu & Scarmeas, 2011). In cluster analysis, subjective choices pertain to variable selection, level of significance and number of clusters to be retained (Newby & Tucker, 2004; Roman-Vinas et al., 2009).

In the context of DP, a relatively novel technique in nutritional epidemiology is reduced-rank regression (or maximum redundancy analysis) which calculates linear combinations of a given set of variables (i.e. food groups) by maximizing the explained variation in a given set of response variables (i.e. biomarkers) (Hoffmann et al., 2004). Reduced-rank regression is a combination of a hypothesis-driven approach based on existing knowledge about diet–disease associations and an exploratory approach using population-specific data. Similar to the other exploratory techniques outlined earlier, reduced-rank regression also entails subjective decisions as regards the clustering of food items into food groups, the number of DP to be retained and the selection of response variables (Hoffmann et al., 2004).

### 2.5.5   DPs and Health

The scientific literature dealing with the relationship between nutrition and health is growing, increasingly relying on holistic approaches (*a priori* and *a posteriori* techniques), as well as on different health outcomes and intermediate end points (Feart et al., 2009; Gu et al., 2010; Kant, 2010; Kant & Graubard, 2005; Newby & Tucker, 2004; Sofi et al., 2013). Both *a priori* and *a posteriori* DPs have been explored in terms of their associations with a myriad of health and disease outcomes, such as anthropometrics, blood pressure/hypertension, metabolic syndrome, blood glucose and insulin measures, bone mineral density, dental caries, type 2 diabetes, cancer, CVD, cognitive impairment, dementia and all-cause mortality (Newby & Tucker, 2004; Sofi et al., 2013). For example, the current (and regularly updated) meta-analysis of cohort studies investigating the association between MeDi and health status reported that a 2-point increase in the MeDi adherence score was associated with an 8% reduction of overall mortality, a 10% reduced risk of CVD and a 4% reduced cancer risk (Sofi et al., 2013). In turn, a recent French study reported that an *alcohol and meat product* DP was positively associated with overweight in both sexes, with abdominal obesity in women and with treated hyperlipidemia and hypertension in men, whereas a *prudent* DP was associated with a smaller waist circumference in women and with hyperlipidemia treatment in men (Kesse-Guyot et al., 2009). As regards *healthy* DP composed of FV, fish, poultry and low-fat food, a statistically significant risk reduction for all-cause mortality, coronary heart disease and certain cancers has been reported (Bertuccio et al., 2013; Kant, 2010; Mozaffarian et al., 2011).

### 2.5.6  DP COVARIATES

The link between a given DP and a given disease might depend on one's age, ethnicity, health risk behaviours (smoking, drinking) and socioeconomic status (Kesse-Guyot et al., 2009; Newby & Tucker, 2004). For example, a study using a multinational sample of elderly participants reported an association between greater adherence to a plant-based diet and all-cause mortality, which was stronger in Greece, Spain, Denmark and the Netherlands, while absent in the United Kingdom and Germany (Bamia et al., 2007). Next, generally more women than men report a healthier DP, which is also associated with higher socioeconomic status (income, education), increased PA and not smoking (Kesse-Guyot et al., 2009; Newby & Tucker, 2004). In turn, adherence to a DP defined predominantly by meat and alcohol consumption has been associated with low education and smoking, whereas a DP characterized by the consumption of convenience foods was inversely related to age (Kesse-Guyot et al., 2009).

## 2.6  ASSOCIATIONS BETWEEN DPS AND COGNITION

Both *a priori* and *a posteriori* DPs (as well as DP based on a combination of hypothesis-driven and exploratory techniques) have been assessed for their relation to cognitive function. Overall, the results of such studies indicate that diets rich in FV, fish, nuts and legumes, coupled with low consumption of meats and high-fat dairy products, have a beneficial influence on cognition in terms of reduced risk of cognitive impairment (Alles et al., 2012; Sofi et al., 2013). However, the current scientific evidence is considered insufficient and more prospective studies and clinical trials seem necessary in order to be able to draw firm conclusions as regards the cause–effect relationship (Gu & Scarmeas, 2011; Otaegui-Arrazola et al., 2014). In the below sections, we give examples of specific findings with both *a priori* and *a posteriori* DPs.

### 2.6.1  ASSOCIATIONS WITH THE MEDITERRANEAN DP

This appears to be the most widely studied DP in reference to brain health and cognitive functioning. In fact, MeDi includes most of the nutrients and food items that have been linked to reduced risk of cognitive decline and MCI/dementia, such as

FV (rich in antioxidants and polyphenols), olive oil (rich of unsaturated fatty acids, vitamin E and polyphenols) and fish (rich in fatty acids, vitamin B12 and selenium) (Alles et al., 2012; Gu et al., 2010; Sofi et al., 2013). Reviews of the research evidence suggest that AD and MCI have increased prevalence among elderly individuals with low adherence to MeDi (Otaegui-Arrazola et al., 2014) and that MeDi could have protective effects in pre-dementia and dementia syndromes (Frisardi et al., 2010; Sofi et al., 2010; Solfrizzi et al., 2011).

A recent prospective study from France evaluated the association between adherence to MeDi and subsequent cognitive function among ageing adults recruited from the general French population (SU.VI.MAX cohort) (Kesse-Guyot et al., 2013). MeDi adherence was estimated with both the MDS and the Mediterranean-style DP score using data from repeated 24 h dietary records. The authors found no association between MeDi measure and cognitive function except for a lower phonemic fluency score with decreasing Mediterranean-style DP score and a lower backward digit span score with decreasing MDS. However, a low MDS was related to a lower composite cognitive score in the small subsample of manual workers who could be hypothesized to have low cognitive reserve (Kesse-Guyot et al., 2013). Another French study using data from the Three-City cohort with healthy elderly did not report any associations between compliance with MeDi (measured with FFQ and 24 h recalls) and risk of incident dementia, after taking into account the impact of sex, age, education, marital status, energy intake, PA, depressive symptoms, medication use, *APOE* genotype and CVD risk factors (Feart et al., 2009). However, higher adherence to MeDi was associated with slower cognitive decline as assessed by the MMSE but not by other cognitive tests (Feart et al., 2009). Finally, a recent Greek study with elderly individuals (aged 65+ years) with moderate MeDi adherence reported that MeDi (and especially intake of pulses, nuts and seeds) was positively associated with MMSE scores, but only in men (Katsiardanis et al., 2013).

The findings on the association between MeDi adherence and risk of cognitive decline, depression, Parkinson's disease and stroke have been summarized in a 2013 meta-analysis (Psaltopoulou et al., 2013). High adherence to MeDi was consistently associated with a 40% reduced risk of cognitive impairment (including MCI, dementia and AD), a 29% reduced risk of stroke and a 32% reduced risk of depression. Moderate adherence was likewise associated with reduced risk of depression and cognitive impairment (Psaltopoulou et al., 2013). Nonetheless, newer systematic reviews in this domain did not show consistent support for a protective effect of MeDi on cognition (Otaegui-Arrazola et al., 2014). For example, evidence from randomized controlled trials is considered incongruent, and there remain many unanswered questions about the role of various confounding factors such as disease stage, other dietary components and food preparation methods (Otaegui-Arrazola et al., 2014).

### 2.6.2 ASSOCIATIONS WITH OTHER A PRIORI DPS

Adherence to the PNNS-GS has been prospectively linked to better performance on a cued recall test and on semantic and phonemic fluency tasks in a sample of ageing adults from the general French population (Kesse-Guyot et al., 2011a). In addition, cross-sectional research with an international sample of elderly has documented that adherence to the healthy diet indicator was associated with better cognitive function (as measured by the MMSE) among men (Huijbregts et al., 1998). In turn, cross-sectional research based on the Nurses' Health Study has shown that diet quality in midlife, assessed via two FFQs and the alternative HEI, was linked to successful ageing overall. Specifically, these authors reported that individuals in the upper versus the lower quintiles of the alternative HEI in midlife had a 34% greater odds of healthy versus usual ageing (i.e. no major limitations in physical function and mental health) (Samieri et al., 2013).

To date, only one dietary programme, the DASH diet, has been evaluated in a randomized controlled trial with respect to its association with cognitive function (Smith et al., 2010). The results of that intervention showed that in a sample of overweight middle-aged individuals, randomization to the DASH diet combined with a behavioural weight-management programme was associated with improved learning and psychomotor speed after a 4-month intervention compared with randomization to a control diet (control group) (Smith et al., 2010).

### 2.6.3   Associations with A Posteriori DPs

A recent comprehensive review of the scientific evidence revealed that most studies in this domain primarily pertained to *a priori* DPs (Alles et al., 2012). Nonetheless, *a posteriori* DPs have also been examined, albeit rarely, with respect to their association with cognitive performance and decline. For example, using data from the French SU.VI.MAX 2 cohort, researchers estimated the DPs among 3,054 individuals with at least three 24 h dietary records provided at baseline (approximately 13 years before the cognitive function assessment) (Kesse-Guyot et al., 2012). Two uncorrelated DPs, *healthy* and *traditional*, based on 34 different food groups were extracted via principal component analysis. The researchers found a positive association between adherence to the *healthy* DP and overall cognitive function (notably verbal memory), with the beneficial effect being the most salient in the subgroup of participants with moderate energy intake (energy intake <2 492 kcal/d in men and <1 805 kcal/day in women) (Kesse-Guyot et al., 2012).

To date, only two studies have investigated the association between DPs derived via reduced-rank regression and risk of cognitive impairment. Using data from the WHICAP cohort, researchers calculated DP based on 30 different food groups. Next, a DP characterized by high intake of omega-3 and omega-6 fatty acids, folate and vitamin E and low intake of saturated fatty acids and vitamin B12 (corresponding to consumption of oil- and vinegar-based salad dressing, nuts, fish, tomatoes, poultry, cruciferous vegetables, fruit and dark and green leafy vegetables, as well as reduced consumption of high-fat dairy products, meat and butter) was strongly associated with lower incident AD risk (Gu et al., 2010). In turn, using data from the SU.VI.MAX cohort, researchers evaluated the cross-time association between a carotenoid-rich DP and subsequent cognitive performance. The DP was extracted via reduced-rank regression on the basis of repeated 24 h dietary records from 381 participants. Then, it was extrapolated to the whole sample (N = 2983) using plasma carotenoid concentrations (lutein, zeaxanthin, β-cryptoxanthin, lycopene, α-carotene, trans-β-carotene and cis-β-carotene) as response variables.

The principal findings revealed that the carotenoid-rich DP was associated with a higher composite cognitive functioning score, after adjustment for sociodemographic, lifestyle and health covariates. Similar results were seen as regards scores on the cued recall task, backward digit span task, trail-making test and the semantic fluency task (Kesse-Guyot et al., 2014).

Next, using data from the Three-City cohort, researchers grouped elderly men and women into five dietary clusters. They found that a *healthy* DP characterized by high consumption of fish in men and FV in women was cross-sectionally related to better cognitive performance measured by MMSE. The authors noted, however, that nutritional data were difficult to cluster into non-overlapping groups (Samieri et al., 2008). Finally, following a Western DP (characterized by consumption of meats, potatoes, processed foods and high-fat dairy products) was associated with more cognitive decline only in individuals with lower educational attainment (Parrott et al., 2013).

## 2.7 POTENTIAL UNDERLYING MECHANISMS

Overall, the epidemiological studies to date provide evidence that DPs are important contributors to cognitive health and age-related cognitive decline (Alles et al., 2012). A number of underlying direct and indirect pathways have been advanced in reference to the link between diet and cognition. Some of the major pathways that have been the subject of extensive research investigation include reduced inflammation and oxidative stress, improved cardiovascular status, improved insulin regulation and neurogenesis. In the following sections, we discuss each of these elements in more detail.

### 2.7.1 INFLAMMATION

Research evidence supports an age-related increase in inflammation (Parrott & Greenwood, 2007). In turn, a number of observational studies, a few prospective studies and some randomized controlled trials have provided support for the impact of DP (especially MeDi) on markers of inflammation (Ahluwalia et al., 2013). In fact, micronutrients play a role in inflammation, either through modulating cytokine production or by scavenging by-products of activated white cells (Julia et al., 2013). For example, scores on an *a posteriori* DP reflecting high intake of vegetables and vegetable oils, hence high intakes of antioxidant micronutrients and essential fatty acids, were inversely associated with risk of elevated C-reactive protein (a marker of inflammation), while a DP reflecting a high omega-6/omega-3 fatty acid intake ratio was positively associated with elevated C-reactive protein (Julia et al., 2013). In addition to their role in cell membrane structure and function and in neurotransmission, findings suggest that omega-3 fatty acids may have anti-inflammatory capabilities by modulating cytokine activity, neurotrophin expression and anti-apoptotic pathways (Parrott & Greenwood, 2007). Omega-3 fatty acids may also play a role in modifying the expression of genes involved in the regulation of inflammatory mechanisms by activating transcription factors (Alles et al., 2012); see Chapter 7 by McNamara. In turn, improvement in inflammatory marker levels has been correlated with improvement in memory functioning (Witte et al., 2009).

## 2.7.2 OXIDATIVE STRESS

The brain is highly susceptible to oxidative stress and oxidative damage due to its high metabolic load, high oxygen consumption rate and its abundance of oxidizable material, such as the long-chain polyunsaturated fatty acids (i.e. docosahexaenoic acid [DHA]) which form the plasma membranes of neural cells (Gomez-Pinilla, 2008). The free radical hypothesis holds that neuronal degeneration may be due to vulnerability to metabolic sources of reactive oxygen species which could damage key constituents in the brain, such as proteins, cell membrane lipids, RNA and DNA (Joseph et al., 2009; Uttara et al., 2009). Micronutrients with antioxidant capacities (vitamin C, vitamin E, selenium, zinc, flavonoids) that have been associated with mitochondrial activity have been shown to influence cognitive function (Gomez-Pinilla, 2008). Antioxidant microelements such as vitamins E and C, β-carotene, polyphenols and selenium play a role in limiting oxidative stress in nervous cells (Uttara et al., 2009). Findings from a sample of 4447 participants in the SU.VI.MAX trial supported the role of an adequate antioxidant nutrient status in the preservation of verbal memory (Kesse-Guyot et al., 2011b). In particular, the participants in that trial received daily vitamin C (120 mg), β-carotene (6 mg), vitamin E (30 mg), selenium (100 mug) and zinc (20 mg) or placebo over 8 years (1994–2002). In 2007–2009, their cognitive performance was assessed. The results showed that verbal memory was improved by antioxidant supplementation especially in individuals who were nonsmokers or who had low serum vitamin C concentrations at baseline (Kesse-Guyot et al., 2011b).

In turn, DHA (a type of omega-3 fatty acid) might enhance cognitive abilities by facilitating synaptic plasticity or enhancing synaptic membrane fluidity via its effects on metabolism (Gomez-Pinilla, 2008). It is known to stimulate glucose utilization and mitochondrial function, reducing oxidative stress (Gomez-Pinilla, 2008). Oxidative stress damage can also be modulated by flavonoids in FV (Casadesus et al., 2002).

## 2.7.3 CARDIOVASCULAR STATUS

Cardiovascular status, including central adiposity, diabetes and hypertension, has been established as a major risk factor for the development of cognitive impairment via direct and indirect mechanisms (Panza et al., 2010). A number of cardiovascular end points have been investigated in relation to DP (Kourlaba et al., 2009). For example, a Portuguese case–control study demonstrated that *a posteriori* DP with lower FV intake in women and a DP characterized by higher consumption of red meat and alcohol (and lower intake of dairy and vegetables) in both sexes were associated with an increased risk of acute myocardial infarction, as well as increased systolic and diastolic blood pressure, C-reactive protein and uric acid levels (Oliveira et al., 2011). In turn, a DP characterized by an increased consumption of vegetable oils, poultry, fish and seafood and low consumption of sweets was associated with better microvascular function (i.e. functional and anatomic capillary density) in a sample of healthy individuals (Karatzi et al., 2014). Next, the prospective relationship of DP with carotid–femoral pulse-wave velocity (a measure of aortic stiffness) and common-carotid-artery intima–media thickness and plaques was investigated in the French SU.VI.MAX cohort (Kesse-Guyot et al., 2010). These authors reported a significant positive association between pulse-wave velocity and a nutritionally poor DP characterized by meat and alcohol consumption, with low intake of fibre, vitamins B9 and C, β-carotene and calcium (Kesse-Guyot et al., 2010). Specifically related to the role of MeDi in cardiovascular health, a review of the scientific evidence has documented MeDi's beneficial impact on lipoprotein levels, endothelium vasodilatation, the incidence of acute myocardial infarction and cardiovascular mortality (Frisardi et al., 2010). In turn, DPs based on DASH with high FV consumption have been associated with lower systolic and diastolic blood pressure (Dauchet et al., 2007). Finally, the link between healthy DP and reduced dementia risk might be partly explained by a reduction in circulating homocysteine levels spurred by vitamin B12, vitamin B6 and folate (Gu & Scarmeas, 2011); see also Chapter 8.

### 2.7.4 INSULIN REGULATION

A number of hormones or peptides, such as leptin, ghrelin, glucagon-like peptide-1 and insulin, have been postulated to influence emotions and cognitive function (Gomez-Pinilla, 2008). There is evidence of independent associations between abnormal metabolism, found in diabetes, obesity and the metabolic syndrome and mental health (Gomez-Pinilla, 2008). Research suggests that cognitive impairment, especially as regards function dependent on the medial temporal lobes, is seen in type 2 diabetes (Parrott & Greenwood, 2007). Moreover, the consumption of rapidly absorbed, carbohydrate-rich foods with a high glycemic index further impairs medial temporal lobe function, with the related increases in oxidative stress and cytokine release partly explaining the association between DP and reduction in cognitive function in individuals with diabetes (Parrott & Greenwood, 2007). Disruptions in insulin-responsive cell signalling in the brain may lead to brain insults and thus to cognitive function impairment (Parrott & Greenwood, 2007); see also Chapter 6 by Sunram-lea. Insulin resistance and hyperinsulinemia could increase systemic inflammatory response and oxidative stress, thus provoking cognitive function deterioration (Parrott & Greenwood, 2007). Other mechanisms associated with glucose or insulin dysregulation include production of glycation end products, endothelial proliferation, amyloid oligomerization and tau phosphorylation, all of which can lead to vascular and neuronal damage (Panza et al., 2012).

### 2.7.5 NEUROGENESIS

Brain structure and function are dependent on nutritional input and energy balance, which influence synaptic plasticity via changes in gene expression of neurotrophic factors (Dauncey, 2009). In fact, the brain requires a disproportionately large amount of energy relative to the rest of the body (Gomez-Pinilla, 2008). Dietary factors can impact a plethora of brain processes by regulating neurotransmitter pathways, synaptic transmission, membrane fluidity and signal-transduction pathways (Gomez-Pinilla, 2008). Apart from its role in learning and memory, the hippocampus is also one of the two brain structures where neurogenesis (i.e. the formation of new neurons) continues into adulthood (Stangl & Thuret, 2009). Research with animal and human subjects has indeed shown the potential to modulate adult hippocampal neurogenesis by diet (Stangl & Thuret, 2009). However, lifestyle, social interaction and stress can also alter the nutritional effects on mental health (Dauncey, 2009). As regards mental and cognitive outcomes, it is critical to protect the neurons from damage and to promote their vitality via management of chronic illnesses (hypertension, high cholesterol, diabetes), engagement in PA, adherence to a balanced, low-calorie micronutrient-rich diets, adequate sleep and stimulating work and social engagement (Institute for the Study of Ageing, 2005; Middleton & Yaffe, 2009). The field of epigenetics, which deals with the triggering of intracellular signalling and DNA changes by lifestyle factors, is now attracting considerable research attention (Gomez-Pinilla, 2008); see also Chapter 3.

## 2.8 IMPORTANCE OF MIDLIFE EXPOSURES

Substantial research evidence has accumulated in support of the critical importance of midlife exposures (DP, lifestyle behaviours, etc.) for cognitive health, especially in the context of ageing (Hughes & Ganguli, 2009; Middleton & Yaffe, 2009). The assessment of dietary and lifestyle exposures early in adulthood is imperative given the very long progression of diseases such as dementia (de la Torre, 2010). Analyses from the Framingham Offspring Cohort Study convincingly showed that midlife hypertension, diabetes, smoking and obesity were significantly associated with an increased rate of progression of vascular brain injury, global and hippocampal atrophy and a decline in executive function a decade later (Debette et al., 2011). The protective effects of a healthy DP (including MeDi) in midlife on late-life risk of cognitive impairment and dementia have also been reported in different study populations (Eskelinen et al., 2011; Samieri et al., 2013), with the effects being especially salient when total energy intake is regulated (Kesse-Guyot et al., 2012). Next, the assessment of midlife dietary intake is important from the point of view of data validity. In the presence of cognitive impairment or dementia, the accuracy of nutrient intake estimation by FFQ has been questioned (Bowman et al., 2011). Specifically, memory deficits have been shown to weaken the validity of FFQ-derived data (Bowman et al., 2011).

It has been highlighted that diet and exercise modifications are most effective for the prevention of nutrition-related disorders when they are instituted early in life, which would also lead to substantially decreased health-care expenditures (Chernoff, 2001). Nonetheless, positive dietary modifications can be implemented at any age. A number of health behaviour modification and education theories have been developed, which can help guide eating change initiation and maintenance (Spahn et al., 2010).

## 2.9 SUCCESSFUL AGEING AND COGNITIVE AGEING

With advancing age, total and resting energy requirements of the body progressively decrease (Roberts & Dallal, 2005), which has largely been attributed to a reduction in energy expenditure and a decline in the basal metabolic rate. Glucose metabolism and blood flow at rest, specifically in the frontal regions and anterior cingulate, have also been postulated to decline with age (Depp et al., 2012). In particular, brain ageing has been hypothesized to result from a progressive inability to counteract oxidative stress and inflammation (Casadesus et al., 2002).

Balanced, varied and adequate nutrition – rich in complex carbohydrates, FV providing antioxidant and functional nutrients, fish providing essential fatty acids and adequate hydration – plays a key role in a healthy lifestyle that maintains bodily and mental functioning (Cannella et al., 2009). Hence, nutrition is regarded as one of the major determinants of healthy ageing (Cannella et al., 2009). The latter has been defined as 'the process of optimizing opportunities for physical, social and mental health to enable older people to take an active part in society without discrimination and to enjoy an independent and good quality of life' (Swedish National Institute of Public Health, 2006). In turn, successful cognitive ageing is a multidimensional construct which encompasses not only performance in different cognitive domains but also socioemotional constructs such as wisdom and resilience (Depp et al., 2012). Functional and structural neuroimaging research suggests multiple pathways to successful cognitive ageing, by way of brain reserve (i.e. the physical ability to withstand damage) and cognitive reserve (i.e. active compensatory function) (Depp et al., 2012). A commonly cited definition of successful cognitive ageing is that proposed by the 2006 National Institutes of Health's Cognitive and Emotional Health Project, which states that the construct pertains to 'not just as the absence of disease, but rather the development and preservation of the multidimensional cognitive structure that allows the older adult to maintain social connectedness, and ongoing sense of purpose, and the abilities to function independently, to permit functional recovery from illness or injury, and to cope with residual cognitive deficits' (Hendrie et al., 2006, p. 13).

Thus, the objective aspects of successful ageing are based on physical health emphasizing freedom from disability and disease, whereas subjective aspects centre on well-being, social connectedness and adaptation (Jeste et al., 2010). In fact, it has been postulated that most older people do not meet the objective criteria for successful ageing, whereas the majority meet the subjective criteria. Evidence-based behavioural and environmental interventions for enhancing successful ageing include PA, calorie restriction, cognitive stimulation, social support and optimization of stress management (Depp et al., 2012; Jeste et al., 2010).

## 2.10  RESEARCH LIMITATIONS AND FUTURE DIRECTIONS

Generally, the reliable and valid retrospective assessment of dietary intake is considered challenging (Alles et al., 2012). Moreover, it should be kept in mind that considerable within-subject variability of dietary intake exists (Gibson, 2005). Reviews of the research evidence also highlight the issue of energy misreporting in dietary surveys (Devlin et al., 2012; Gibson, 2005). For example, energy underreporting occurs when the individual denies ever eating the food, fails to report the correct portion size consumed or fails to report the number of times the food was consumed (Devlin et al., 2012). Some authors report that the magnitude of underreporting of energy intake is fairly independent of the dietary assessment method used and affects about 30% of studied individuals (Poslusna et al., 2009), whereas others note that misreporting differs by DP (Devlin et al., 2012). Women and over-weight individuals might be more likely to under-report intake (Thompson & Byers, 1994). Whereas statistical correction via the residual method of energy adjustment is useful in decreasing the influence of misreporting (Poslusna et al., 2009), it is important for future studies to explore in more detail the actual effects of energy misreporting (Devlin et al., 2012) as well as the effect of dietary measurement error on DP interpretation (Kant, 2010).

With respect to *a priori* DPs, such as MeDi, some authors have raised questions about internal and external validity, given that two individuals with the same score may have different diets and also that similar MeDi scores do not necessarily cor-respond to similar quantities of foods consumed (Alles et al., 2012). Other concerns about MDS pertain to lack of information on the actual amount of food consumed (only its ranking relative to the sample median), use of different tools for dietary assessment and reliance on dichotomous (beneficial versus detrimental) food groups (Alles et al., 2012). Authors have also noted that *a priori* indices are typically based on current (or slightly outdated) conceptions and might not reflect new knowledge about healthy diets (Remig et al., 2010). For example, fish was not part of the initial HEI, whereas trans-fatty acids have not yet been accounted for by diet quality scores (Remig et al., 2010). With respect to *a posteriori* DPs, some authors have noted that cluster analysis might present more limitations compared with principal compo-nent analysis (Bountziouka et al., 2011) and that such DPs often reflect a number of subjective choices (regarding food groupings, number of DPs retained, pretreatment of nutritional data and variable selection) (Moeller et al., 2007). In addition, factor analysis scores might not be easy to interpret given that a person's diet might load onto more than one factor (Hearty & Gibney, 2009). Nonetheless, there are recur-rent DPs identified in different populations and different contexts. For example, the *healthy/prudent* and the Western DPs have been identified in 30% and 19% of the reviewed studies, respectively (Moeller et al., 2007). Given the current challenges in DP analysis, future research ought to advance methodological guidelines that could streamline and validate DP extraction strategies and thus permit their comparison and synthesis in meta-analyses.

As regards cognitive function, a major limitation concerns the fact that interpre-tation of results and comparisons across studies might be challenging owing to the lack of uniformity in measures of cognition (Alles et al., 2012). It is not possible to draw parallels among studies which focus on global cognitive function, individual cognitive domains or incident cases of MCI and AD (Alles et al., 2012); see Chapters 4 and 8 also. In addition, research evidence suggests that FV, for example, might have a differential effect on cognition according to specific groups of FV and to the type of cognitive function studied (Peneau et al., 2011). Next, further research on the role of MeDi in cognition is needed in a variety of settings because much of the existing evidence is derived from few population samples (Kesse-Guyot et al., 2013; Sofi et al., 2010). Authors have also highlighted the need for additional mechanistic evidence in order to understand whether the potential effects of antioxidants, B vita-mins, long-chain omega-3 fatty acids and MeDi-type DP are indirect via vascular pathways or are directly neuroprotective or anti-amyloidogenic or both (Otaegui-Arrazola et al., 2014). Future research with younger populations (aged 40–65 years);

use of biomarkers, accounting for potentially harmful dietary components; and use of neuroimaging data is also critical (Otaegui-Arrazola et al., 2014). Finally, the presence of publication bias has been evoked, given that no published study to date has reported the absence of associations between *a posteriori* DP and cognitive decline (Alles et al., 2012).

## 2.11  CONCLUDING REMARKS

Investigating the role of a single nutrient or food item in health is challenging because of the marked synergies and interactions among nutrients in the food matrix. Also, the effect of a single nutrient may be too small to be identified, whereas the cumulative effects of a variety of nutrients included in a DP may be sufficiently large to detect. Nutrition is probably one of the major determinants of successful ageing and a key modifiable lifestyle factor which merits increased attention for the primary prevention of cognitive impairment. It has been pointed out that the global ageing of the worldwide population entails an emerging epidemic of age-related cognitive decline and dementia. Current evidence suggests that a MeDi-type diet rich in FV, plant-derived products and seafood rich in long-chain omega-3 fatty acids, with low or moderate alcohol intake and low intakes of meat, saturated fatty acids and added sugar, could be protective against cognitive decline. Beginning early in life, individuals can help reduce their risk of physical and mental impairment in the course of ageing by following a well-balanced, nutritious dietary regimen, maintaining a healthy weight and being physically active.

### TOP 5 SUMMARY POINTS FROM THIS CHAPTER

- The worldwide population ageing portends serious consequences in all areas of life. Researchers forecast an unprecedented rise in age-related morbidity, including cognitive impairment and dementia and associated health-care costs, concomitant with marked declines in the quality of life of the elderly. Hence, urgent and concerted public health action aimed at preserving the physical and mental health and autonomy of the elderly is needed.
- Despite substantial heterogeneity among individuals, normal ageing generally leads to a reduction in brain volume, decreasing number of synapses and decreased integrity of white matter tracts, all leading to potential cognitive impairment. The latter represents a continuum of subjective and objective symptoms, ranging from normal (healthy) cognitive ageing; extending to subjective memory complaints, MCI and preclinical dementia; and ending with AD.
- Given the current lack of dementia cure, prioritizing prevention is critical. The roles of various modifiable lifestyle factors, such as healthy diets, prevention of nutritional deficiencies, engagement in PA and social interaction, have been identified as paramount prevention strategies.

- Nutrition-based strategies – focused on individual nutrients and especially on overall DPs (such as MeDi and DASH) – merit particular attention as prevention options regarding cognitive ageing and cognitive decline, with a potentially far-reaching public health impact.
- Current research evidence suggests that DPs rich in fruit, vegetables, fish, nuts, complex carbohydrates and legumes, coupled with a low consumption of meats, added sugar and high-fat dairy products, might have a beneficial direct and indirect (via reduced inflammation and oxidative stress, improved cardiovascular status, etc.) impact on cognition.

### WHERE TO FROM HERE?

- Future research ought to advance methodological guidelines that could streamline and validate DP extraction strategies and thus permit their comparison and synthesis in meta-analyses.
- Additional mechanistic evidence is needed with respect to the potential direct and indirect effects of a number of nutrients and foods, including antioxidants, B vitamins, long-chain omega-3 fatty acids and Mediterranean-type DPs.
- Future research with younger populations (aged 40–65 years), use of sensitive and novel nutrient status biomarkers and use of neuroimaging data is critical.

## ABBREVIATIONS

AD, Alzheimer's disease
CVD, cardiovascular disease
DASH, Dietary Approaches to Stop Hypertension
DP, dietary pattern(s)
FFQ, food frequency questionnaire(s)
FV, fruit and vegetables
HEI, Healthy Eating Index
MCI, mild cognitive impairment
MDS, Mediterranean diet score
MeDi, Mediterranean diet
MMSE, mini-mental state examination
MRI, magnetic resonance imaging
PA, physical activity
PNNS, Programme National Nutrition Santé
PNNS-GS, Programme National Nutrition Santé Guideline Score

## REFERENCES

Ahluwalia, N., Andreeva, V. A., Kesse-Guyot, E., & Hercberg, S. (2013). Dietary patterns, inflammation and the metabolic syndrome. *Diabetes & Metabolism, 39*(2), 99–110.

Akin, J. S., Guilkey, D. K., Popkin, B. M., & Fanelli, M. T. (1986). Cluster analysis of food consumption patterns of older Americans. *Journal of the American Dietetic Association, 86*(5), 616–624.

Alles, B., Samieri, C., Feart, C., Jutand, M. A., Laurin, D., & Barberger-Gateau, P. (2012). Dietary patterns: A novel approach to examine the link between nutrition and cognitive function in older individuals. *Nutrition Research Reviews, 25*(2), 207–222.

American Psychiatric Association. (2013). *Diagnostic and statistical manual of mental disorders* (5th ed.) *(DSM-5)*. Washington, DC: American Psychiatric Association.

Amieva, H., Jacqmin-Gadda, H., Orgogozo, J. M., Le Carret, N., Helmer, C., Letenneur, L., ... Dartigues, J. F. (2005). The 9 year cognitive decline before dementia of the Alzheimer type: A prospective population-based study. *Brain, 128*(Pt 5), 1093–1101.

Amieva, H., Le Goff, M., Millet, X., Orgogozo, J. M., Peres, K., Barberger-Gateau, P., ... Dartigues, J. F. (2008). Prodromal Alzheimer's disease: Successive emergence of the clinical symptoms. *Annals of Neurology, 64*(5), 492–498.

Appel, L. J., Moore, T. J., Obarzanek, E., Vollmer, W. M., Svetkey, L. P., Sacks, F. M., ... Karanja, N. (1997). A clinical trial of the effects of dietary patterns on blood pressure. DASH Collaborative Research Group. *The New England Journal of Medicine, 336*(16), 1117–1124.

Bamia, C., Trichopoulos, D., Ferrari, P., Overvad, K., Bjerregaard, L., Tjonneland, A., ... Trichopoulou, A. (2007). Dietary patterns and survival of older Europeans: The EPIC-Elderly Study (European Prospective Investigation into Cancer and Nutrition). *Public Health Nutrition, 10*(6), 590–598.

Bernstein, M., & Munoz, N. (2012). Position of the Academy of Nutrition and Dietetics: Food and nutrition for older adults: Promoting health and wellness. *Journal of the Academy of Nutrition and Dietetics, 112*(8), 1255–1277.

Bertuccio, P., Rosato, V., Andreano, A., Ferraroni, M., Decarli, A., Edefonti, V., & La Vecchia, C. (2013). Dietary patterns and gastric cancer risk: A systematic review and meta-analysis. *Annals of Oncology, 24*(6), 1450–1458.

Borsch-Supan, A. (1992). Population ageing, social security design, and early retirement. *Journal of Institutional and Theoretical Economics, 148*(4), 533–557.

Bountziouka, V., Tzavelas, G., Polychronopoulos, E., Constantinidis, T. C., & Panagiotakos, D. B. (2011). Validity of dietary patterns derived in nutrition surveys using a priori and a posteriori multivariate statistical methods. *International Journal of Food Sciences and Nutrition, 62*(6), 617–627.

Bowman, G. L., Shannon, J., Ho, E., Traber, M. G., Frei, B., Oken, B. S., ... Quinn, J. F. (2011). Reliability and validity of food frequency questionnaire and nutrient biomarkers in elders with and without mild cognitive impairment. *Alzheimer Disease and Associated Disorders, 25*(1), 49–57.

Brodaty, H., Heffernan, M., Kochan, N. A., Draper, B., Trollor, J. N., Reppermund, S., ... Sachdev, P. S. (2013). Mild cognitive impairment in a community sample: The Sydney Memory and Ageing Study. *Alzheimer's & Dementia, 9*(3), 310–317, e311.

Cannella, C., Savina, C., & Donini, L. M. (2009). Nutrition, longevity and behavior. *Archives of Gerontology and Geriatrics, 49*(Suppl. 1), 19–27.

Casadesus, G., Shukitt-Hale, B., & Joseph, J. A. (2002). Qualitative versus quantitative caloric intake: Are they equivalent paths to successful ageing? *Neurobiology of Aging, 23*(5), 747–769.

Chernoff, R. (2001). Nutrition and health promotion in older adults. *The Journals of Gerontology Series A: Biological Sciences and Medical Sciences, 56*(Spec No 2), 47–53.

Cheung, B. H., Ho, I. C., Chan, R. S., Sea, M. M., & Woo, J. (2014). Current evidence on dietary pattern and cognitive function. *Advances in Food and Nutrition Research, 71*, 137–163.

Dauchet, L., Kesse-Guyot, E., Czernichow, S., Bertrais, S., Estaquio, C., Peneau, S., … Hercberg, S. (2007). Dietary patterns and blood pressure change over 5-y follow-up in the SU.VI.MAX cohort. *The American Journal of Clinical Nutrition, 85*(6), 1650–1656.

Dauncey, M. J. (2009). New insights into nutrition and cognitive neuroscience. *Proceedings of the Nutrition Society, 68*(4), 408–415.

Daviglus, M. L., Plassman, B. L., Pirzada, A., Bell, C. C., Bowen, P. E., Burke, J. R., … Williams, J. W., Jr. (2011). Risk factors and preventive interventions for Alzheimer disease: State of the science. *Archives of Neurology, 68*(9), 1185–1190.

de la Torre, J. C. (2010). Alzheimer's disease is incurable but preventable. *Journal of Alzheimer's Disease, 20*(3), 861–870.

Debette, S., Seshadri, S., Beiser, A., Au, R., Himali, J. J., Palumbo, C., … DeCarli, C. (2011). Midlife vascular risk factor exposure accelerates structural brain ageing and cognitive decline. *Neurology, 77*(5), 461–468.

Depp, C. A., Harmell, A., & Vahia, I. V. (2012). Successful cognitive ageing. *Current Topics in Behavioral Neurosciences, 10*, 35–50.

Devlin, U. M., McNulty, B. A., Nugent, A. P., & Gibney, M. J. (2012). The use of cluster analysis to derive dietary patterns: Methodological considerations, reproducibility, validity and the effect of energy mis-reporting. *Proceedings of the Nutrition Society, 71*(4), 599–609.

Drexler, E. I., Voss, B., Amunts, K., Schneider, F., & Habel, U. (2013). Mild cognitive impairment: Advantages of a comprehensive neuropsychological assessment. *Current Alzheimer Research, 10*(10), 1098–1106.

Eskelinen, M. H., Ngandu, T., Tuomilehto, J., Soininen, H., & Kivipelto, M. (2011). Midlife healthy-diet index and late-life dementia and Alzheimer's disease. *Dementia and Geriatric Disorders Extra, 1*(1), 103–112.

Estaquio, C., Kesse-Guyot, E., Deschamps, V., Bertrais, S., Dauchet, L., Galan, P., … Castetbon, K. (2009). Adherence to the French Programme National Nutrition Sante Guideline Score is associated with better nutrient intake and nutritional status. *Journal of the American Dietetic Association, 109*(6), 1031–1041.

Feart, C., Samieri, C., Rondeau, V., Amieva, H., Portet, F., Dartigues, J. F., … Barberger-Gateau, P. (2009). Adherence to a Mediterranean diet, cognitive decline, and risk of dementia. *JAMA, 302*(6), 638–648.

Folstein, M. F., Folstein, S. E., & McHugh, P. R. (1975). "Mini-mental state". A practical method for grading the cognitive state of patients for the clinician. *Journal of Psychiatric Research, 12*(3), 189–198.

Freeman, W. D., Vatz, K. A., Griggs, R. C., & Pedley, T. (2013). The Workforce Task Force report: Clinical implications for neurology. *Neurology, 81*(5), 479–486.

Frisardi, V., Panza, F., Seripa, D., Imbimbo, B. P., Vendemiale, G., Pilotto, A., & Solfrizzi, V. (2010). Nutraceutical properties of Mediterranean diet and cognitive decline: Possible underlying mechanisms. *Journal of Alzheimer's Disease, 22*(3), 715–740.

Gibson, R. S. (2005). *Principles of nutritional assessment* (2nd ed.). New York: Oxford University Press.

Gillette-Guyonnet, S., Secher, M., & Vellas, B. (2013). Nutrition and neurodegeneration: Epidemiological evidence and challenges for future research. *British Journal of Clinical Pharmacology, 75*(3), 738–755.

Gomez-Pinilla, F. (2008). Brain foods: The effects of nutrients on brain function. *Nature Reviews Neuroscience, 9*(7), 568–578.

Gu, Y., Luchsinger, J. A., Stern, Y., & Scarmeas, N. (2010). Mediterranean diet, inflammatory and metabolic biomarkers, and risk of Alzheimer's disease. *Journal of Alzheimer's Disease, 22*(2), 483–492.

Gu, Y., Nieves, J. W., Stern, Y., Luchsinger, J. A., & Scarmeas, N. (2010). Food combi-
    nation and Alzheimer disease risk: A protective diet. *Archives of Neurology, 67*(6),
    699–706.
Gu, Y., & Scarmeas, N. (2011). Dietary patterns in Alzheimer's disease and cognitive ageing.
    *Current Alzheimer Research, 8*(5), 510–519.
Harada, C. N., Natelson Love, M. C., & Triebel, K. L. (2013). Normal cognitive ageing.
    *Clinics in Geriatric Medicine, 29*(4), 737–752.
Hearty, A. P., & Gibney, M. J. (2009). Comparison of cluster and principal component analysis
    techniques to derive dietary patterns in Irish adults. *British Journal of Nutrition, 101*(4),
    598–608.
Hendrie, H. C., Albert, M. S., Butters, M. A., Gao, S., Knopman, D. S., Launer, L. J., …
    Wagster, M. V. (2006). The NIH Cognitive and Emotional Health Project. Report of the
    critical evaluation study committee. *Alzheimer's Dement, 2*(1), 12–32.
Hercberg, S., Chat-Yung, S., & Chaulia, M. (2008). The French National Nutrition and Health
    Program: 2001–2006–2010. *International Journal of Public Health, 53*(2), 68–77.
Hoffmann, K., Schulze, M. B., Schienkiewitz, A., Nothlings, U., & Boeing, H. (2004).
    Application of a new statistical method to derive dietary patterns in nutritional epidemi-
    ology. *American Journal of Epidemiology, 159*(10), 935–944.
Hu, F. B. (2002). Dietary pattern analysis: A new direction in nutritional epidemiology.
    *Current Opinion in Lipidology, 13*(1), 3–9.
Hughes, T. F., & Ganguli, M. (2009). Modifiable midlife risk factors for late-life cognitive
    impairment and dementia. *Current Psychiatry Reviews, 5*(2), 73–92.
Huijbregts, P., Feskens, E., Rasanen, L., Fidanza, F., Nissinen, A., Menotti, A., & Kromhout,
    D. (1997). Dietary pattern and 20 year mortality in elderly men in Finland, Italy, and The
    Netherlands: Longitudinal cohort study. *BMJ, 315*(7099), 13–17.
Huijbregts, P. P., Feskens, E. J., Rasanen, L., Fidanza, F., Alberti-Fidanza, A., Nissinen, A., …
    Kromhout, D. (1998). Dietary patterns and cognitive function in elderly men in Finland,
    Italy and The Netherlands. *European Journal of Clinical Nutrition, 52*(11), 826–831.
Institute for the Study of Ageing. (2005). *A practical guide to achieving and maintaining cog-
    nitive vitality with ageing.* New York: Institute for the Study of Ageing, Ltd.
Issa, C., Darmon, N., Salameh, P., Maillot, M., Batal, M., & Lairon, D. (2011). A Mediterranean
    diet pattern with low consumption of liquid sweets and refined cereals is negatively
    associated with adiposity in adults from rural Lebanon. *International Journal of Obesity
    (London), 35*(2), 251–258.
Jacobs, D. M., Sano, M., Dooneief, G., Marder, K., Bell, K. L., & Stern, Y. (1995).
    Neuropsychological detection and characterization of preclinical Alzheimer's disease.
    *Neurology, 45*(5), 957–962.
Jacobs, D. R., Jr., Gross, M. D., & Tapsell, L. C. (2009). Food synergy: An operational con-
    cept for understanding nutrition. *The American Journal of Clinical Nutrition, 89*(5),
    1543S–1548S.
Jeste, D. V., Depp, C. A., & Vahia, I. V. (2010). Successful cognitive and emotional ageing.
    *World Psychiatry, 9*(2), 78–84.
Jonker, C., Geerlings, M. I., & Schmand, B. (2000). Are memory complaints predictive for
    dementia? A review of clinical and population-based studies. *International Journal of
    Geriatric Psychiatry, 15*(11), 983–991.
Joseph, J., Cole, G., Head, E., & Ingram, D. (2009). Nutrition, brain ageing, and neurodegen-
    eration. *The Journal of Neuroscience, 29*(41), 12795–12801.
Julia, C., Meunier, N., Touvier, M., Ahluwalia, N., Sapin, V., Papet, I., … Kesse-Guyot, E.
    (2013). Dietary patterns and risk of elevated C-reactive protein concentrations 12 years
    later. *British Journal of Nutrition, 110*(4), 747–754.
Kant, A. K. (1996). Indexes of overall diet quality: A review. *Journal of the American Dietetic
    Association, 96*(8), 785–791.

Kant, A. K. (2010). Dietary patterns: Biomarkers and chronic disease risk. *Applied Physiology, Nutrition, and Metabolism, 35*(2), 199–206.

Kant, A. K., & Graubard, B. I. (2005). A comparison of three dietary pattern indexes for predicting biomarkers of diet and disease. *Journal of the American College of Nutrition, 24*(4), 294–303.

Karatzi, K., Protogerou, A., Kesse-Guyot, E., Fezeu, L. K., Carette, C., Blacher, J., ... Czernichow, S. (2014). Associations between dietary patterns and skin microcirculation in healthy subjects. *Arteriosclerosis, Thrombosis, and Vascular Biology, 34*(2), 463–469.

Katsiardanis, K., Diamantaras, A. A., Dessypris, N., Michelakos, T., Anastasiou, A., Katsiardani, K. P., ... Petridou, E. T. (2013). Cognitive impairment and dietary habits among elders: The Velestino Study. *Journal of Medicinal Food, 16*(4), 343–350.

Kennedy, E. T., Ohls, J., Carlson, S., & Fleming, K. (1995). The Healthy Eating Index: Design and applications. *Journal of the American Dietetic Association, 95*(10), 1103–1108.

Kesse-Guyot, E., Amieva, H., Castetbon, K., Henegar, A., Ferry, M., Jeandel, C., ... SU.VI. MAX 2 Research Group. (2011a). Adherence to nutritional recommendations and subsequent cognitive performance: Findings from the prospective Supplementation with Antioxidant Vitamins and Minerals 2 (SU.VI.MAX 2) study. *The American Journal of Clinical Nutrition, 93*(1), 200–210.

Kesse-Guyot, E., Andreeva, V. A., Ducros, V., Jeandel, C., Julia, C., Hercberg, S., & Galan, P. (2014). Carotenoid-rich dietary patterns during midlife and subsequent cognitive function. *British Journal of Nutrition, 111*(5):915–923.

Kesse-Guyot, E., Andreeva, V. A., Jeandel, C., Ferry, M., Hercberg, S., & Galan, P. (2012). A healthy dietary pattern at midlife is associated with subsequent cognitive performance. *Journal of Nutrition, 142*(5), 909–915.

Kesse-Guyot, E., Andreeva, V. A., Lassale, C., Ferry, M., Jeandel, C., Hercberg, S., & Barberger-Gateau, P. (2013). Mediterranean diet and cognitive function: A French study. *The American Journal of Clinical Nutrition, 97*(2), 369–376.

Kesse-Guyot, E., Bertrais, S., Peneau, S., Estaquio, C., Dauchet, L., Vergnaud, A. C., ... Bellisle, F. (2009). Dietary patterns and their sociodemographic and behavioural correlates in French middle-aged adults from the SU.VI.MAX cohort. *European Journal of Clinical Nutrition, 63*(4), 521–528.

Kesse-Guyot, E., Fezeu, L., Jeandel, C., Ferry, M., Andreeva, V., Amieva, H., ... Galan, P. (2011b). French adults' cognitive performance after daily supplementation with antioxidant vitamins and minerals at nutritional doses: A post hoc analysis of the Supplementation in Vitamins and Mineral Antioxidants (SU.VI.MAX) trial. *The American Journal of Clinical Nutrition, 94*(3), 892–899.

Kesse-Guyot, E., Vergnaud, A. C., Fezeu, L., Zureik, M., Blacher, J., Peneau, S., ... Czernichow, S. (2010). Associations between dietary patterns and arterial stiffness, carotid artery intima-media thickness and atherosclerosis. *European Journal of Cardiovascular Prevention and Rehabilitation, 17*(6), 718–724.

Korczyc, E., Laco, M., Vincelette, G. A., Cuaresma, J. C., & Loichinger, E. (2013). *EU11 regular economic report No. 26. Macroeconomic report: Faltering recovery. Special topic: The economic growth implications of an ageing European Union* (No. #74822). Washington, DC: The World Bank.

Kourlaba, G., Polychronopoulos, E., Zampelas, A., Lionis, C., & Panagiotakos, D. B. (2009). Development of a diet index for older adults and its relation to cardiovascular disease risk factors: The Elderly Dietary Index. *Journal of the American Dietetic Association, 109*(6), 1022–1030.

Lezak, M. D., Howieson, D. B., Bigler, E. D., & Tranel, D. (2012). *Neuropsychological assessment* (5th ed.). New York: Oxford University Press.

Masdeu, J. C., Kreisl, W. C., & Berman, K. F. (2012). The neurobiology of Alzheimer disease defined by neuroimaging. *Current Opinion in Neurology, 25*(4), 410–420.

McCullough, M. L., Feskanich, D., Stampfer, M. J., Giovannucci, E. L., Rimm, E. B., Hu, F. B., ... Willett, W. C. (2002). Diet quality and major chronic disease risk in men and women: Moving toward improved dietary guidance. *The American Journal of Clinical Nutrition, 76*(6), 1261–1271.

Middleton, L. E., & Yaffe, K. (2009). Promising strategies for the prevention of dementia. *Archives of Neurology, 66*(10), 1210–1215.

Moeller, S. M., Reedy, J., Millen, A. E., Dixon, L. B., Newby, P. K., Tucker, K. L., ... Guenther, P. M. (2007). Dietary patterns: Challenges and opportunities in dietary patterns research an Experimental Biology workshop, April 1, 2006. *Journal of the American Dietetic Association, 107*(7), 1233–1239.

Mozaffarian, D., Appel, L. J., & Van Horn, L. (2011). Components of a cardioprotective diet: New insights. *Circulation, 123*(24), 2870–2891.

Newby, P. K., & Tucker, K. L. (2004). Empirically derived eating patterns using factor or cluster analysis: A review. *Nutrition Reviews, 62*(5), 177–203.

Ngo, J., Engelen, A., Molag, M., Roesle, J., Garcia-Segovia, P., & Serra-Majem, L. (2009). A review of the use of information and communication technologies for dietary assessment. *British Journal of Nutrition, 101 Suppl. 2*, S102–112.

Oliveira, A., Rodriguez-Artalejo, F., Gaio, R., Santos, A. C., Ramos, E., & Lopes, C. (2011). Major habitual dietary patterns are associated with acute myocardial infarction and cardiovascular risk markers in a southern European population. *Journal of the American Dietetic Association, 111*(2), 241–250.

Ortiz-Andrellucchi, A., Sanchez-Villegas, A., Doreste-Alonso, J., de Vries, J., de Groot, L., & Serra-Majem, L. (2009). Dietary assessment methods for micronutrient intake in elderly people: A systematic review. *British Journal of Nutrition, 102*(Suppl. 1), S118–S149.

Otaegui-Arrazola, A., Amiano, P., Elbusto, A., Urdaneta, E., & Martinez-Lage, P. (2014). Diet, cognition, and Alzheimer's disease: Food for thought. *European Journal of Nutrition, 53*(1), 1–23.

Pandya, A., Gaziano, T. A., Weinstein, M. C., & Cutler, D. (2013). More Americans living longer with cardiovascular disease will increase costs while lowering quality of life. *Health Affairs (Millwood), 32*(10), 1706–1714.

Panza, F., Frisardi, V., Capurso, C., Imbimbo, B. P., Vendemiale, G., Santamato, A., ... Solfrizzi, V. (2010). Metabolic syndrome and cognitive impairment: Current epidemiology and possible underlying mechanisms. *Journal of Alzheimer's Disease, 21*(3), 691–724.

Panza, F., Solfrizzi, V., Logroscino, G., Maggi, S., Santamato, A., Seripa, D., & Pilotto, A. (2012). Current epidemiological approaches to the metabolic-cognitive syndrome. *Journal of Alzheimer's Disease, 30*(Suppl. 2), S31–S75.

Parrott, M. D., & Greenwood, C. E. (2007). Dietary influences on cognitive function with ageing: From high-fat diets to healthful eating. *Annals of the New York Academy of Sciences, 1114*, 389–397.

Parrott, M. D., Shatenstein, B., Ferland, G., Payette, H., Morais, J. A., Belleville, S., ... Greenwood, C. E. (2013). Relationship between diet quality and cognition depends on socioeconomic position in healthy older adults. *Journal of Nutrition, 143*(11), 1767–1773.

Patterson, R. E., Haines, P. S., & Popkin, B. M. (1994). Diet quality index: Capturing a multi-dimensional behavior. *Journal of the American Dietetic Association, 94*(1), 57–64.

Peneau, S., Galan, P., Jeandel, C., Ferry, M., Andreeva, V., Hercberg, S., ... SU.VI.MAX 2 Research Group. (2011). Fruit and vegetable intake and cognitive function in the SU.VI.MAX 2 prospective study. *The American Journal of Clinical Nutrition, 94*(5), 1295–1303.

Perez-Lopez, F. R., Chedraui, P., Haya, J., & Cuadros, J. L. (2009). Effects of the Mediterranean diet on longevity and age-related morbid conditions. *Maturitas, 64*(2), 67–79.

Poslusna, K., Ruprich, J., de Vries, J. H., Jakubikova, M., & van't Veer, P. (2009). Misreporting of energy and micronutrient intake estimated by food records and 24 hour recalls, control and adjustment methods in practice. *British Journal of Nutrition, 101*(Suppl. 2), S73–S85.

Psaltopoulou, T., Sergentanis, T. N., Panagiotakos, D. B., Sergentanis, I. N., Kosti, R., & Scarmeas, N. (2013). Mediterranean diet, stroke, cognitive impairment, and depression: A meta-analysis. *Annals of Neurology, 74*(4), 580–591.

Querfurth, H. W., & LaFerla, F. M. (2010). Alzheimer's disease. *The New England Journal of Medicine, 362*(4), 329–344.

Reichman, W. E., Fiocco, A. J., & Rose, N. S. (2010). Exercising the brain to avoid cognitive decline: Examining the evidence. *Ageing Health, 6*(5), 565–584.

Remig, V., Franklin, B., Margolis, S., Kostas, G., Nece, T., & Street, J. C. (2010). Trans fats in America: A review of their use, consumption, health implications, and regulation. *Journal of the American Dietetic Association, 110*(4), 585–592.

Ritchie, K., Artero, S., & Touchon, J. (2001). Classification criteria for mild cognitive impairment: A population-based validation study. *Neurology, 56*(1), 37–42.

Roberts, S. B., & Dallal, G. E. (2005). Energy requirements and ageing. *Public Health Nutrition, 8*(7A), 1028–1036.

Roman, G. C. (2003). Vascular dementia: Distinguishing characteristics, treatment, and prevention. *Journal of the American Geriatrics Society, 51*(5 Suppl. Dementia), S296–S304.

Roman-Vinas, B., Ribas Barba, L., Ngo, J., Martinez-Gonzalez, M. A., Wijnhoven, T. M., & Serra-Majem, L. (2009). Validity of dietary patterns to assess nutrient intake adequacy. *British Journal of Nutrition, 101*(Suppl. 2), S12–S20.

Rumawas, M. E., Meigs, J. B., Dwyer, J. T., McKeown, N. M., & Jacques, P. F. (2009). Mediterranean-style dietary pattern, reduced risk of metabolic syndrome traits, and incidence in the Framingham Offspring Cohort. *The American Journal of Clinical Nutrition, 90*(6), 1608–1614.

Samieri, C., Jutand, M. A., Feart, C., Capuron, L., Letenneur, L., & Barberger-Gateau, P. (2008). Dietary patterns derived by hybrid clustering method in older people: Association with cognition, mood, and self-rated health. *Journal of the American Dietetic Association, 108*(9), 1461–1471.

Samieri, C., Sun, Q., Townsend, M. K., Chiuve, S. E., Okereke, O. I., Willett, W. C., … Grodstein, F. (2013). The association between dietary patterns at midlife and health in ageing: An observational study. *Annals of Internal Medicine, 159*(9), 584–591.

Shankle, W. R., Romney, A. K., Hara, J., Fortier, D., Dick, M. B., Chen, J. M., … Sun, X. (2005). Methods to improve the detection of mild cognitive impairment. *Proceedings of the National Academy of Sciences of the United States of America, 102*(13), 4919–4924.

Shatenstein, B., Ferland, G., Belleville, S., Gray-Donald, K., Kergoat, M. J., Morais, J., … Greenwood, C. (2012). Diet quality and cognition among older adults from the NuAge study. *Experimental Gerontology, 47*(5), 353–360.

Smith, P. J., Blumenthal, J. A., Babyak, M. A., Craighead, L., Welsh-Bohmer, K. A., Browndyke, J. N., … Sherwood, A. (2010). Effects of the dietary approaches to stop hypertension diet, exercise, and caloric restriction on neurocognition in overweight adults with high blood pressure. *Hypertension, 55*(6), 1331–1338.

Sofi, F., Macchi, C., Abbate, R., Gensini, G. F., & Casini, A. (2010). Effectiveness of the Mediterranean diet: Can it help delay or prevent Alzheimer's disease? *Journal of Alzheimer's Disease, 20*(3), 795–801.

Sofi, F., Macchi, C., Abbate, R., Gensini, G. F., & Casini, A. (2013). Mediterranean diet and health status: An updated meta-analysis and a proposal for a literature-based adherence score. *Public Health Nutrition.* doi:http://dx.doi.org/10.1017/S1368980013003169

Solfrizzi, V., Capurso, C., D'Introno, A., Colacicco, A. M., Santamato, A., Ranieri, M., … Panza, F. (2008). Lifestyle-related factors in predementia and dementia syndromes. *Expert Review of Neurotherapeutics, 8*(1), 133–158.

Solfrizzi, V., Frisardi, V., Seripa, D., Logroscino, G., Imbimbo, B. P., D'Onofrio, G., ... Panza, F. (2011). Mediterranean diet in predementia and dementia syndromes. *Current Alzheimer Research, 8*(5), 520–542.

Spahn, J. M., Reeves, R. S., Keim, K. S., Laquatra, I., Kellogg, M., Jortberg, B., & Clark, N. A. (2010). State of the evidence regarding behavior change theories and strategies in nutrition counseling to facilitate health and food behavior change. *Journal of the American Dietetic Association, 110*(6), 879–891.

Stangl, D., & Thuret, S. (2009). Impact of diet on adult hippocampal neurogenesis. *Genes & Nutrition, 4*(4), 271–282.

Swedish National Institute of Public Health. (2006). *Healthy ageing: A challenge for Europe.* Stockholm, Sweden: Swedish National Institute of Public Health.

Teng, E. L., & Chui, H. C. (1987). The Modified Mini-Mental State (3MS) examination. *Journal of Clinical Psychiatry, 48*(8), 314–318.

Thomann, P. A., Seidl, U., Brinkmann, J., Hirjak, D., Traeger, T., Wolf, R. C., ... Schroder, J. (2012). Hippocampal morphology and autobiographic memory in mild cognitive impairment and Alzheimer's disease. *Current Alzheimer Research, 9*(4), 507–515.

Thompson, F. E., & Byers, T. (1994). Dietary assessment resource manual. *Journal of Nutrition, 124*(11 Suppl.), 2245S–2317S.

Trichopoulou, A., Costacou, T., Bamia, C., & Trichopoulos, D. (2003). Adherence to a Mediterranean diet and survival in a Greek population. *The New England Journal of Medicine, 348*(26), 2599–2608.

United Nations. (2002). *World population ageing: 1950–2050.* New York: United Nations, Department of Economic and Social Affairs.

U.S. Census Bureau Population Division. Projection of the population by age and sex for the United States: 2010 to 2050 (NP2008-T12). Washington, DC: U.S. Census Bureau. Released on August 14, 2008.

Uttara, B., Singh, A. V., Zamboni, P., & Mahajan, R. T. (2009). Oxidative stress and neurodegenerative diseases: A review of upstream and downstream antioxidant therapeutic options. *Current Neuropharmacology, 7*(1), 65–74.

Waijers, P. M., Feskens, E. J., & Ocke, M. C. (2007). A critical review of predefined diet quality scores. *British Journal of Nutrition, 97*(2), 219–231.

Willett, W. (1998). *Nutritional epidemiology* (2nd ed.). Oxford, U.K.: Oxford University Press.

Willett, W. C., Sacks, F., Trichopoulou, A., Drescher, G., Ferro-Luzzi, A., Helsing, E., & Trichopoulos, D. (1995). Mediterranean diet pyramid: A cultural model for healthy eating. *The American Journal of Clinical Nutrition, 61*(6 Suppl.), 1402S–1406S.

Witte, A. V., Fobker, M., Gellner, R., Knecht, S., & Floel, A. (2009). Caloric restriction improves memory in elderly humans. *Proceedings of the National Academy of Sciences of the United States of America, 106*(4), 1255–1260.

Woo, J. (2011). Nutritional strategies for successful ageing. *Medical Clinics of North America, 95*(3), 477–493, ix–x.

World Health Organization. (2014). *Definition of an older or elderly person.* Geneva, Switzerland: WHO.

# 3 Genetics of Brain and Cognition and Their Interactions with Dietary and Environmental Factors

*Jose M. Ordovas*

## CONTENTS

## SUMMARY

Genetic, epigenetic and dietary factors and their interactions play a major role in brain development and the balance between its health and disease status. The dramatic developments in genomic and neuroimaging techniques are enabling researchers to study these interactions with new breadth and depth. This chapter provides a definition of key terms used to examine the relationship between genetics, diet, metabolism and brain function. Both TCF7L2 and *APOE* will be discussed and current knowledge regarding genetics and brain architecture and function will be reviewed.

## 3.1   INTRODUCTION

A distinctive feature of the modern human is its brain size. Humans have developed an energetically costly brain that needs a constant influx of energy and other nutrients. It has been hypothesized that the current brain size and function of contemporary humans has been achieved thanks to a nutritional shift towards high-quality diets that included, among other things, more meat and energy-dense foods (Armelagos, 2014). To this purpose, the controlled use of fire and the possibility of cooking, as well as other types of food processing, are exclusive human features that increased our ability to extract more calories from the food as well as the use of new food sources. These changes have required significant metabolic adaptations to new foods and environments that have been driven by recent genetic positive selection (Jeong & DiRienzo, 2014) such as those represented by the variable number of copies of the amylase gene (Santos et al., 2012) or lactase persistency (Brüssow, 2013; Gerbault et al., 2013), both driven by the nutritional environment. In general, dietary factors exert their effects on the brain by affecting molecular events related to the management of energy metabolism and synaptic plasticity. Energy metabolism influences neuronal function, neuronal signalling and synaptic plasticity, ultimately affecting mental health (Gomez-Pinilla & Tyagi, 2013). Among the dietary factors involved, dietary docosahexaenoic acid (DHA) seems crucial for supporting plasma membrane function, interneuronal signalling and cognition (see Chapter 7 from McNamara and Valentine). Thus, it has been proposed that the adoption by our ancestors of a *shore* diet was crucial for the evolutionary development of our brain (Duarte, 2014).

The new genomic tools are providing us with some evidence to understand the genetic changes supporting these recent human adaptations. In fact, those genes related to metabolism display some of the strongest signals of positive natural selection (Brown, 2012), particularly, those involved in protein, carbohydrate, lipid and phosphate metabolism. However, food has not been the only changing environment since our ancestors exited Africa and recent research has provided evidence for genes involved in metabolic adaptation to cold (i.e. *ME2*, *ME3*, *LEPR*, *PON1*, *UCP1* and *UCP3*) and high altitude (i.e. *EGLN1*, *EPAS1*, *PRKAA1*, *NOS2A* and *PPARA*). However, for our purpose, we will focus on those associated directly with nutrient metabolism and with nutrition-related metabolic disorders. In this regard, signatures of positive selection have been found for *PCSK9*, encoding a serine protease known to degrade the low-density lipoprotein receptor; *ANGPTL4*, a gene involved in the regulation of glucose and lipid metabolism that contains variants known to affect triglyceride and HDL levels; *ALMS1*, a gene involved in ciliogenesis and also associated with obesity and type 2 diabetes; *TCF7L2*, a transcription factor with a well-known association with type 2 diabetes; and *APOE*, the most studied of all, which is involved in binding, uptake and catabolism of lipoproteins. Specifically, the *APOE4* allele has been associated with increased total cholesterol, low-density lipoprotein cholesterol, cholesterol absorption and responsiveness to dietary fats and with cognition and Alzheimer's disease (AD), making this locus the most interesting candidate gene to examine the relationship between genetics, diet, metabolism and brain function. Both TCF7L2 and *APOE* will be discussed in more detail in Sections 3.3 and 3.5, respectively, but before we get to them, we will review our current knowledge regarding genetics and brain architecture and function.

## 3.2 GENES RELATED TO BRAIN ARCHITECTURE AND FUNCTION

Regarding brain anatomy, the current evidence indicates that the different features examined are highly heritable, with the genetic component accounting for up to 80% of its variability. However, the genetic variants identified so far using genome-wide association studies (GWASs) and traditional phenotypes can explain merely 5% of the variance. A more recent study has investigated the genomic architecture of human neuroanatomical diversity (Toro et al., 2014) using neuroimaging and whole-genome genotyping data from 1765 subjects. The investigators show that up to 54% of the heritability is captured by large numbers of single-nucleotide polymorphisms (SNPs) of small-effect spread throughout the genome, especially within genes and close regulatory regions. Table 3.1 illustrates the loci identified using this approach (Baranzini et al., 2009; Jahanshad et al., 2013; Kim & Webster, 2011; Paus et al., 2012; Potkin et al., 2009; Shen et al., 2010; Stein et al., 2010a, 2010b, 2012). The traits that have shown statistically significant associations at the GWAS level ($p < 5 \times 10^{-8}$) include *brain connectivity* and *brain structure*. For other traits, such as *brain development*, *brain cytoarchitecture*, *brain imaging* and *brain lesion load*, none of the association signals reached the threshold for GWAS significance.

For brain connectivity, the published GWAS investigated a relatively small number of subjects (n = 331). Therefore, the results should be interpreted with caution and need validation. The most significant findings include regions on chromosome 20 (encompassing endosulfine alpha pseudogene 1 [*ENSAP1*] and peptidylprolyl isomerase A [cyclophilin A] pseudogene 17 [*PPIAP17*]), chromosome 6 (cytochrome C, somatic pseudogene 17 [*CYCSP17*]) and chromosome 3 (including keratin 8 pseudogene 25 [*KRT8P25*] and apolipoprotein O pseudogene 2 [*APOOP2*]). The fact that all these loci include pseudogenes hinders the biological interpretation of the findings. Nevertheless, other signals fall within or near genes with closer neurological ties. This is the case of the neural precursor cell-expressed, developmentally down-regulated 4, E3 ubiquitin protein ligase (*NEDD4*) gene on chromosome 15. This gene is expressed in brain and it has been associated with several functions, including its membership on a signalling complex that includes also RAP2A and TNIK, which regulates neuronal dendrite extension and arborization during development; the ubiquitin-conjugating enzyme E2A (*UBE2A*), on chromosome X, has been previously associated with several diseases including mental retardation; the leucine-rich repeat-containing 20 (*LRRC20*) gene, on chromosome 10, has not been well characterized but it is expressed also in different regions of the brain. The tachykinin receptor 1 (*TACR1*), on chromosome 2, has been associated with causalgia, a rare pain syndrome related to partial peripheral nerve injuries, and with social phobia. It has tachykinin receptor activity and substance P receptor activity. This family of receptors is thought to mediate central stress reactions, mood control, excitatory neurotransmission, immune modulation and airway and lung function. Its expression has been localized in high concentrations in the CNS (particularly the striatum, amygdala and some hypothalamic and thalamic nuclei) and peripheral tissues. Spondin 1, extracellular matrix protein (*SPON1*), on chromosome 11, functions as a cell adhesion protein that promotes the attachment of spinal cord and sensory neuron cells and the outgrowth

**TABLE 3.1**

**Results of GWAS Related to Brain Features**

| First Author | Disease/Trait | Initial Sample Size | Region | Mapped Gene | SNPs | p-Value |
|---|---|---|---|---|---|---|
| Jahanshad, N. | Brain connectivity | 331 European ancestry individuals | 20p12.1 | ENSAP1 – PPIAP17 | rs16997087 | 1E−10 |
| | | | 15q21.3 | NEDD4 | rs17819300 | 1E−10 |
| | | | Xq24 | UBE2A | rs7879933 | 2E−10 |
| | | | 10q22.1 | LRRC20 | rs4747011 | 9E−10 |
| | | | 6q16.1 | TSG1 – CYCSP17 | rs2224003 | 1E−9 |
| | | | 3p26.2 | CNTN4 | rs17024684 | 2E−9 |
| | | | 20p12.1 | ENSAP1 – PPIAP17 | rs16997087 | 2E−9 |
| | | | 3p11.2 | KRT8P25 – APOOP2 | rs9834692 | 3E−9 |
| | | | 3p11.2 | KRT8P25 – APOOP2 | rs9883474 | 3E−9 |
| | | | 2p12 | TACR1 | rs3771863 | 3E−9 |
| | | | 6q16.1 | TSG1 – CYCSP17 | rs10485022 | 5E−9 |
| | | | 11p15.2 | SPON1 | rs2618516 | 6E−10 |
| Stein, J. L. | Brain structure | 2020 European ancestry neuropsychiatric disorder cases, 5775 European ancestry controls (1) | 12q24.22 | HRK – RPL36P15 | rs7294919 | 7E−16 |
| | | | 12q14.3 | HMGA2 | rs10784502 | 1E−12 |
| Paus, T. | Brain development | 557 French Canadian female adolescent individuals (2) | NR | — | NR | NS |
| Kim, S. | Brain cytoarchitecture | 14 European ancestry bipolar cases, 15 European ancestry depression cases, 13 European ancestry schizophrenia cases, 14 European ancestry controls | 5q22.2 | MCC | rs6594713 | 2E−6 |
| | | | 2q33.1 | PLCL1 – SATB2 | rs11893063 | 2E−6 |
| Stein, J. L. | Brain structure (hippocampal volume) | 162 European ancestry AD cases, 343 European ancestry amnestic MCI cases, 193 European ancestry healthy elderly controls | 1p22.2 | ZNF326 – BARHL2 | rs2813746 | 2E−6 |
| | | | 10p12.31 | AIFM1P1 – MALRD1 | rs16917919 | 8E−6 |
| | | | 12q23.2 | UTP20 | rs2290720 | 3E−6 |
| | | | 16q21 | LOC101927580 | rs8056650 | 1E−6 |

*(Continued)*

**TABLE 3.1 (*Continued*)**

**Results of GWAS Related to Brain Features**

| First Author | Disease/Trait | Initial Sample Size | Region | Mapped Gene | SNPs | p-Value |
|---|---|---|---|---|---|---|
| Stein, J. L. | Brain structure (temporal lobe volume) | 173 European ancestry AD cases, 361 European ancestry MCI cases, 208 European ancestry controls | 3p22.1 | NFU1P1 – MYRIP | rs9832461 | 4E–6 |
| | | | 4p15.1 | MAPRE1P2 – RPL31P31 | rs1448284 | 2E–6 |
| | | | 12p13.1 | GRIN2B | rs11055612 | 3E–6 |
| | | | 14q24.3 | NRXN3 | rs7155434 | 8E–6 |
| | | | 15q22.2 | TLN2; LOC102724972 | rs2456930 | 3E–7 |
| Stein, J. L. | Brain structure | 740 European ancestry individuals | 6q16.2 | BDH2P1 – FAXC | rs2132683 | 1E–6 |
| | | | 6q15 | MAP3K7 – MIR4643 | rs713155 | 5E–7 |
| | | | 1p35.1 | CSMD2 | rs476463 | 1E–6 |
| | | | 7q31.32 | CADPS2 | rs2429582 | 6E–7 |
| | | | 3p21.31 | CCR3 – UQCRC2P1 | rs9990343 | 4E–7 |
| | | | 11q23.3 | RPL15P15 – BUD13 | rs490592 | 1E–6 |
| | | | 20q13.12 | RPL5P2 – SPINT3 | rs11696501 | 9E–7 |
| | | | 3p12.1 | SRRM1P2 – LINC00971 | rs10511089 | 7E–7 |
| | | | 8q23.1 | PGAM1P13 – RNA5SP275 | rs4534106 | 1E–6 |
| | | | 6q12 | NUFIP1P – RNA5SP208 | rs11970254 | 6E–7 |
| | | | 9p13.2 | SHB | rs7873102 | 6E–7 |
| | | | 1p36.13 | EMC1 | rs710865 | 1E–7 |
| | | | 20p12.1 | LOC101929486 | rs2073233 | 1E–6 |
| | | | 2q37.3 | BOK | rs12479254 | 6E–7 |
| | | | 16p12.1 | CACNG3 – RBBP6 | rs11643520 | 6E–7 |
| | | | 5p12 | RPL29P12 – FGF10 | rs4296809 | 9E–7 |
| | | | 13q32.2 | FARP1 | rs688872 | 1E–6 |
| | | | 14q22.1 | FRMD6; FRMD6-AS2 | rs7140150 | 5E–7 |
| | | | 6p12.3 | GLYATL3 | rs9473582 | 8E–7 |

(*Continued*)

**TABLE 3.1 (Continued)**

**Results of GWAS Related to Brain Features**

| First Author | Disease/Trait | Initial Sample Size | Region | Mapped Gene | SNPs | p-Value |
|---|---|---|---|---|---|---|
| Shen, L. | Brain imaging | 175 European ancestry AD cases, 354 European ancestry amnestic MCI cases, 204 European ancestry controls | 2q36.1 | — | rs10932886 | E |
| | | | 19q13.32 | — | rs429358 | NS |
| | | | 3q28 | — | rs7610017 | NS |
| | | | 7p21.3 | — | rs6463843 | NS |
| | | | 19q13.32 | — | rs2075650 | NS |
| | | | 10q21.1 | — | rs16912145 | NS |
| | | | 7q35 | — | rs12531488 | NS |
| | | | 1p31.3 | — | rs7526034 | NS |
| | | | 3p14.1 | — | rs7647307 | NS |
| | | | 4p15.1 | — | rs4692256 | E |
| Potkin, S. G. | Brain imaging in schizophrenia (interaction) | 46 European ancestry cases, 60 European ancestry controls, 18 cases, 14 controls | 3p12.3 | VDAC1P7 – MRPS17P3 | rs9836484 | 4E–6 |
| | | | 3q26.31 | TNIK | rs2088885 | 6E–6 |
| | | | 5q23.2 | LINC01183 | rs245201 | 9E–8 |
| | | | 2q37.3 | OTOS – GPC1 | rs1574192 | 4E–6 |
| | | | 14q32.32 | TRAF3 | rs10133111 | 5E–6 |
| | | | 6q16.1 | EIF4EBP2P3 – POU3F2 | rs9491640 | 9E–6 |
| Baranzini, S. E. | Brain lesion load | 791 European ancestry cases, 883 European ancestry controls | 2q37.1 | UGT1A | rs2602397 | 4E–6 |
| | | | 14q12 | NUBPL – ARHGAP5-AS1 | rs2039485 | 6E–6 |
| | | | 6q25.3 | IGF2R | rs6917747 | 7E–6 |
| | | | 19p13.11 | CPAMD8 | rs11666377 | 7E–6 |

Bolded genes indicate statistically significant association at GWAS level ($<5 \times$ E–8).

*Replication sample sizes when available:* (1) 599 European ancestry neuropsychiatric disorder cases, 11,915 European ancestry controls, 143 European ancestry and African American neuropsychiatric disorder cases, 94 European ancestry and African American controls, 605 Hispanic controls; (2) 2601 European ancestry adolescent individuals. NS, not significant; NR, not reported.

of neurites in vitro, and it may contribute to the growth and guidance of axons in both the spinal cord and the PNS. Tumour suppressor TSG1 (*TSG1*) on chromosome 6 is an RNA gene and is affiliated with the lncRNA class. Its function and potential relation with the neural system is unknown. Finally, the contactin 4 (CNTN4) gene on chromosome 3 encodes a member of the contactin family of immunoglobulins. Contactins are axon-associated cell adhesion molecules that function in neuronal network formation and plasticity. The encoded protein may play a role in the formation of axon connections in the developing nervous system. Deletion or mutation of this gene may play a role in 3p deletion syndrome and autism spectrum disorders.

Despite the larger number of subjects included in the GWAS for brain structure (2020 cases and 5775 controls), the yield of genes/loci from its analysis is more limited. It includes also a pseudogene on chromosome 12 (ribosomal protein L36 pseudogene 15 [*RPL36P15*]; *HRK*, a gene that encodes a member of the BCL-2 protein family involved in activating or inhibiting apoptosis; and the HMGA2 gene, encoding a protein that belongs to the non-histone chromosomal high-mobility group protein family that has been previously related to obesity).

The findings from GWAS investigation cognition-related traits are humbling; see Table 3.2 (Cirulli et al., 2010; Davies et al., 2014; Davis et al., 2010; DeJager et al., 2012; Hashimoto et al., 2013; LeBlanc et al., 2012; Need et al., 2009; Seshadri et al., 2007; Zhang & Pierce, 2014). The results did not reveal many new loci at the GWAS significant level. In fact, most signals related to cognitive decline fall in the region of chromosome 19 harbouring the *APOE* gene. Nevertheless, some new genomic regions provided significant signals. These include the *PTPRO* gene on chromosome 12 and a region of chromosome 15 encompassing the eukaryotic translation elongation factor 1 alpha 1 pseudogene 22 (*EEF1A1P22*) and WD repeat domain 72 (*WDR72*) loci. None of these loci have been previously associated with cognition-related traits. *PTPRO* encodes the protein tyrosine phosphatase, receptor type O, which possesses tyrosine phosphatase activity. PTPRO appears to play a role in regulating the glomerular pressure/filtration rate relationship through an effect on podocyte structure and function. The *WDR72* gene encodes a protein with eight WD-40 repeats. Mutations in this gene have been associated with amelogenesis imperfecta hypomaturation type 2A3, a disorder of tooth development. Finally, the *EEF1A1P22* has no previous phenotype associated. Paradoxically, obvious candidate genes such as brain-derived neurotrophic factor (BDNF) did not show in any of the GWAS analyzed.

The current gaps in knowledge regarding the missing heritability of brain architecture and function will be progressively filled up thanks to the fact that brain imaging studies are increasing in size and scope. The ongoing imaging studies involving consortia including tens of thousands of people are providing the statistical power to discover new genetic variants. Moreover, the traditional variables used in previous association studies are extended to test genetic associations with signals at millions of locations in the brain, and connectome-wide, genome-wide scans can jointly screen brain circuits and genomes. In addition, the field is rapidly advancing with ultra-high-resolution imaging and whole-genome sequencing that will provide a more complete genetic picture of the brain and hopefully of the cognitive-related traits, as well as their interactions with behavioural and environmental factors (Medland et al., 2014).

**TABLE 3.2**

**Results of GWAS Related to Cognition Traits**

| First Author Reference | Disease/Trait | Initial Sample Size | Region | Mapped Gene | SNPs | p-Value |
|---|---|---|---|---|---|---|
| Zhang, C. | Cognitive decline (age related) | 5765 European ancestry individuals, 890 African American individuals | 19q13.32 | *APOE* | **rs769449** | **5E−19** |
| | | | 19q13.32 | **TOMM40** | **rs115881343** | **4E−9** |
| | | | 5q21.1 | SLCO6A1 | rs10073892 | 7E−7 |
| | | | 21q22.11 | USF1P1 − IFNGR2 | rs9980664 | 3E−6 |
| | | | 11q14.1 | MIR5579 − ARL6IP1P3 | rs11231991 | 4E−6 |
| | | | 7p15.3 | DNAH11 | rs2390593 | 4E−6 |
| | | | 4q31.1 | LINC00499 − CCRN4L | rs77803164 | 4E−6 |
| | | | 2q34 | MIR548F2 − PCED1CP | rs10497985 | 4E−6 |
| | | | 7q33 | DGKI | rs6978230 | 6E−6 |
| | | | 2q36.1 | KCNE4 − TRNAK39P | rs895767 | 7E−6 |
| | | | 5q23.2 | KRT18P16 − HMGB1P29 | rs1021769 | 7E−6 |
| Hashimoto, R. | Cognitive decline | 166 Japanese ancestry schizophrenia cases, 323 Japanese ancestry controls (1) | NR | − | NR | NS |
| Davies, G. | Cognitive decline | 3280 European ancestry individuals (2) | 19q13.32 | **TOMM40** | **rs2075650** | **2E−8** |
| De Jager, P. L. | Cognitive decline | 749 European ancestry individuals (3) | 19q13.32 | **APOC1** | **rs4420638** | **4E−27** |
| LeBlanc, M. | Cognitive function | 190 European ancestry schizophrenia cases, 157 European ancestry bipolar disorder cases, 353 European ancestry controls | 12p12.3 | **PTPRO** | **rs2300290** | **1E−8** |
| | | | 15q21.3 | **EEF1A1P22 − WDR72** | **rs719714** | **4E−8** |
| Davis, O. S. | Cognitive ability | 860 European ancestry children (4) | NR | − | NR | NS |

*(Continued)*

**TABLE 3.2 (Continued)**
**Results of GWAS Related to Cognition Traits**

| First Author Reference | Disease/Trait | Initial Sample Size | Region | Mapped Gene | SNPs | p-Value |
|---|---|---|---|---|---|---|
| Cirulli, E. T. | Cognitive performance | Up to 813 European ancestry individuals, up to 167 East Asian ancestry individuals, up to 7 Hispanic/Latin American ancestry individuals, up to 74 South Asian ancestry individuals | 1p34.3 | ACTN4P2 – MANEAL | rs12117544 | 8E-6 |
| | | | 1p13.2 | KCND3-IT1 – TXNP3 | rs7555668 | 3E-6 |
| | | | 1q21.2 | LOC102723321 | rs1891498 | 9E-6 |
| | | | 2p25.3 | FAM150B – TMEM18 | rs4643574 | 5E-6 |
| | | | 2p25.1 | KCNF1 – FLJ33534 | rs6739054 | 2E-6 |
| | | | 2p24.2 | NT5C1B – FLJ41481 | rs1876040 | 6E-8 |
| | | | 2q37.1 | HMGB1P3 – TPM3P8 | rs17275498 | 8E-6 |
| | | | 3q13.2 | PLCXD2 | rs4450776 | 5E-6 |
| | | | 4q12 | SRIP1 – MIR548AG1 | rs10517437 | 4E-6 |
| | | | 4q21.22 | RPS6P6 – LINC00575 | rs7658637 | 6E-7 |
| | | | 4q35.2 | LINC01060 – HSPA8P12 | rs7659062 | 8E-6 |
| | | | 4q35.2 | LINC01060 – HSPA8P12 | rs7659062 | 9E-6 |
| | | | 4q35.2 | LINC01060 – HSPA8P12 | rs7662358 | 8E-6 |
| | | | 4q35.2 | LINC01060 – HSPA8P12 | rs7662358 | 9E-6 |
| | | | 5p15.33 | CTD-2194D22.4 – IRX2 | rs17586674 | 5E-6 |
| | | | 5p15.33 | IRX1 – LINC01020 | rs492478 | 4E-6 |
| | | | 5q23.2 | RPSAP37 – GRAMD3 | rs13169113 | 9E-6 |
| | | | 6q13 | KRT19P1 – RIMS1 | rs10455248 | 4E-6 |
| | | | 6q15 | BACH2 | rs2289577 | 9E-6 |
| | | | 6q16.1 | ATF1P1 – COPS5P1 | rs2506933 | 6E-6 |
| | | | 6q22.31 | COX6A1P3 – TBC1D32 | rs1343075 | 2E-6 |
| | | | 7q31.2 | CAPZA2 – RNA5SP239 | rs7782376 | 8E-6 |
| | | | 8p23.2 | CSMD1 | rs2616984 | 4E-6 |
| | | | 8p23.1 | C8orf12 | rs2002030 | 5E-6 |

(Continued)

**TABLE 3.2 (Continued)**

**Results of GWAS Related to Cognition Traits**

| First Author Reference | Disease/Trait | Initial Sample Size | Region | Mapped Gene | SNPs | p-Value |
|---|---|---|---|---|---|---|
| | | | 8p12 | GTF2E2; SMIM18 | rs2978263 | 8E–6 |
| | | | 8q13.3 | KCNB2 | rs2247572 | 1E–6 |
| | | | 8q21.3 | RNA5SP272 – RIPK2 | rs4397449 | 3E–6 |
| | | | 8q22.3 | NCALD | rs517811 | 5E–6 |
| | | | 8q24.23 | FLJ45872 | rs9657451 | 2E–6 |
| | | | 8q24.23 | FAM135B | rs11166827 | 5E–6 |
| | | | 9q31.2 | TAL2 – TMEM38B | rs1463984 | 3E–6 |
| | | | 9q33.3 | LHX2 – NEK6 | rs2807580 | 3E–6 |
| | | | 10p12.1 | KIAA1217 | rs2484873 | 4E–7 |
| | | | 10q25.3 | AFAP1L2 | rs4751674 | 4E–6 |
| | | | 10q26.2 | LINC01163 – MGMT | rs9804317 | 7E–6 |
| | | | 11q14.1 | LOC101928964 | rs11232369 | 8E–6 |
| | | | 11q23.3 | GRIK4 | rs12797755 | 8E–6 |
| | | | 12p13.32 | EFCAB4B – PARP11 | rs2058350 | 8E–6 |
| | | | 12q14.3 | TBC1D30 | rs939876 | 2E–6 |
| | | | 12q21.1 | CHCHD3P2 – RPL31P48 | rs10879517 | 4E–6 |
| | | | 13q31.1 | RPL21P111 – LINC00331 | rs17070284 | 3E–6 |
| | | | 14q21.3 | LINC00648 – RPL18P1 | rs7151223 | 1E–6 |
| | | | 14q21.3 | CDKL1 | rs1265879 | 4E–6 |
| | | | 14q22.1 | MAP4K5 | rs17718580 | 8E–7 |
| | | | 14q22.1 | ATL1 | rs17122693 | 3E–7 |
| | | | 14q22.1 | ZFP64P1 | rs8020441 | 5E–7 |
| | | | 14q24.3 | NRXN3 | rs6574433 | 6E–6 |
| | | | 15q21.2 | TNFAIP8L3 | rs1124769 | 9E–6 |

*(Continued)*

**TABLE 3.2 (Continued)**
**Results of GWAS Related to Cognition Traits**

| First Author Reference | Disease/Trait | Initial Sample Size | Region | Mapped Gene | SNPs | p-Value |
|---|---|---|---|---|---|---|
| | | | 15q21.3 | LOC102724766 | rs4775031 | 2E–6 |
| | | | 15q23 | RNU6-1 – PIAS1 | rs448720 | 5E–6 |
| | | | 15q26.2 | RPL26P5 – LINC01197 | rs6496074 | 3E–6 |
| | | | 16q23.3 | CDH13 | rs3784962 | 3E–6 |
| | | | 16q23.3 | CDH13 | rs3784962 | 6E–6 |
| | | | 18q12.1 | ARIH2P1 – HSPA9P2 | rs4145170 | 3E–6 |
| | | | 19p13.2 | ZNF788 | rs17638629 | 7E–6 |
| | | | 20p12.3 | PLCB1 | rs6118083 | 7E–6 |
| | | | 20p11.21 | ACSS1 | rs6050267 | 9E–6 |
| | | | 20q13.12 | OSER1-AS1 | rs6017291 | 6E–6 |
| | | | 21q22.3 | PKNOX1 | rs234720 | 2E–7 |
| | | | 6p22.1 | TRIM31 | rs34704616 | 6E–6 |
| | | | Xq21.31 | TGIF2LX – USP12PX | rs5941436 | 5E–6 |
| | | | Xq28 | IDS | rs530501 | 4E–6 |
| Need AC | Cognitive performance | Up to 1295 individuals | 2p16.3 | LOC730100 | rs1206397 | 3E–7 |
| | | | 3q26.32 | LOC102724550 | rs7612209 | 4E–6 |
| | | | 16q23.3 | MPHOSPH6 – CDH13 | rs4082514 | 3E–6 |
| | | | 12p12.3 | LOC101928387 | rs6486986 | 8E–6 |
| | | | 5p15.31 | RNA5SP176 – ADCY2 | rs7729273 | 1E–6 |
| | | | 16p12.1 | HSPE1P16 – C16orf82 | rs2203512 | 3E–7 |
| | | | 17q21.32 | LOC101060400 | rs2326017 | 3E–7 |
| | | | Xq28 | KRT8P8 – GABRQ | rs10856240 | 9E–6 |
| | | | 3q23 | PXYLP1 | rs16851254 | 8E–6 |
| | | | 13q31.2 | TET1P1 – RPL29P29 | rs969962 | 9E–6 |

(Continued)

**TABLE 3.2 (Continued)**
**Results of GWAS Related to Cognition Traits**

| First Author Reference | Disease/Trait | Initial Sample Size | Region | Mapped Gene | SNPs | p-Value |
|---|---|---|---|---|---|---|
| | | | 13q21.33 | RNA5SP32 – RPL18AP17 | rs4083578 | 8E–6 |
| | | | 11p12 | RPL9P23 – HNRNPKP3 | rs10501293 | 5E–6 |
| | | | 3p22.3 | RPL36AP17 – RFC3P1 | rs6799705 | 2E–7 |
| | | | 12q23.3 | SETP7 – BTBD11 | rs1820460 | 8E–6 |
| | | | 11q14.2 | C11orf73 | rs6592284 | 2E–6 |
| | | | 18q22.1 | RPL31P9 – DSEL | rs2124349 | 4E–6 |
| | | | 6p21.2 | CCDC167 | rs904251 | 7E–6 |
| | | | 11q13.5 | CAPN5 | rs3781684 | 7E–6 |
| | | | 12q24.23 | CCDC64 | rs11064994 | 6E–6 |
| | | | 15q23 | CORO2B | rs11856323 | 1E–7 |
| | | | 7p14.3 | CPVL; LOC100506497 | rs2252521 | 5E–6 |
| | | | 13q14.11 | DNAJC15 – MOCS3P2 | rs1324015 | 9E–6 |
| | | | 3q27.2 | EHHADH | rs7374394 | 2E–6 |
| | | | 1p36.13 | FAM131C | rs9442235 | 6E–6 |
| | | | 1q41 | FAM177B | rs6683071 | 4E–6 |
| | | | 8q24.13 | FAM91A1 – FER1L6 | rs10481151 | 4E–7 |
| | | | 4q28.1 | MIR2054 | rs12639834 | 6E–6 |
| | | | 3q13.33 | FBXO40 | rs3772130 | 6E–6 |
| | | | 13q12.3 | FLT1 | rs17086609 | 5E–6 |
| | | | 15q12 | GABRB3 | rs8043440 | 2E–6 |
| | | | 2q31.1 | GORASP2 | rs4668356 | 1E–6 |
| | | | 12p13.1 | GRIN2B | rs2160519 | 2E–6 |
| | | | 3p25.1 | SLC6A6; GRIP2 | rs9036 | 3E–6 |
| | | | Xp22.2 | MID1 | rs5934953 | 1E–7 |

*(Continued)*

**TABLE 3.2 (Continued)**
**Results of GWAS Related to Cognition Traits**

| First Author Reference | Disease/Trait | Initial Sample Size | Region | Mapped Gene | SNPs | p-Value |
|---|---|---|---|---|---|---|
| | | | 7q31.1 | IMMP2L | rs10279573 | 3E–6 |
| | | | 9p22.2 | PABPC1P11 – PUS7P1 | rs4284125 | 8E–6 |
| | | | 21q21.3 | MRPL39 – JAM2 | rs17001239 | 2E–6 |
| | | | 1p32.1 | LINC01135 | rs4601609 | 5E–6 |
| | | | 13q21.33 | KLHL1 | rs7984606 | 8E–6 |
| | | | 11p13 | FBXO3 – LMO2 | rs11032423 | 8E–6 |
| | | | 1q32.1 | MDM4 | rs12143943 | 5E–6 |
| | | | 3p22.1 | MOBP | rs816488 | 4E–6 |
| | | | 14q23.3 | MTHFD1 | rs10498514 | 8E–7 |
| | | | 12q24.31 | NCOR2 | rs12423712 | 7E–6 |
| | | | 21q11.2 | NRIP1 | rs2229741 | 6E–7 |
| | | | 20p12.3 | PLCB1 | rs6056209 | 2E–6 |
| | | | 18q12.3 | RNA5SP454 – RIT2 | rs8085804 | 8E–6 |
| | | | 13q34 | RPL21P107 – LINC00346 | rs767210 | 3E–7 |
| | | | 17q25.2 | SEC14L1 | rs3744064 | 7E–7 |
| | | | 9p22.2 | PABPC1P11 – PUS7P1 | rs10810865 | 4E–6 |
| | | | 9p22.1 | SLC24A2 | rs4258076 | 4E–6 |
| | | | 8q12.1 | RPS26P7 – TOX | rs960089 | 6E–6 |
| | | | 19q12 | TSHZ3 | rs1078373 | 6E–6 |
| | | | 4p13 | UCHL1 – LIMCH1 | rs461096 | 9E–6 |
| | | | 15q21.3 | UNC13C | rs1897031 | 1E–6 |
| | | | 1q23.2 | VANGL2 – SLAMF6 | rs16832015 | 2E–6 |
| | | | Xp22.31 | VCX2 – VCX3B | rs7892812 | 8E–6 |

*(Continued)*

**TABLE 3.2 (Continued)**

**Results of GWAS Related to Cognition Traits**

| First Author Reference | Disease/Trait | Initial Sample Size | Region | Mapped Gene | SNPs | p-Value |
|---|---|---|---|---|---|---|
| Seshadri, S. | Cognitive test performance | 694 European ancestry individuals | 7p14.1 | VPS41 | rs11984145 | 6E–6 |
| | | | 6p21.2 | FLJ45825 | rs1757171 | 7E–6 |
| | | | 1p22.2 | LMO4 – RPL36AP10 | rs2179965 | 1E–6 |
| | | | 4q13.2 | RPS23P3 – CENPC | rs1155865 | 2E–6 |
| | | | 21q21.3 | LOC102724420 | rs2832077 | 2E–6 |
| | | | 14q21.3 | RPL18P1 – ATP5G2P2 | rs2352904 | 2E–6 |
| | | | 6p23 | LINC01108 – RPL6P17 | rs6914079 | 2E–6 |
| | | | 5q32 | PPP2R2B | rs9325032 | 3E–6 |
| | | | 12q23.3 | LOC100287944 | rs3891355 | 3E–6 |
| | | | 11q14.1 | TENM4 | rs530965 | 4E–6 |
| | | | 17q22 | PPM1E | rs9303401 | 5E–6 |
| | | | 11q25 | NCAPD3 | rs1031381 | 6E–6 |
| | | | 1q42.2 | TARBP1 | rs10489896 | 6E–6 |
| | | | 12p11.1 | ST13P9 – ALG10 | rs9300212 | 8E–6 |
| | | | 9q22.2 | DIRAS2 – OR7E109P | rs1831521 | 8E–6 |
| | | | 2q22.1 | UBBP1 – THSD7B | rs934299 | 9E–6 |

Bolded genes indicate statistically significant association at GWAS level ($<5 \times E{-}8$).

*Replication sample sizes when available:* (1) 339 schizophrenia cases; (2) 1367 European ancestry individuals; (3) 1562 European ancestry individuals, 717 cases; (4) 2619 European ancestry children.

## 3.3 GENE–DIET INTERACTIONS RELATED TO BRAIN STRUCTURE, FUNCTION AND COGNITIVE DECLINE

Molecular mechanisms underlying brain structure and function are affected by nutrition throughout the life cycle, with profound implications for health and disease. Responses to nutrition are in turn influenced by individual differences in multiple target genes. Recent advances in genomics and epigenomics are increasing understanding of mechanisms by which nutrition and genes interact. This review starts with a short account of current knowledge on nutrition–gene interactions, focusing on the significance of epigenetics to nutritional regulation of gene expression and the roles of SNP and copy number variants (CNVs) in determining individual responses to nutrition. A critical assessment is then provided of recent advances in nutrition–gene interactions, and especially energy status, in three related areas: (1) mental health and well-being, (2) mental disorders and schizophrenia and (3) neurological (neurodevelopmental and neurodegenerative) disorders and AD. Optimal energy status, including physical activity, has a positive role in mental health. By contrast, suboptimal energy status, including undernutrition and overnutrition, is implicated in many disorders of mental health and neurology. These actions are mediated by changes in energy metabolism and multiple signalling molecules, for example, BDNF. They often involve epigenetic mechanisms, including DNA methylation and histone modifications. Recent advances show that many brain disorders result from a sophisticated network of interactions between numerous environmental and genetic factors (Dauncey, 2012).

None of the loci identified for cognitive function has shown gene–environment interactions or evidence of being regulated by dietary factors. However, as indicated earlier, the GWAS signals detected using cognitive decline as phenotype fall within the neighbourhood of the *APOE* gene. This gene has been studied for several decades and it has shown associations with cardiovascular diseases, ageing, longevity and cognition in humans (Deelen, 2011; Garatachea et al., 2014; Kathiresan & Srivastava, 2012; Khan et al., 2013b; Lindahl-Jacobsen et al., 2013; McKay et al., 2011b; Novelli et al., 2008; Schächter et al., 1994). In fact, carrying the *APOE4* allele is the most important genetic risk for AD, making this gene the archetypal to demonstrate interactions between different biological systems and the environment.

The common polymorphism defined by the alleles E2/E3/E4 has been the most studied. It is defined by two base changes in the DNA that give rise, respectively, to two amino acid changes of the following characteristics: rs429358 (Cys112Arg; E4) and rs7412 (Arg136Cys; E2). The E4 allele was initially associated with higher low-density lipoproteins-cholesterol (LDL-C) concentrations and total cholesterol (Sing & Davignon, 1985), and this association has remained consistently replicated by hundreds of studies. Although the E4 allele was also associated with greater cardio-vascular disease risk (Bennet & Di Angelantonio, 2007; Song et al., 2004; Stengård et al., 1996), the evidence on this association was lower than that observed for LDL-C concentrations (Khan et al., 2013a; Yin et al., 2013). At the same time, evidence began to accumulate on the association between the E4 allele and the greater risk of dementia and, in particular, ADs (Liddell et al., 1994; Poirier et al., 1993). With the advent of GWAS, these studies soon confirmed the consistent association between the *APOE* genotype and LDL-C concentrations (Global Lipids Genetics Consortium et al., 2013; Teslovich et al., 2010), as well as their association with AD (Coon et al., 2007). Meta-analyses of GWAS have also shown the association of the *APOE* genotype with cardiovascular diseases (Willer et al., 2013), although weaker than the previously mentioned associations. With regard to ageing, studies of candidate genes have consistently shown the association of the E4 allele with lesser longevity (Garatachea et al., 2014; McKay et al., 2011a; Novelli et al., 2008; Schupf et al., 2013), so reflecting the greater risk of cardiovascular disease and neurodegenerative diseases. In addition, several gene–environment interactions between the *APOE* polymorphism and environmental factors including tobacco smoking and physical activity in determining intermediate and disease phenotypes have been reported (Bernstein et al., 2002; Corella et al., 2001; Grammer et al., 2013; Gustavsson et al., 2012; Humphries et al., 2001; Pezzini et al., 2004; Talmud et al., 2005). Among these, it is interesting to note that Grammer et al. analyzed the association between the *APOE* polymorphism, smoking, angiographic coronary artery disease and mortality in participants of the Ludwigshafen Risk and Cardiovascular Health Study. They found that the presence of the E4 allele in current smokers increased cardiovascular and all-cause mortality. Although the *APOE*-smoking interaction in cardiovascular diseases has been previously reported in other studies (Humphries et al., 2001; Pezzini et al., 2004; Talmud et al., 2005), more evidence is still needed.

More puzzling are the reported interactions between the *APOE* gene, n-3 polyunsaturated fatty acids (PUFAs) and cognition-related traits. n-3 PUFAs have been suggested to decrease cognitive decline and potentially delay the onset of AD; however, despite an extended popular belief for a beneficial effect of dietary intake of n-3 PUFAs and age-related cognitive decline, the scientific evidence supporting the benefits is inconsistent. These inconsistencies parallel those related to the heterogeneity of plasma lipid responses to a cholesterol-lowering diet, and these interindividual differences in response may be explained in part by genetic factors. In the later case, we have previously shown that subjects carrying the *APOE4* allele had higher baseline plasma LDL-C levels, but they had, on average, greater LDL-C decreases following a low-fat, low-cholesterol diet. In this case, those who were at greater risk for hypercholesterolemia achieved greater benefit from the prudent diet. However, regarding the *APOE4*-n3 PUFA interactions related to cognition, the emerging picture is rather different. Several studies, using different experimental approaches, have consistently shown that a benefit of n3 PUFA on cognition-related measures may be present only in the absence of the *APOE4* allele; see Table 3.3 (Barberger-Gateau et al., 2007; Beydoun et al., 2007; Eskelinen et al., 2008; Huang et al., 2005; Martínez-Lapiscina et al., 2014; Samieri et al., 2011, 2013; Whalley et al., 2008). In fact, only one of the studies showed a better outcome for subjects with the *APOE4* allele consuming higher amount of n-3 PUFA, and this was restricted to visual working memory. This is a very important observation with significant implications for public health and clinical practice. Therefore, more studies are needed to further replicate the current observations. Some additional knowledge could come from existing studies that have examined the relation between diet- and cognition-related traits; however, these studies treated *APOE* as a

**TABLE 3.3**

**Association between n-3 PUFA and Cognitive Outcomes Stratified by APOE Status**

| Study | Population | Objectives | Description | Findings |
|---|---|---|---|---|
| Whalley et al. (2008) | 120 volunteers, born in 1936, with IQs available at age 11 years were followed up at ages of 64, 66 and 68 years. | To determine the contribution of erythrocyte n-3 PUFA content to cognitive ageing in the presence or absence of the APOE4 allele. | At the first follow-up, APOE genotype and PUFA composition of erythrocyte membranes were determined. Cognitive tests were administered at all follow-ups. Cognitive performance at 64 years old and cognitive changes from 64 to 68 years old to erythrocyte n-3 PUFA composition on recruitment and to APOE4 allele status were investigated. | Cognitive benefits were associated with higher erythrocyte n-3 PUFA content but were significant only in the absence of the APOE epsilon4 allele. |
| Samieri et al. (2013) | 1135 participants from the Three-City study aged 65 years and over, of whom 19% were APOE4 carriers. | To investigate the association between dietary fat and plasma concentrations of (EPA) and DHA in elderly persons, taking the APOE4 genotype into account. | Plasma fatty acids were measured and APOE genotype was determined. | A positive association was found between fish consumption and plasma DHA, but it was stronger in APOE4 noncarriers. Plasma DHA increased significantly with age (P = 0.009) in APOE4 noncarriers only. |
| Huang et al. (2005) | 2233 subjects participating in the cardiovascular health cognition study (CHCS). | To compare associations of lean fish versus fatty fish intake with dementia, AD and VaD and in relation to APOE4 status. | Fish intake was assessed by FFQ. Incident dementia, AD and VaD were determined through a series of cognitive tests, physician's assessment and committee consensus. | In CHCS, consumption of fatty fish was associated with a reduced risk of dementia and AD for those without the APOE4 allele. |

*(Continued)*

**TABLE 3.3 (*Continued*)**

**Association between n-3 PUFA and Cognitive Outcomes Stratified by *APOE* Status**

| Study | Population | Objectives | Description | Findings |
|---|---|---|---|---|
| Samieri et al. (2011) | Prospective population-based cohort (with participants aged ≥65 years, n = 1228 nondemented at baseline). | EPA and DHA may slow cognitive decline. The *APOE4* allele may modify this relationship. | Estimation of the associations between EPA and DHA plasma levels and subsequent cognitive decline over 7 years, taking into account *APOE4* status and depression. | EPA and DHA may contribute to delaying decline in visual working memory in *APOE-ε4* carriers. |
| Potkin et al. (2009) | 28 subjects. | To determine whether the plasma fatty acid response to a dietary supplement of EPA + DHA was altered in carriers of L162V and/ or E4. | This was an add-on project; in the original study, men were selected based on whether or not they were carriers of L162V. E4 status was determined afterwards. All subjects received an EPA + DHA supplement for 6 weeks. | When the groups were separated based on the presence of E4, baseline EPA and DHA in plasma TAG were 67 and 60% higher, respectively, in E4 carriers. After the supplementation, there were significant gene × diet interactions in which only noncarriers had increased EPA and DHA in plasma NEFA and TAG, respectively. |
| Barberger-Gateau et al. (2007) | 8085 nondemented participants aged 65 and over were included in the Three-City cohort study. | To analyze the relationship between dietary patterns and risk of dementia or AD, adjusting for sociodemographic and vascular risk factors and taking into account the *APOE* genotype. | Subjects were examined in 1999–2000 and had at least one re-examination over 4 years (rate of follow-up 89.1%). A committee of neurologists validated 281 incident cases of dementia (including 183 AD). | Frequent consumption of fruits and vegetables, fish and omega-3-rich oils may decrease the risk of dementia and AD, especially among *APOE4* noncarriers. |

*(Continued)*

**TABLE 3.3 (Continued)**
**Association between n-3 PUFA and Cognitive Outcomes Stratified by APOE Status**

| Study | Population | Objectives | Description | Findings |
|---|---|---|---|---|
| Beydoun et al. (2007) | 2251 participants in the Atherosclerosis Risk in Communities (ARIC) Study. | To prospectively study the association between plasma fatty acids and cognitive decline in adults aged 50–65 years at baseline and conduct a subgroup analysis. | Plasma fatty acids in cholesteryl esters and phospholipids were analyzed. Three neuropsychological tests in the domains of delayed word recall, psychomotor speed and verbal fluency were administered. | EPA and DHA in plasma cholesteryl esters were associated with less cognitive decline on the Word Fluency Test in APOE4 noncarrier subjects. |
| Eskelinen et al. (2008) | A longitudinal population based in Kuopio and Joensuu, Eastern Finland. After an average follow-up of 21 years, a total of 1449 (72%) individuals aged 65–80 years participated in the re-examination in 1998. Altogether, 82 (5.7%) people were diagnosed with MCI. | To investigate the association of midlife dietary fat intake to cognitive performance and to the occurrence of clinical MCI later in life in a nondemented population. | Dietary information was collected with a structured questionnaire and an interview at midlife. Main outcome measures included MCI, global cognitive and executive functions; episodic, semantic and prospective memory; and psychomotor speed. | In the analyses stratified by the APOE4, midlife total fat intake was associated with MCI only among APOE4 noncarriers odds ratio (OR) (OR 2.05), and the association between SFA intake and MCI was found only among APOE4 carriers (OR 5.06). |
| Martinez-Lapiscina et al. (2014) | 522 participants (67 ± 6 years at baseline) enrolled in the PREDIMED-NAVARRA. | To investigate MedDiet–gene interactions for cognition and assess the effect of the MedDiet on cognition across different genetic profiles. | Randomly allocated to one of three diets: two MedDiets (supplemented with either extra-virgin olive oil or nuts) or a low-fat diet. They were evaluated with the mini-mental state examination and the clock-drawing test (CDT) after 6.5 years of intervention. Subjects were genotyped for CR1-rs3818361, CLU-rs11136000, PICALM-rs3851179 and APOE genes. | Cognitive performance was better for non-APOE4 and for APOE4 carriers of MedDiet groups compared to controls, but for CDT performance, we only found statistical significant differences for non-APOE4 carriers. |

potential confounder and did not provide information stratified by *APOE* genotype (Danthiir et al., 2014; Eskelinen et al., 2008; Féart et al., 2009). Therefore, the current knowledge supports a gene by environment interaction in which unlike *APOE4* noncarriers, *APOE4* carriers seem not to be protected against AD when consuming fish. This knowledge is relevant to the analysis of trials of n-3 PUFA supplements in cognitive ageing and dementia prevention. This interaction of n-3 PUFAs and *APOE4* genotype should be considered when designing interventions to increase n-3 PUFA blood levels in older people.

The consistency of the findings and the potential of this knowledge to improve cognition and decrease its age-related decline call for a better understanding of the mechanisms involved on the differential effect of n-3 PUFA according to *APOE* allele. In this regard, a recent work in human and animal models is revealing that the differential transport of essential fatty acids to the brain may be responsible for the lack of response of *APOE4* carriers to dietary n-3 PUFAs. Recent work (Chouinard-Watkins et al., 2013) indicates that DHA metabolism is significantly different in *APOE4* carriers compared with noncarriers. These investigators examined [$^{13}$C] DHA metabolism over 4 weeks in 40 subjects, *APOE4* carriers (n = 6) and noncarriers (n = 34). In *APOE4* carriers, mean plasma [$^{13}$C]DHA was 31% lower than that in *APOE4* noncarriers, and cumulative beta-oxidation of [$^{13}$C]DHA was higher than that in noncarriers. The whole-body half-life of [$^{13}$C]DHA was 77% lower in *APOE4* carriers compared with noncarriers. These results strongly support the notion that DHA metabolism depends, in part, on *APOE* genotype and may help explain why there is no association between DHA levels in plasma and cognition in *APOE4* carriers. However, the mechanism by with *APOE4* affects DHA metabolism in the brain cannot be determined from the experimental design of this study. For this purpose, other investigators have used experimental models. Thus, Vandal et al. (2014) evaluated plasma and brain fatty acid profiles and uptake of [$^{14}$C]-DHA using in situ cerebral perfusion through the blood–brain barrier in 4- and 13-month-old male and female *APOE*-targeted replacement mice (*APOE2*, *APOE3* and *APOE4*), fed with a DHA-depleted diet. Cortical and plasma DHAs were 9% lower and 34% higher in *APOE4* compared to *APOE2* mice, respectively. Brain uptake of [$^{14}$C]-DHA was 24% lower in *APOE4* versus *APOE2* mice. A significant relationship was established between DHA and *APOE* concentrations in the cortex of mice and AD patients. Altogether, these results suggest that lower brain uptake of DHA in *APOE4* than in *APOE2* mice may limit the accumulation of DHA in cerebral tissues. These data provide mechanistic support for the lack of benefit of DHA in *APOE4* carriers on cognitive function and the risk of AD.

A dietary intervention study in humans has also attempted to elucidate some of the mechanisms of differential response. In this case, the authors (Hanson et al., 2013) built on the knowledge that lipid-depleted (LD) apolipoproteins are less effective at binding and clearing Aβ and LD Aβ peptides are more toxic to neurons. However, the lack of access to neurons brought them to characterize the lipidation states of Aβ peptides and *APOE* in the cerebrospinal fluid in adults with respect to cognitive diagnosis and *APOE4* allele carrier status and after a dietary intervention. Twenty older adults with normal cognition (mean age, 69 years) and 27 with amnesic mild cognitive impairment (MCI) (mean age, 67 years) participated in this study, and they were randomized to a diet high in saturated fat content with a high glycemic index (high diet; 45% of energy from fat [>25% saturated fat], 35%–40% from carbohydrates with a mean glycemic index >70 and 15%–20% from protein) or a diet low in saturated fat content and with a low glycemic index (low diet; 25% of energy from fat [<7% saturated fat], 55%–60% from carbohydrates with a mean glycemic index <55 and 15%–20% from protein). Baseline levels of LD Aβ were greater for adults with MCI compared with adults with normal cognition. These findings were magnified in adults with MCI and the *APOE4* allele, who had higher LD *APOE* levels irrespective of cognitive diagnosis. The low diet tended to decrease LD Aβ levels, whereas the high diet increased these fractions. Therefore, the lipidation states of apolipoproteins and Aβ peptides in the brain differ depending on *APOE* genotype and cognitive diagnosis. Moreover, these effects can be modulated by diet. Therefore, the mechanistic studies lend support to the *APOE4* by n-3 PUFA interactions demonstrated in epidemiological studies providing some ground for more personalized approaches to dietary prevention and therapy for cognition decline and AD.

## 3.4 BRAIN-DERIVED NEUROTROPHIC FACTOR GENE, A MISSING CANDIDATE FROM GWAS

The BDNF gene codes for a protein that is a member of the nerve growth factor family. It is induced by cortical neurons and is necessary for survival of striatal neurons in the brain. Expression of this gene is reduced in both AD and Huntington disease patients. This gene may play a role in the regulation of stress response and in the biology of mood disorders. Despite being absent from the list of genes related to brain architecture and cognition identified through GWAS, this gene has been repeatedly associated in individual studies using the candidate gene approach. Specifically, a common SNP has been identified in the human BDNF gene (BDNF Val66Met) that leads to decreased BDNF secretion and impairments in specific forms of learning and a variable influence on brain morphology and cognition in humans (Dincheva et al., 2012; Forde et al., 2014; Teh et al., 2012). Nevertheless, a meta-analysis that included 23 publications containing 31 independent samples comprised of 7095 individuals did not establish significant genetic associations between the Val66Met polymorphism and a wide variety of cognitive functions including indicators of general cognitive ability, memory, executive function, visual processing skills and cognitive fluency (Mandelman & Grigorenko, 2012). However, this meta-analysis captured only a small fraction of the hundreds of studies carried out around the BDNF Val66Met SNP. In fact, another meta-analysis of seven studies (n = 399) investigating the association between Val66Met BDNF polymorphism and hippocampal volumes in healthy subjects (Hajek et al., 2012) showed a significant bilateral hippocampal volume reduction. These conflicting results in BDNF genetic studies as well as its absence from the results from GWAS may result from confounding or modifying factors such as age, gender, stress, other environmental factors, sample size, ethnicity and phenotype assessment (Hong et al., 2011).

In relation to stress, the relationship between life stress and the BDNF Val66Met has been reviewed, and the results from a meta-analysis suggest that the Met allele of BDNF Val66Met significantly moderates the relationship between life stress and depression. More specifically, the interaction between BDNF and life stress in depression is stronger for stressful life events rather than for childhood adversity (Hosang et al., 2014). However, the most interesting interactions, with greater public health relevance, relate to physical activity. Physical activity enhances cognitive performance, yet there are significant interindividual differences regarding the effectiveness of and motivation to exercise that limit the success of exercise in the prevention and therapy of age-related diseases including cognitive decline and AD. Genetic differences might be one source of this variation. Regarding motivation to exercise, there is evidence suggesting that those with at least one copy of the met allele in the BDNF Val66Met SNP (rs6265) had greater increases in positive mood and lower perceived exertion during exercise (Caldwell-Hooper et al., 2014).

In terms of effectiveness of exercise on cognition-/mood-related functions, the working hypothesis has been that carriers of the methionine-specifying (Met) allele of the Val66Met polymorphism have reduced secretion of BDNF and poorer memory, whereas physical activity increases BDNF levels. Therefore, the BDNF polymorphism could moderate the association of physical activity with cognitive functioning or, alternatively, the deleterious effect of the Met allele at this polymorphism could be compensated for by physical activity or worsened by physical inactivity (Brown et al., 2014; Cárdenas-Morales et al., 2014; Erickson et al., 2013; Kim et al., 2011; Mata et al., 2010; Nascimento et al., 2014). Of interest for future research is the fact that interactions with other environmental/behavioural factors have not been properly studied. Thus, despite some reports associating BDNF activity with appetite and obesity (Rosas-Vargas et al., 2011), there are no reports of gene by diet interactions related to the BDNF gene. In fact, the dual action of BDNF in neuronal metabolism and synaptic plasticity is crucial for activating signalling cascades under the action of diet and other environmental factors, using, among others, mechanisms of epigenetic regulation.

## 3.5   TCF7L2 GENE: ASSOCIATION WITH DIABETES AND STROKE AND MODULATION BY DIET

TCF7L2 is a component of the Wnt signalling pathway. This pathway controls almost every aspect of embryonic development and mediates homeostatic regeneration in adult tissues (Clevers & Nusse, 2012). A common genetic variant within the TCF7L2 gene (rs7903146) has been consistently associated with diabetes (Guinan, 2012; Peng et al., 2013), CVD (Bielinski et al., 2008; Kucharska-Newton et al., 2010; Muendlein et al., 2011; Sousa et al., 2009) and longevity (Garagnani et al., 2013). Of interest for our discussion is the fact that conditions such as hypertension, diabetes (Ryan et al., 2014), atrial fibrillation, ischemic heart disease, dyslipidaemia and obesity have propensity to induce strokes, which increase risk of dementia up to fivefold in the elderly, and more than 30% of stroke survivors will develop dementia within 2 years. Moreover, a link between vascular diseases and clinical AD also exists (Kalaria, 2012). Thus, this connection between metabolic disorders, stroke and cognition provides relevance to our recent findings describing an important gene–diet interaction between the rs7903146-TCF7L2 polymorphism and intervention with Mediterranean diet on stroke incidence (Corella et al., 2013). This showed that TT individuals have a higher risk of stroke when consuming a control diet, whereas intervention with Mediterranean diet is capable of counteracting the genetic risk of stroke. Moreover, we observed that this interaction with Mediterranean diet could also be observed in intermediate phenotypes of cardiovascular risk. Thus, TT individuals who had low adherence to the Mediterranean diet presented higher fasting glucose concentrations, total cholesterol, LDL-C and triglycerides than C-carriers. Nevertheless, with high adherence to Mediterranean diet, these parameters became normal and no statistically significant differences between genotypes were detected. Our results together with those obtained in longevity by the Italian group underline the importance of the TCF7L2 gene and of the Wnt signalling pathway as an important hub for the genetics cardiovascular diseases and longevity in which relevant gene–diet interactions also have an influence. Therefore, new research revealing the effects of the interaction between the TCF7L2 gene and Mediterranean diet on cognitive decline and healthy ageing is needed.

## 3.6   EPIGENOMICS, BRAIN AND COGNITION

In this discussion, we cannot ignore the epigenome, which is likely to play a critical role in the maintenance of brain health and function throughout the entire lifespan. Therefore, its study is critical in ageing. The term epigenomics is used to describe a variety of modifications to the genome that do not involve changes in DNA sequence and can result in alteration of gene expression permitting differential expression of common genetic information (Tammen et al., 2013).

The epigenetic marks are reversible and allow a rapid adaptation to the environment. There are three main categories of epigenetic alterations (Klironomos, 2013; Varley et al., 2013): DNA methylation, histone modification and noncoding RNA (although it is still debated whether noncoding RNA can be included). Evidence that dietary and pharmacological interventions have the potential to reverse environment-induced modification of epigenetic states (e.g. early-life experience, nutrition, medication, infection) has provided an additional stimulus for understanding the biological basis of individual differences in cognitive abilities and disorders of the brain. The main challenge for epigenetics in neurological traits is to determine how experiences and environmental signals effect the expression of neuronal genes to produce individual differences in behaviour, cognition, personality and mental health.

To this end, focusing on DNA and histone modifications and their initiators, mediators and readers may provide new inroads for understanding the molecular basis of phenotypic plasticity and disorders of the brain. In relation to diet, it has been demonstrated that diet affects DNA methylation (Blusztajn & Mellott, 2012; Sable et al., 2013; Villamor et al., 2012), contributing to the idea that nutrition may affect neurological process through epigenetic mechanisms. To this end, epigenetic regulation of neuronal plasticity appears as an important mechanism by which foods can prolong their effects on long-term neuronal plasticity. This has been demonstrated primarily in animal models. Thus, Sable et al. (2013) linked maternal nutrition with brain methylation patterns in the offspring and, interestingly, the modulation of these effects by n-3 PUFA. These investigators used Wistar rats as a model. Pregnant rats were divided into control and five treatment groups at two levels of folic acid (normal and excess folate) in the presence and absence of vitamin B12. n-3 PUFA supplementation was given to vitamin B12–deficient groups. Following delivery, eight dams from each group were shifted to control diet and the remaining continued on the same treatment diet. The offspring were examined at three time points (at birth, postnatal day 21 and 3 months of age). Their results demonstrate that maternal micronutrient imbalance results in global hypomethylation in the offspring brain at birth. At adult age, the cortex of the offspring displayed hypermethylation as compared with controls, in spite of the postnatal control diet. In contrast, prenatal n-3 PUFA supplementation was able to normalize methylation at 3 months of age. These findings provide new evidence for the role of n-3 PUFA in reversing methylation patterns, thereby highlighting its contribution in neuroprotection and cognition. This epigenetic mechanism could explain the relation between maternal intake of methyl-donor nutrients (methyl-donor nutrients are substrates for methylation reactions involved in these neurodevelopment processes) and child cognition early in life. On the other side of the spectrum of age, a recent study documented that in a cohort of normal elderly people, verbal and visual memory function correlated positively with the amount of dietary choline consumption. However, it is not known whether these actions of choline on human cognition are mediated by epigenomic mechanisms or by its influence on acetylcholine or phospholipid synthesis.

## 3.7   CONCLUDING SUMMARY

Genetic, epigenetic and dietary factors and their interactions play a major role in brain development and the balance between its health and disease status. The dramatic developments in genomic and neuroimaging techniques are enabling researchers to study these interactions with new breadth and depth. Thus, the structural and functional integrity of the living brain can be assessed using neuroimaging, enabling large-scale epidemiological studies to identify factors that help or harm the brain. These data can be analyzed against the entire genome and epigenome to identify associations between brain architecture, genetic variations and dietary factors such as n-3 PUFA, among others. This knowledge will provide us with practical tools to predict disease and achieve better prevention through personalization.

---

**DEFINITIONS OF KEY TERMS**

*Genome*: A genome is an organism's complete set of DNA, including all of its genes. In humans, a copy of the entire genome – more than 3 billion DNA base pairs – is contained in all cells that have a nucleus.

*Epigenome*: The epigenome comprises all of the chemical compounds that have been added to the entirety of one's DNA (genome) as a way to regulate the activity (expression) of the genes within the genome.

*SNP*: SNPs are the most common type of genetic variation among people. Each SNP represents a difference in a single DNA building block, called a nucleotide.

*GWAS*: GWASs are used to identify genes involved in human phenotypes and diseases. This method searches the genome for SNPs that occur more frequently in people with a particular phenotype or disease than in people without the phenotype or disease. Each study can look at millions of SNPs simultaneously.

*CNV*: A CNV is when the number of copies of a particular gene varies from one individual to the next.

*Allele*: An allele is one of two or more versions of a gene. An individual inherits two alleles for each gene, one from each parent. If the two alleles are the same, the individual is homozygous for that gene. If the alleles are different, the individual is heterozygous. It is also used for noncoding regions of the genome.

*Gene expression*: Gene expression is the process by which the information encoded in a gene is used to direct the assembly of a protein molecule.

*Epigenomics*: The systematic study of the global gene expression changes due to epigenetic processes and not due to DNA base sequence changes.

*Epigenetic*: Changes in the regulation of the expression of gene activity without alteration of genetic structure.

*DNA methylation*: The attachment of methyl (CH3-) groups to DNA at cytosine (C) bases; correlated with reduced transcription of a gene.

*Histone modification*: Histones are small chromosomal proteins (approximately 12–20 kD) attached to the DNA in cell nuclei by ionic linkages. Their modification by acyl or methyl groups is involved in the regulation of gene expression.

*Noncoding RNA*: The most common form of RNA (called messenger RNA) is considered protein-coding RNA, because it acts as the template for making proteins. Noncoding RNAs, however, do not carry (encode) information for producing proteins, although they do have other important functions in cells.

*Phenotype*: The observable physical and/or biochemical characteristics of the expression of a gene.

*Polymorphism*: Natural variations in a DNA sequence that occur with fairly high frequency in the general population (>1%).

*Aβ*: Amyloid-beta (Aβ or Abeta) refers to peptides of 36–43 amino acids that are involved in AD as the main component of the amyloid plaques found in the brains of Alzheimer's patients.

*C13-DHA*: Carbon-13 ($^{13}$C) is a natural, stable isotope of carbon. It is used for isotopic labelling, a technique used to track the passage of the isotope through a reaction, metabolic pathway or cell. The reactant, in this case the fatty acid DHA, is *labelled* by replacing specific atoms, usually C12, by their isotope (C13). The reactant is then allowed to undergo the reaction. The position of the isotopes in the products is measured to determine the sequence the isotopic atom followed in the reaction or the cell's metabolic pathway.

## REFERENCES

Armelagos, C. J. (2014). Brain evolution, the determinates of food choice, and the omnivore's dilemma. *Critical Reviews in Food Science and Nutrition, 54*(10), 1330–1341.

Baranzini, S. E., Wang, J., Gibson R. A., Galwey, N., Naegelin, Y., Barkhof, F., ... Oksenberg, J. R. (2009). Genome-wide association analysis of susceptibility and clinical phenotype in multiple sclerosis. *Human Molecular Genetics, 18*(4), 767–778.

Barberger-Gateau, P., Raffaitin, C., Letenneur, L., Berr, C., Tzourio, C., Dartigues, J. F., & Alpérovitch, A. (2007). Dietary patterns and risk of dementia: The Three-City cohort study. *Neurology, 69*(20), 1921–1930.

Bennet, A. M., Di Angelantonio, E., Ye, Z., Wensley, F., Dahlin, A., Ahlbom, A., ... Danesh, J. (2007). Association of apolipoprotein E genotypes with lipid levels and coronary risk. *JAMA, 298,* 1300–1311.

Bernstein, M. S., Costanza, M. C., James, R. W., Morris, M. A., Cambien, F., Raoux, S., & Morabia, A. (2002). Physical activity may modulate effects of *APOE* genotype on lipid profile. *Arteriosclerosis, Thrombosis, and Vascular Biology, 22*(1), 133–140.

Beydoun, M. A., Kaufman, J. S., Satia, J. A., Rosamond, W., & Folsom, A. R. (2007). Plasma n-3 fatty acids and the risk of cognitive decline in older adults: The Atherosclerosis Risk in Communities Study. *The American Journal of Clinical Nutrition, 85*(4), 1103–1111.

Bielinski, S. J., Pankow, J. S., Folsom, A. R., North, K. E., & Boerwinkle, E. (2008). TCF7L2 single nucleotide polymorphisms, cardiovascular disease and all-cause mortality: The Atherosclerosis Risk in Communities (ARIC) study. *Diabetologia, 51*(6), 968–970.

Blusztajn, J., & Mellott, T. (2012). Choline nutrition programs brain development via DNA and histone methylation. *Central Nervous System Agents in Medicinal Chemistry, 12*(2), 82–94.

Brown, B., Bourgeat, P., Peiffer, J., Burnham, S., Laws, S., Rainey-Smith, S., ... Martins, R. (2014). For the AIBL Research Group. Influence of BDNF Val66Met on the relationship between physical activity and brain volume. *Neurology, 83,* 1345–1352. doi:10.1212/WNL.0000000000000867

Brown, E. A. (2012). Genetic explorations of recent human metabolic adaptations: Hypotheses and evidence. *Biological Reviews of the Cambridge Philosophical Society, 87*(4), 838–855.

Brüssow, H. (2013). Nutrition, population growth and disease: A short history of lactose. *Environmental Microbiology, 15*(8), 2154–2161.

Caldwell-Hooper, A., Bryan, A., & Hagger, M. (2014). What keeps a body moving? The brain-derived neurotrophic factor val66met polymorphism and intrinsic motivation to exercise in humans. *Journal of Behavioural Medicine, 37*(6), 1180–1192.

Cárdenas-Morales, L., Grön, G., Sim, E. J., Stingl, J. C., & Kammer, T. (2014). Neural activation in humans during a simple motor task differs between BDNF polymorphisms. *PLoS One, 9*(5), e96722.

Chouinard-Watkins, R., Rioux-Perreault, C., Fortier, M., Tremblay-Mercier, J., Zhang, Y., Lawrence, P., ... Plourde, M. (2013). Disturbance in uniformly 13C-labelled DHA metabolism in elderly human subjects carrying the *APOE* ε4 allele. *British Journal of Nutrition, 110*(10), 1751–1759.

Cirulli, E. T., Kasperaviciūte, D., Attix, D. K., Need, A. C., Ge, D., Gibson, G., & Goldstein, D. B. (2010). Common genetic variation and performance on standardized cognitive tests. *European Journal of Human Genetics, 18*(7), 815–820.

Clevers, H., & Nusse, R. (2012). Wnt/β-catenin signaling and disease. *Cell, 149*(6), 1192–1205.

Coon, K.D., Myers, A.J., Craig, D.W., Webster, J.A., Pearson, J.V., Lince, D.H., ... Stephan, D.A. (April 2007). A high-density whole-genome association study reveals that *APOE* is the major susceptibility gene for sporadic late-onset Alzheimer's disease. *Journal of Clinical Psychiatry, 68*(4), 613–618.

Corella, D., Carrasco, P., Sorlí, J., Estruch, R., Rico-Sanz, J., Martínez-González, M., ... Ordovás, J. M. (2013). Mediterranean diet reduces the adverse effect of the TCF7L2-rs7903146 polymorphism on cardiovascular risk factors and stroke incidence: A randomized controlled trial in a high-cardiovascular-risk population. *Diabetes Care, 36*(11), 3803–3811.

Corella, D., Guillén, M., Sáiz, C., Portolés, O., Sabater, A., Cortina, S., ... Ordovas, J. M. (2001). Environmental factors modulate the effect of the *APOE* genetic polymorphism on plasma lipid concentrations: Ecogenetic studies in a Mediterranean Spanish population. *Metabolism, 50*(8), 936–944.

Danthiir, V., Hosking, D., Burns, N., Wilson, C., Nettelbeck, T., Calvaresi, E., ... Wittert, G. (2014). Cognitive performance in older adults is inversely associated with fish consumption but not erythrocyte membrane n-3 fatty acids. *Journal of Nutrition, 144*(3), 311–320.

Dauncey, M. J. (2012). Recent advances in nutrition, genes and brain health. *Proceedings of the Nutrition Society, 71*(4), 581–591.

Davies, G., Harris, S., Reynolds, C., Payton, A., Knight, H., Liewald, D., ... Deary, I. (2014). A genome-wide association study implicates the *APOE* locus in nonpathological cognitive ageing. *Molecular Psychiatry, 19*(1), 76–87.

Davis, O. S., Butcher, L. M., Docherty, S., Meaburn, E. L., Curtis, C. J., Simpson, M. A., ... Plomin, R. (2010). A three-stage genome-wide association study of general cognitive ability: Hunting the small effects. *Behavior Genetic, 40*(6), 759–767.

De Jager, P., Shulman, J., Chibnik, L. B., Keenan, B. T., Raj, T., Wilson, R. S., ... Evans, D. A. (2012). A genome-wide scan for common variants affecting the rate of age-related cognitive decline. *Neurobiology of Aging, 33*(5), 1017.e1011–1015.

Deelen, J. E. A. (2011). Genome-wide association study identifies a single major locus contributing to survival into old age; the *APOE* locus revisited. *Aging Cell, 10*, 686–698.

Dincheva, I., Glatt, C. E., & Lee, F. S. (2012). Impact of the BDNF Val66Met polymorphism on cognition: Implications for behavioral genetics. *Neuroscientist, 18*(5), 439–451.

Duarte, C. M. (2014). Red ochre and shells: Clues to human evolution. *Trends in Ecology & Evolution, 29*(10), 560–565.

Erickson, K. I., Banducci, S. E., Weinstein, A. M., Macdonald, A. R., Ferrell, R., Halder, I., ... Manuck, S. (2013). The brain-derived neurotrophic factor Val66Met polymorphism moderates an effect of physical activity on working memory performance. *Psychological Science, 24*(9), 1770–1779.

Eskelinen, M. H., Ngandu, T., Helkala, E. L., Tuomilehto, J., Nissinen, A., Soininen, H., & Kivipelto, M. (2008). Fat intake at midlife and cognitive impairment later in life: A population-based CAIDE study. *International Journal of Geriatric Psychiatry, 23*(7), 741–747.

Féart, C., Samieri, C., Rondeau, V., Amieva, H., Portet, F., Dartigues, J., ... Barberger-Gateau, P. (2009). Adherence to a Mediterranean diet, cognitive decline, and risk of dementia. *JAMA, 302*(6), 638–648.

Forde, N., Ronan, L., Suckling, J., Scanlon, C., Neary, S., Holleran, L., ... Cannon, D. (2014). Structural neuroimaging correlates of allelic variation of the BDNF val66met polymorphism. *Neuroimage, 15*(90), 280–289.

Garagnani, P., Giuliani, C., Pirazzini, C., Olivieri, F., Bacalini, M., Ostan, R., ... Franceschi, C. (2013). Centenarians as super-controls to assess the biological relevance of genetic risk factors for common age-related diseases: A proof of principle on type 2 diabetes. *Aging (Albany NY), 5*(5), 373–385.

Garatachea, N., Emanuele, E., Calero, M., Fuku, N., Arai, Y., Abe, Y., ... Lucia, A. (2014). *APOE* gene and exceptional longevity: Insights from three independent cohorts. *Experimental Gerontology, 53*, 16–23.

Garatachea, N., Emanuele, E., Calero, M., Fuku, N., Arai, Y., Abe, Y., ... Lucia, A. (2014). *APOE* gene and exceptional longevity: Insights from three independent cohorts. *Experimental Gerontology, 53C*, 16–23.

Gerbault, P., Roffet-Salque, M., Evershed, R. P., & Thomas, M. G. (2013). How long have adult humans been consuming milk? *IUBMB Life, 65*(12), 983–990.

Global Lipids Genetics Consortium, Willer, C. J., Schmidt, E. M., Sengupta, S., Peloso, G. M., Gustafsson, S., ... Abecasis, G. R. (2013). Discovery and refinement of loci associated with lipid levels. *Nature Genetics, 45*(11), 1274–1283.

Gomez-Pinilla, F., & Tyagi, E. (2013). Diet and cognition: Interplay between cell metabolism and neuronal plasticity. *Current Opinion in Clinical Nutrition and Metabolic Care, 16*(6), 726–733.

Grammer, T. B., Hoffmann, M. M., Scharnagl, H., Kleber, M. E., Silbernagel, G., Pilz, S., ... März, W. (2013). Smoking, apolipoprotein E genotypes, and mortality (the Ludwigshafen RIsk and Cardiovascular Health study). *European Heart Journal, 34*(17), 1298–1305.

Guinan, K. (2012). Worldwide distribution of type II diabetes-associated TCF7L2 SNPs: Evidence for stratification in Europe. *Biochemical Genetics, 50*(3–4), 159–179.

Gustavsson, J., Mehlig, K., Leander, K., Strandhagen, E., Björck, L., Thelle, D., ... Nyberg, F. (2012). Interaction of apolipoprotein E genotype with smoking and physical inactivity on coronary heart disease risk in men and women. *Atherosclerosis, 220*(2), 486–492.

Hajek, T., Kopecek, M., & Höschl, C. (2012). Reduced hippocampal volumes in healthy carriers of brain-derived neurotrophic factor Val66Met polymorphism: Meta-analysis. *The World Journal of Biological Psychiatry, 13*(3), 178–187.

Hanson, A., Bayer-Carter, J., Green, P., Montine, T., Wilkinson, C., Baker, L., ... Craft, S. (2013). Effect of apolipoprotein E genotype and diet on apolipoprotein E lipidation and amyloid peptides: Randomized clinical trial. *JAMA Neurology, 70*(8), 972–980.

Hashimoto, R., Ikeda, M., Ohi, K., Yasuda, Y., Yamamori, H., Fukumoto, M., ... Takeda, M. (2013). Genome-wide association study of cognitive decline in schizophrenia. *American Journal of Psychiatry, 170*(6), 683–684.

Hong, C., Liou, Y., & Tsai, S. (2011). Effects of BDNF polymorphisms on brain function and behavior in health and disease. *Brain Research Bulletin, 86*(5–6), 287–297.

Hosang, G., Shiles, C., Tansey, K., McGuffin, P., & Uher, R. (2014). Interaction between stress and the BDNF Val66Met polymorphism in depression: A systematic review and meta-analysis. *BMC Medical, 16*, 12–17.

Huang, T. L., Zandi, P. P., Tucker, K. L., Fitzpatrick, A. L., Kuller, L. H., Fried, L. P., ... Carlson, M. C. (2005). Benefits of fatty fish on dementia risk are stronger for those without *APOE* epsilon4. *Neurology, 65*(9), 1409–1414.

Humphries, S. E., Talmud, P., Hawe, E., Bolla, M., Day, I. N., & Miller, G. J. (2001). Apolipoprotein E4 and coronary heart disease in middle-aged men who smoke: A prospective study. *Lancet, 358*(9276), 115–119.

Jahanshad, N., Rajagopalan, P., Hua, X., Hibar, D. P., Nir, T. M., Toga, A. W., ... Thompson, P. M. (2013). Alzheimer's Disease Neuroimaging Initiative. Genome-wide scan of healthy human connectome discovers SPON1 gene variant influencing dementia severity. *Proceedings of the National Academy of Sciences of the United States of America, 110*(2), 4768–4773.

Jeong, C., & Di Rienzo, A. (2014). Adaptations to local environments in modern human populations. *Current Opinion in Genetics & Development, 14*(29c), 108.

Kalaria, R. N. (2012). Risk factors and neurodegenerative mechanisms in stroke related dementia. *Panminerva Medica, 54*(3), 139–148.

Kathiresan, S., & Srivastava, D. (2012). Genetics of human cardiovascular disease. *Cell, 148*(1242–57).

Khan, T. A., Shah, T., Prieto, D., Zhang, W., Price, J., Fowkes, G., ... Casas, J. (2013a). Apolipoprotein E genotype, cardiovascular biomarkers and risk of stroke: Systematic review and meta-analysis of 14,015 stroke cases and pooled analysis of primary biomarker data from up to 60,883 individuals. *International Journal of Epidemiology, 42*(2), 475–492.

Khan, T. A., Shah, T., Prieto, D., Zhang, W., Price, J., Fowkes, G., ... Casas, J. (2013b). Apolipoprotein E genotype, cardiovascular biomarkers and risk of stroke: Systematic review and meta-analysis of 14,015 stroke cases and pooled analysis of primary biomarker data from up to 60,883 individuals. *International Journal of Epidemiology, 42*, 475–492.

Kim, J. M., Stewart, R., Bae, K. Y., Kim, S. W., Yang, S. J., Park, K. H., ... Yoon, J. S. (2011). Role of BDNF val66met polymorphism on the association between physical activity and incident dementia. *Neurobiology of Aging, 32*(3), 551.e555–512.

Kim, S., & Webster, M. J. (2011). Integrative genome-wide association analysis of cytoarchitectural abnormalities in the prefrontal cortex of psychiatric disorders. *Molecular Psychiatry, 16*(4), 452–461.

Klironomos, F. D. E. A. (2013). How epigenetic mutations can affect genetic evolution: Model and mechanism. *Bioessays, 35*(571–578).

Kucharska-Newton, A. M., Monda, K. L., Bielinski, S., Boerwinkle, E., Rea, T., Rosamond, W., ... North, K. (2010). Role of BMI in the Association of the TCF7L2 rs7903146 Variant with Coronary Heart Disease: The Atherosclerosis Risk in Communities (ARIC) Study. *Journal of Obesity, 2010*, pii: 651903.

LeBlanc, M., Kulle, B., Sundet, K., Agartz, I., Melle, I., Djurovic, S., ... Andreassen, O. (2012). Genome-wide study identifies PTPRO and WDR72 and FOXQ1-SUMO1P1 interaction associated with neurocognitive function. *Journal of Psychiatric Research, 46*(2), 271–278.

Liddell, M., Williams, J., Bayer, A., Kaiser, F., & Owen, M. (1994). Confirmation of association between the e4 allele of apolipoprotein E and Alzheimer's disease. *Journal of Medical Genetics, 31*(3), 197–200.

Lindahl-Jacobsen, R., Tan, Q., Mengel-From, J., Christensen, K., Nebel, A., & Christiansen, L. (2013). Effects of the *APOE* e2 allele on mortality and cognitive function in the oldest old. *The Journals of Gerontology Series A: Biological Sciences and Medical Sciences, 68*, 389–394.

Mandelman, S. D., & Grigorenko, E. L. (2012). Genes BDNF Val66Met and cognition: All, none, or some? A meta-analysis of the genetic association. *Brain Behaviour, 11*(2), 127–136.

Martínez-Lapiscina, E., H, Galbete, C., Corella, D., Toledo, E., Buil-Cosiales, P., Salas-Salvado, J., ... Martinez-Gonzalez, M. A. (2014). Genotype patterns at CLU, CR1, PICALM and *APOE*, cognition and Mediterranean diet: The PREDIMED-NAVARRA trial. *Genes & Nutrition, 9*(3), 393.

Mata, J., Thompson, R., & Gotlib, I. (2010). BDNF genotype moderates the relation between physical activity and depressive symptoms. *Health Psychology, 29*(2), 130–133. doi:10.1037/a0017261

McKay, G. J., Silvestri, G., Chakravarthy, U., Dasari, S., Fritsche, L., Weber, B., ... Patterson, C. (2011a). Variations in apolipoprotein E frequency with age in a pooled analysis of a large group of older people. *American Journal of Epidemiology, 173*(12), 1357–1364.

McKay, G. J., Silvestri, G., Chakravarthy, U., Dasari, S., Fritsche, L., Weber, B., ... Patterson, C. (2011b). Variations in apolipoprotein E frequency with age in a pooled analysis of a large group of older people. *American Journal of Epidemiology, 173*, 1357–1364.

Medland, S. E., Jahanshad, N., Neale, B. M., & Thompson, P. M. (2014). Whole-genome analyses of whole-brain data: Working within an expanded search space. *Nature Neuroscience, 17*(6), 791–800.

Muendlein, A., Saely, C., Geller-Rhomberg, S., Sonderegger, G., Rein, P., Winder, T., ... Drexel, H. (2011). Single nucleotide polymorphisms of TCF7L2 are linked to diabetic coronary atherosclerosis. *PLoS One, 6*(3), e17978.

Nascimento, C. M., Pereira, J. R., Pires de Andrade, L., Garuffi, M., Ayan, C., Kerr, D., ... Stella, F. (2014). Physical exercise improves peripheral BDNF levels and cognitive functions in elderly mild cognitive impairment individuals with different BDNF Val66Met genotypes. *Journal of Alzheimer's Disease.*

Need, A. C., Attix, D. K., McEvoy, J. M., Cirulli, E. T., Linney, K. L., Hunt, P., ...
    Goldstein, D. B. (2009). A genome-wide study of common SNPs and CNVs in cogni-
    tive performance in the CANTAB. *Human Molecular Genetics, 18*(23), 4650–4661.
Novelli, V., Viviani Anselmi, C., Roncarati, R., Guffanti, G., Malovini, A., Piluso, G., &
    Puca, A. A. (2008). Lack of replication of genetic associations with human longevity.
    *Biogerontology, 9*, 85–92.
Paus, T., Bernard, M., Chakravarty, M. M., Davey Smith, G., Gillis, J., Lourdusamy, A., ...
    Pausova, Z. (2012). KCTD8 gene and brain growth in adverse intrauterine environment:
    A genome-wide association study. *Cerebral Cortex, 22*(11), 2634–2642.
Peng, S., Zhu, Y., Lü, B., Xu, F., Li, X., & Lai, M. (2013). TCF7L2 gene polymorphisms and
    type 2 diabetes risk: A comprehensive and updated meta-analysis involving 121,174
    subjects. *Mutagenesis, 28*(1), 25–37.
Pezzini, A., Grassi, M., Del Zotto, E., Bazzoli, E., Archetti, S., Assanelli, D., ... Padovani, A.
    (2004). Synergistic effect of apolipoprotein E polymorphisms and cigarette smoking on
    risk of ischemic stroke in young adults. *Stroke, 35*(2), 438–442.
Poirier, J., Davignon, J., Bouthillier, D., Kogan, S., Bertrand, P., & Gauthier, S. (1993).
    Apolipoprotein E polymorphism and Alzheimer's disease. *Lancet, 342*(8873), 697–699.
Potkin, S. G., Turner, J. A., Guffanti, G., Lakatos, A., Fallon, J., Nguyen, D., ... Macciardi, F.
    (2009). FBIRN. A genome-wide association study of schizophrenia using brain activa-
    tion as a quantitative phenotype. *Schizophrenia Bulletin, 35*(1), 96–108.
Rosas-Vargas, H., Martínez-Ezquerro, J., & Bienvenu, T. (2011). Brain-derived neurotrophic
    factor, food intake regulation, and obesity. *Archives of Medical Research, 42*(6), 484–494.
Ryan, J., Fine, D., & Rosano, C. (2014). Type 2 diabetes and cognitive impairment: Contributions
    from neuroimaging. *Journal of Geriatric Psychiatry and Neurology, 27*(1), 47–55.
Sable, P., Randhir, K., Kale, A., Chavan-Gautam, P., & Joshi, S. (2013). Maternal micronu-
    trients and brain global methylation patterns in the offspring. *Nutritional Neuroscience,
    18*(1), 30–36.
Samieri, C., Féart, C., Proust-Lima, C., Peuchant, E., Dartigues, J. F., Amieva, H., & Barberger-
    Gateau, P. (2011). ω-3 fatty acids and cognitive decline: Modulation by *APOEε*4 allele
    and depression. *Neurobiology of Aging, 32*(12), 2317.e2313–2322.
Samieri, C., Lorrain, S., Buaud, B., Vaysse, C., Berr, C., Peuchant, E., ... Barberger-Gateau,
    P. (2013). Relationship between diet and plasma long-chain n-3 PUFAs in older people:
    Impact of apolipoprotein E genotype. *The Journal of Lipid Research, 54*(9), 2559–2567.
Santos, J. L., Saus, E., Smalley, S., Cataldo, L., Alberti, G., Parada, J., ... Estivill, X. (2012).
    Copy number polymorphism of the salivary amylase gene: Implications in human nutri-
    tion research. *Journal of Nutrigenetics and Nutrigenomics, 5*(3), 117–131.
Schächter, F., Faure-Delanef, L., Guénot, F., Rouger, H., Froguel, P., Lesueur-Ginot, L., &
    Cohen, D. (1994). Genetic associations with human longevity at the *APOE* and ACE
    loci. *Nature Genetics, 6*, 29–32.
Schupf, N., Barral, S., Perls, T., Newman, A., Christensen, K., Thyagarajan, B., ... Mayeux, R.
    (2013). Apolipoprotein E and familial longevity. *Neurobiology of Aging, 34*(4), 1287–1291.
Seshadri, S., DeStefano, A., Au, R., Massaro, J., Beiser, A., Kelly-Hayes, M., ... Wolf, P. (2007).
    Genetic correlates of brain aging on MRI and cognitive test measures: A genome-wide
    association and linkage analysis in the Framingham Study. *BMC Medical Genetics,
    8*(Suppl. 1), S15.
Shen, L., Kim, S., Risacher, S. L., Nho, K., Swaminathan, S., West, J. D., ... Saykin, A. J.
    (2010). Alzheimer's Disease Neuroimaging Initiative: Whole genome association study
    of brain-wide imaging phenotypes for identifying quantitative trait loci in MCI and AD:
    A study of the ADNI cohort. *Neuroimage, 53*(3), 1051–1063.
Sing, C. F., & Davignon, J. (1985). Role of the apolipoprotein E polymorphism in determin-
    ing normal plasma lipid and lipoprotein variation. *The American Journal of Human
    Genetics, 37*(268–85).

Song, Y., Stampfer, M. J., & Liu, S. (2004). Meta-analysis: Apolipoprotein E genotypes and risk for coronary heart disease. *Annals of Internal Medicine, 141*(2), 137–147.

Sousa, A., Marquezine, G., Lemos, P., Martinez, E., Lopes, N., Hueb, W., ... Pereira, A. (2009). TCF7L2 polymorphism rs7903146 is associated with coronary artery disease severity and mortality. *PLoS One, 11*(4), e7696.

Stein, J., Hua, X., Lee, S., Ho, A., Leow, A., Toga, A., ... Initiative, A. S. D. N. (2010a). Voxelwise genome-wide association study (vGWAS). *Neuroimage, 53*(3), 1160–1174.

Stein, J., Hua, X., Morra, J., Lee, S., Hibar, D. P., Ho, A. J., ... Initiative, A. S. D. N. (2010b). Genome-wide analysis reveals novel genes influencing temporal lobe structure with relevance to neurodegeneration in Alzheimer's disease. *Neuroimage, 51*(2), 542–554.

Stein, J., Medland, S. E., Vasquez, A. A., Hibar, D. P., Senstad, R. E., Winkler, A. M., ... Thompson, P. M. (2012). Enhancing Neuro Imaging Genetics through Meta-Analysis Consortium. Identification of common variants associated with human hippocampal and intracranial volumes. *Nature Genetics, 44*(5), 552–561.

Stengård, J. H., Pekkanen, J., Ehnholm, C., Nissinen, A., & Sing, C. F. (1996). Genotypes with the apolipoprotein epsilon4 allele are predictors of coronary heart disease mortality in a longitudinal study of elderly Finnish men. *Human Genetics, 97*(677–84).

Talmud, P., Stephens, J., Hawe, E., Demissie, S., Cupples, L., Hurel, S., ... Ordovas, J. (2005). The significant increase in cardiovascular disease risk in *APOE*epsilon4 carriers is evident only in men who smoke: Potential relationship between reduced antioxidant status and *APOE4*. *Annuals of Human Genetics, 69*(Pt6), 613–622.

Tammen, S. A., Friso, S., & Choi, S. W. (2013). Epigenetics: The link between nature and nurture. *Molecular Aspects of Medicine, 34*(4), 753–764.

Teh, C., Lee, T., Kuchibhatla, M., Ashley-Koch, A., Macfall, J., Krishnan, R., & Beyer, J. (2012). Bipolar disorder, brain-derived neurotrophic factor (BDNF) Val66Met polymorphism and brain morphology. *PLoS One, 7*(7), e38469.

Teslovich, T. M., Musunuru, K., Smith, A. V., Edmondson, A. C., Stylianou, I. M, Koseki, M., ... Kathiresan, S. (2010). Biological, clinical and population relevance of 95 loci for blood lipids. *Nature, 466*(7307), 707–713.

Toro, R., Poline, J. B., Huguet, G., Loth, E., Frouin, V., Banaschewski, T., ... Bourgeron, T. (2014). Genomic architecture of human neuroanatomical diversity. *Molecular Psychiatry, 16*. doi:10.1038/mp.2014.99

Vandal, M., Alata, W., Tremblay, C., Rioux-Perreault, C., Salem, N. J., Calon, F., & Plourde, M. (2014). Reduction in DHA transport to the brain of mice expressing human *APOE4* compared to *APOE2*. *Journal of Neurochemistry, 129*(3), 516–526.

Varley, K. E., Gertz, J., Bowling, K. M., Parker, S. L, Reddy, T. E., Pauli-Behn, F., ... Myers, R. M. (2013). Dynamic DNA methylation across diverse human cell lines and tissues. *Genome Research, 23*, 555–567.

Villamor, E., Rifas-Shiman, S. L., Gillman, M. W., & Oken, E. (2012). Maternal intake of methyl-donor nutrients and child cognition at 3 years of age. *Paediatric and Perinatal Epidemiology, 26*(4), 328–335. doi:10.1111/j.1365-3016.2012.01264.x

Whalley, L. J., Deary, I. J., Starr, J. M., Wahle, K. W., Rance, K. A., Bourne, V. J., & Fox, H. C. (2008). n-3 Fatty acid erythrocyte membrane content, *APOE* varepsilon4, and cognitive variation: An observational follow-up study in late adulthood. *The American Journal of Clinical Nutrition, 87*(2), 449–445.

Yin, Y. W., Sun, Q. Q., Zhang, B. B., Hu, A. M., Liu, H. L., Wang, Q., & Hou, Z. Z. (2013). Association between apolipoprotein E gene polymorphism and the risk of coronary artery disease in Chinese population: Evidence from a meta-analysis of 40 studies. *PLoS One, 8*(6), e66924.

Zhang, C., & Pierce, B. L. (2014). Genetic susceptibility to accelerated cognitive decline in the US Health and Retirement Study. *Neurobiology of Aging, 35*(6), 1512.e1511–1518.

# Section II

Process and Methods for
Measuring Brain Function
and Cognition

# 4 Cognitive Assessment
## *Principles, Paradigms and Pitfalls*

### Samrah Ahmed and Celeste A. De Jager

## CONTENTS

## SUMMARY

An accruing body of research in a range of healthy and diseased populations has begun to show that nutrition can have an effect on cognitive function. The detection of a relationship between nutrition and cognitive health requires careful selection of cognitive assessments to identify participants for enrolment into studies of potential treatments and to monitor and detect subtle or more overt changes in cognition as a result of intervention. A plethora of cognitive instruments are available to measure cognition, but not all will be most efficient for the task at hand. The decision to include tests into a battery will be based on a number of considerations. This chapter will discuss the key considerations in identifying and administering cognitive assessments that are appropriate for use in trials assessing nutrient interventions, taking into account the primary outcomes as well as the participant populations involved. With these fundamentals considered, we will briefly propose a practical structure for cognitive assessment in nutrition research.

## 4.1 METHODOLOGY: KEY CONSIDERATIONS IN THE PSYCHOMETRIC PROPERTIES OF COGNITIVE TESTS

Accurate interpretation of cognitive tests is based on a set of key methodological premises. Only with these psychometric properties intact can the test be used to support clinical inferences made about the presence or absence of cognitive impairment secondary to nutritional intervention. As such, the researcher can trust that the given scores represent a true measure of performance before and after intervention.

### 4.1.1 SENSITIVITY AND SPECIFICITY

Sensitivity and specificity measurements provide indications as to what proportion of individuals can be correctly classified as suffering from a disease (sensitivity) and what proportion can be shown to be healthy (specificity), based on a given test score. Selecting optimally sensitive and specific measures to detect nutrition-induced changes is imperative to be able to draw an accurate inference from the results. Without optimal measures, a number of errors may be introduced. A null result may not reflect the true absence of an effect of nutrition, but rather the lack of sensitivity of a test (a type 2 error). Conversely, inappropriate test selection may lead to an effect being inferred where no true relationship exists (type 1 error).

More often than not, a trade-off will be necessary, given that perfect sensitivity and specificity values for a test are not at all common. To address sensitivity and specificity issues, researchers can compute receiver operator characteristic (ROC) curves in order to assess the accuracy of a cognitive test. This statistic provides an index of the ability to make a decision about a patient's clinical status when given a score acquired from a particular test. An ROC curve provides a graphical representation of the trade-off between the rates of true-positive classification (i.e. people who had the disease and who were correctly classified as having so) and the rate of false-positive classification (i.e. those people who did not have the disease and who were incorrectly classified as having so). The diagnostic accuracy of a given cognitive test for deciding which of a group of tests is most accurate for diagnosis of the condition of interest can be empirically determined by calculating the area under the curve (AUC), shown in Figures 4.1 and 4.2.

### 4.1.2 IMPAIRMENT CRITERIA

In order to determine when performance on a given test represents impairment, an impairment criterion should be employed. Tests will be scored up and compared to appropriate normative data, after which a decision is required as to whether the pattern of the patient's performance reflects impairment. Impairment criteria are necessary

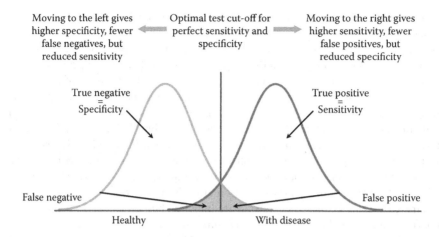

FIGURE 4.1 Factors in determining optimal sensitivity and specificity of cognitive assessments.

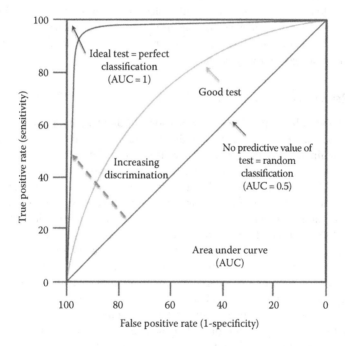

FIGURE 4.2 ROC curves can be used to quantify the diagnostic ability of cognitive assessments.

to determine whether a low score on a cognitive test is low enough to substantiate a claim of impairment consistent with a particular diagnosis or disease process or whether the score is within a normative range. Poor performance may reflect lifelong difficulties in a particular area, such as reading or arithmetic, or may indicate that the patient was not well motivated or anxious during testing. Given these possible confounds, it is becoming increasingly important to be able to determine a patient's premorbid level of functioning in order to more accurately determine if a person's performance truly reflects impairment. Where prior test data are not available, tests such as the widely used National Adult Reading Test (NART) (Bright et al., 2002) may be employed. A change of 1.5 or 2 standard deviations from this estimate of premorbid functioning is typically used to as a criterion to determine the likelihood that performance on cognitive tests is impaired. Selecting the stringency of impairment criterion is another key consideration. When criterion are less stringent, that is, 1–1.5 standard deviations below test means, then the false-positive rate will be higher, that is, those people with no impairment will be considered impaired, although the true-positive rate will be higher, that is, those people who are impaired and correctly identified as being so. Conversely, if the impairment criterion is set too high, the false-negative rate increases, that is, those people who are impaired but are judged as being within a normal range. A balance needs to be acquired so that accurate conclusions can be drawn about the utility of a given intervention. Many nutritional interventions have shown some benefit, but poorly selected impairment criteria have either prevented a positive conclusion from being drawn or indeed an effect has been concluded where there is little to report. This issue also underlines the importance of using a battery of well-selected tests, rather than basing conclusions on one test criterion alone. A single aberrant score, regardless of how well considered a test may be for a particular cognitive domain, must not be relied upon.

### 4.1.3  RELIABILITY AND VALIDITY

Reliability and validity provide the foundation of cognitive assessment. Reliability can be defined as how consistent or stable test scores are after repeated observations are obtained from an individual over time, or in different testing conditions. Reliable tests should therefore give similar results when repeated under similar circumstances. Assessment of clinical change is essential to a nutritional intervention trial where the major premise is that any change from baseline cognitive scores to a retest session at a later time signals the benefit incurred by the nutritional intervention. Therefore, accurate detection of changes in test scores is critical.

Of course, it is not often that exact test scores are obtained on every testing session due to several factors that can contribute. For example, random factors may impact reliability, such as the individuals' motivation at the time of testing or the noise or temperature in the room. There may be inherent difficulties in the cognitive test, such as the use of complex language or grammatical constructs that may disadvantage those individuals not formally educated. Accepting that no cognitive test is error-free, a reliable test is one that is able to maximally assess a given cognitive domain, while minimizing the effects of extraneous variables. Table 4.3 provides some options for reliable tests. As a general rule, cognitive tests assessing verbal, visual and personality-based domains are highly reliable (Anastasi, 1968). However, attention and memory tests are more susceptible to confounding variables such as anxiety and fatigue (Franzen, 2000). It is advisable to take this into account and introduce ample opportunity for breaks as well as clear explanation and support to manage any test anxiety.

Validity can be defined as how well a cognitive test measures what it purports to measure. The researcher must first be confident that the test is free from random errors, that is, that the test's reliability has first been established. The content of the test must then (1) provide an accurate depiction of the cognitive domain in question and (2) be comparable to other, well-established tests for assessing that cognitive domain. Further evidence for validity of a given task may be acquired using brain imaging, to show that the test correlates with brain areas that subserve the cognitive function in question (see Chapter 12 by Camfield).

### 4.1.4   NORMATIVE DATA

Normative data, that is, data acquired from a healthy population and/or a population that has not been given a particular nutritional intervention, are necessary to be able to interpret scores in populations who have been given an intervention. The majority of cognitive tests do not separate normative data for different age groups, genders, education levels, etc., although there are a few widely used tests that do take into account some of these differences (see Mitrushina et al., 2005). The majority of tests do have normative data for the geographic population, that is, British tests are standardized for the British population. This results in normative data that have been acquired, most often, from an adult population that ranges in age from young adulthood to senior years. In most cases this is actually not an issue and these norms tend to serve their purpose. However, issues may arise in the extremes of a population, for example, in participants with no formal education or different cultures or different languages. Referring to standard normative data often leads to false positives or false negatives in such populations. It is essential, therefore, to either ensure that inclusion and exclusion criteria for participant recruitment to a study match the normative sample or that new normative data are acquired for the population being studied (Table 4.1).

---

**TABLE 4.1**
**Summary of Section 4.1**

**Methodology: Key Considerations in the Psychometric Properties of Cognitive Tests**

The sensitivity of a test indicates what proportion of individuals can be correctly classified as suffering from a disease.

The specificity of a test describes what proportion of individuals can be shown to be healthy.

A trade-off between sensitivity and specificity is often the case, and ROC curves can be computed to assess the accuracy of a cognitive test.

Impairment criteria are necessary to determine whether a low score on a cognitive test indicates impairment consistent with a particular diagnosis or disease process or whether the score is within a normative range.

Reliability and validity are the foundation of a good cognitive test. Reliability is how consistent or stable test scores are after repeated observations are obtained from an individual over time or in different testing conditions. Validity is how well a cognitive test measures what it purports to measure.

Normative data are needed to be able to interpret scores in populations who have been given an intervention. The normative and test populations must be matched as closely as possible.

---

## 4.2 CAUTIONS IN ASSESSING COGNITIVE FUNCTION

Methodological quality is clearly the foundation of accurate assessment of cognition; however, a second set of equally important considerations is in the practical administration of assessments. The key issue to remember is that the point of cognitive assessment is to extract the best possible performance from a participant, such that any change in cognition over time can be attributed accurately and confidently to a given nutritional intervention and not to potential confounds.

### 4.2.1 PRACTICE EFFECTS

Repeat cognitive assessment using the same cognitive indices is essential when determining the impact of a nutritional intervention. With repeated testing however, healthy participants and many patient populations are susceptible to practice effects. In particular, tests that have components of speed testing or have a single solution to the question being asked can be easily remembered and are more likely to show practice effects (Basso et al., 1999).

Practice effects are also a particular problem in tests of memory. Memory tests are usually based on the premise of learning a small set of verbal or visual material, and many tests are without validated parallel versions. As a result, many participants, bar those with severe memory impairment, are able to learn some aspect of the material and recall this at a subsequent assessment (Wilson et al., 2000). There is also evidence to suggest that participants achieve a more general test-taking benefit, such that cognitive performance is enhanced after repeated assessments, even where different test stimuli are employed (Wilson et al., 2000).

In order to get around this problem, a number of methods may be considered. First, tests can be chosen that have sufficiently validated parallel forms, where available, although the number of cognitive tests with validated forms is limited. It is imperative that the researcher is confident of interform reliability between alternate versions of tests, as if the level of difficulty differs between each version, then this can introduce errors in assessment. Second, sufficient time should be left between each assessment. This will vary depending on the tests used and requires a survey of existing literature examining practice effects in the tests chosen. Such literature may not always exist, particularly for newer tests or test versions, and the judgment of a clinician or researcher who frequently uses the tests of interest may be the best solution. Third, where time and resources permit, the study can be designed to take into account practice effects. Evidence suggests that practice effects are greatest between the first and second assessment (Ivnik et al., 1999). A researcher may then consider providing at least two baseline assessments before introducing the experimental assessment (McCaffrey & Westervelt, 1995).

### 4.2.2 PARTICIPANT CHARACTERISTICS

Poor evaluation of the needs of a given population may mean that cognitive change is over- or underestimated. As such, all populations of interest should be given a tailored cognitive assessment. It should not be automatically assumed that tests suitable or showing a significant effect of change in one population will be applicable to all other populations without further validation. For example, a test of reaction time may be shown to be sensitive to change in young adults but may be too demanding in an elderly population and require different normative data to take into account age-related changes in processing speed. From our own work in dementia and, therefore, a largely elderly population, a number of guidelines can be extracted, which have empirical supporting evidence. Of course, many of these will apply to any population and can, therefore, be considered a general set of rules:

1. The testing environment
   a. The temperature of the room should be comfortable for the participant.
   b. Lighting should be adequate, that is, not too bright or in direct sunlight, which may also create glare on computer equipment being used, and not too dark so as the participant is unable to see what they are doing.
   c. Free from noise and distractions, away from other people and other activities.
   d. Seating that allows the participant to position themselves comfortably at an appropriate height and distance from the computer screen/test stimuli.
2. The participant
   a. The assessment should be conducted at the pace set by the individual.
   b. All assessments should be properly introduced and explained to put the participant at ease.
   c. Good judgment should be employed throughout the assessment such that if a person appears distressed by a particular task that may be tapping cognitive impairments, testing should be postponed or abandoned. Similarly, if the participant appears fatigued. Overall testing time and breaks should be scheduled according to the individual.
   d. Participants should be asked whether they suffer from any sensory deficits prior to testing. For example, participants with visual or hearing deficits should be reminded to bring their glasses or hearing aid with them to the assessment. The researcher should also check again at the time of assessment that these aids are sufficient in order to complete the tests being administered. Colour blindness may also need to be assessed for some tests.
   e. Any motor deficits or diminished praxis as results of age or medical conditions not being studied (e.g. arthritic conditions) should be determined, so that errors on visuospatial tasks or processing speed/reaction time are not inaccurately attributed to the disease being studied when in fact they are affected by co-morbidities.
   f. A full list of medications being taken by the participant should be acquired. Medications may have effects on cognitive performance, which will confound the impact of any nutritional intervention. Researchers should also be aware that it may take several weeks for a person to fully adjust to a newly prescribed medication and the interim period may not be the best time to administer cognitive tests. Hence, time on treatment may need to be recorded.

---

**TABLE 4.2**

**Summary of Section 4.2**

**Cautions in Assessing Cognitive Function**

Practice effects are a common problem where repeat cognitive assessment is required. Choose tests with parallel forms or leave sufficient time between each assessment.

Particular characteristics of the population being tested need to be taken into account such as the stability of the testing environment, the participant's needs and the timing of the assessment, to achieve the most accurate reflection of the participants' abilities at a given time point.

---

3. Timing of assessment
   a. Select a mutually convenient time for assessment, when the participant feels their cognitive abilities are at their best. For example, this may be in the morning or afternoon.
   b. Where possible, avoid assessments after medical, particularly invasive, procedures.
   c. Avoid assessments in the presence of pain or discomfort that the participant may be feeling due to existing medical problems or anything that may arise during assessment, for example, headache or sore eyes.
   d. Control for previous food/beverage intake especially caffeine and sugar levels, either by keeping to participants' usual intake or by standardizing intake before assessments (Table 4.2).

## 4.3  PRACTICAL GUIDE TO COGNITIVE ASSESSMENT

It is important to note that no single test will be entirely sufficient to draw a conclusion as to the efficacy of an intervention nor would it be advisable to rely on one test alone. As a general rule, cognitive assessments should not be used in isolation. For example, significant improvement on a verbal memory test does not indicate if the improvement is due to improved memory function alone or due to improvements in language or to attentional factors. Similarly, a non-significant result may mask that the participant was not attending, fatigued or unmotivated at the time of that particular test. A much more advisable course of action is to develop a stepwise assessment procedure beginning with cognitive screening and which incorporates tests of all primary cognitive domains with two or more tests in each domain, as well as additional sources of collateral information about the patient from themselves, family members and caregivers. This protocol will then assist in looking for inconsistencies in cognitive performance as exhibited in variations across a range of tests and information sources.

### 4.3.1  COGNITIVE SCREENING

To begin with, sensitive cognitive screening tools are needed to identify patients for enrolment into studies of potential nutritional interventions. A number of screening tools are available and selection will depend on some of the previously mentioned factors, such as the population being tested. Recent reviews of available screening instruments (Cullen et al., 2007) have shown that certain cognitive scales have a degree of redundancy that masks the true level of impairment and can waste time in diagnostic assessment. Time is a familiar constraint, and in a large clinical trial or research study, what is needed is a screening tool to provide focus and offer direction as to the cognitive domains that need to be specifically addressed with more detailed neuropsychological assessment; neuropsychiatric assessment of mood, anxiety and apathy; imaging and other investigations.

A number of global scales have been developed for screening of cognitive impairment. A few examples are the following:

1. The Mini–Mental State Examination (MMSE) (Folstein et al., 1975) has traditionally been used as a screening tool in research studies and clinical practice and as an outcome measure in clinical trials (Shulman et al., 2006). The MMSE consists of 30 items, taking approximately 10 min to administer. While it has been extensively used, it is not a detailed screen and has been shown to be less sensitive in mildly impaired populations, such as in the prodromal stages of Alzheimer's disease (Ahmed et al., 2012; Saka et al., 2006; Slavin et al., 2007) and is thus better suited to assessing patients with moderate to severe impairments. The MMSE is also unsuitable as an outcome measure for nutritional intervention studies as it is unlikely to show significant change in those with mild impairment or normal cognitive function (de Jager et al., 2014).
2. The Addenbrooke's Cognitive Examination (ACE III) (Hsieh et al., 2015) is a global index, which consists of 100 items, and takes approximately 20 min to complete. It has been used largely to detect dementia syndromes; however, it does provide a more comprehensive screen than the MMSE including the domains of memory, attention and orientation, fluency, language and visuospatial skills.
3. The Montreal Cognitive Assessment (MoCA) (Nasreddine et al., 2005) is a short, 30-point test, which takes approximately 10 min to administer. Studies have shown that the MoCA is a more difficult test than the MMSE and thus better able to detect mild impairment (Ahmed et al., 2012; Nasreddine et al., 2005).

### 4.3.2 Detailed Cognitive Assessment

A large number of cognitive tests have been developed and finding the *right* tests for the job can be a daunting task. As a general rule, a detailed and comprehensive assessment should sample a number of different areas of cognitive ability, in particular the primary cognitive domains of memory, language, attention and visuospatial skills. Selection of tests may be based on literature searches to determine which tests have been shown to be sensitive to nutrient-induced cognitive change. Table 4.3 provides a review of cognitive tests employed in completed randomized control trials

**TABLE 4.3**

**Cognitive Tests Shown to Be Sensitive to Cognitive Change in Trials of Nutrient Interventions**

| Cognitive Domain | Studies | Tests Sensitive to Cognitive Change Secondary to Nutrient Intervention |
|---|---|---|
| *Verbal memory* | Krikorian et al. (2010) | California verbal learning test (CVLT) |
| | Karr et al. (2012) | Rey auditory verbal learning test (RAVLT) |
| | Gleason et al. (2009) | Common objects recall test |
| | Fioravanti et al. (1998) | Randt memory test |
| | Bryan et al. (2002) and Deijen et al. (1992) | Selective reminding test |
| | Krikorian et al. (2010) | Verbal paired associate learning (VPAL) |
| | File et al. (2001) and Kritz-Silverstein et al. (2003) | WMS paragraph recall |
| | de Jager et al. (2012) | Hopkins verbal learning test (HVLT) |
| *Spatial memory* | File et al. (2005) | CANTAB delayed matching to sample test (DMST) |
| | Lewerin et al. (2005) | Identical pictures test |
| | Thorp et al. (2009) | Novel spatial working memory test |
| | Gleason et al. (2009) | Rey complex figure test |
| | Yurko-Mauro et al. (2010) | CANTAB paired associate learning (PAL) |
| | Pipingas et al. (2008) | Spatial pattern recognition |
| | Pipingas et al. (2008) | Spatial working memory |
| | Ryan et al. (2008) | CDR spatial working memory |
| | Gleason et al. (2009) | Visual spatial learning test |
| | Field et al. (2011) | Visual spatial memory |
| | Duffy et al. (2003) and File et al. (2001) | Long-term episodic memory |
| | Gleason et al. (2009) | Rey complex figure test |
| | Lee et al. (2013) | WMS visual 2 test |
| *Executive function* | de Jager et al. (2012); Deijen et al. (1992); File et al. (2001); Gleason et al. (2009); and Kritz-Silverstein et al. (2003) | Verbal fluency |
| | Kritz-Silverstein et al. (2003) and Thorp et al. (2009) | Trail making test A and B |
| | File et al. (2001, 2005) and Gleason et al. (2009) | CANTAB intradimensional/ extradimensional shift |

*(Continued)*

**TABLE 4.3 (Continued)**

**Cognitive Tests Shown to Be Sensitive to Cognitive Change in Trials of Nutrient Interventions**

| Cognitive Domain | Studies | Tests Sensitive to Cognitive Change Secondary to Nutrient Intervention |
|---|---|---|
| | Duffy et al. (2003) and File et al. (2001, 2005) | CANTAB Stockings of Cambridge |
| *Working memory* | Casini et al. (2006) and Lee et al. (2013) | Digit span |
| | Scholey et al. (2010) | Serial subtraction by 3s |
| *Attention and information processing speed* | Crews et al. (2008) | Stroop colour test |
| | Field et al. (2011) | Choice reaction time |
| | File et al. (2001) | Paced auditory serial addition test |
| | Scholey et al. (2010) | Rapid visual information processing (RVIP) |
| | Crews et al. (2008) | WAIS digit symbol |
| *Language* | Ryan et al. (2008) and van Asselt et al. (2001) | Peabody picture vocabulary |
| *Psychomotor skills* | Gleason et al. (2009) | Grooved pegboard test |
| *Global screening test* | Stott et al. (2005) and Walker et al. (2012) | Telephone inventory for cognitive status – modified (TICS-M) |

WMS, Wechsler Memory Scale; CANTAB, Cambridge Neuropsychological Test Automated Battery; CDR, Cognitive Drug Research; WAIS, Wechsler Adult Intelligence Scale.

that have studied the effects of nutrients on cognitive function and that have been shown to be sensitive to cognitive change. The table is meant as a useful point of reference for the selection of tests already shown to be sensitive to each of the primary cognitive domains.

### 4.3.3 INFORMANT INTERVIEW

Interviewing a family member or caregiver can give an added, valuable perspective to any change in cognition. In some situations, mild changes may not be detected or may be insufficient to achieve significance on formal cognitive assessment, but asking an informant about the patient's abilities and mood in different situations may reflect a more significant and meaningful change. For example, memory as an overall function may be perceived as unimpaired and may not lead to a complaint, whereas questioning about memory in relation to specific activities might reveal more information about particular difficulties (Ahmed et al., 2008a). Formal measures are available, such as the informant interview from the Cambridge Mental Disorders of the Elderly Examination interview (CAMDEX) (Roth et al., 1986), the Cambridge Behavioural Inventory (CBI) (Wedderburn et al., 2008) and the Informant Questionnaire on Cognitive Decline in the Elderly (IQCODE) (Jorm, 2004).

### 4.3.4 FUNCTIONAL IMPAIRMENT

The impact that cognitive impairment and subsequent intervention may have on activities of daily living (ADLs), such as cooking, washing and personal hygiene, can be illuminating, again where formal cognitive assessment may not be significant, but also as it reflects the *real-world* impact of an intervention. ADLs can be assessed using formal scales such as the subsection of the informant interview in the CAMDEX, the CBI or scales specifically designed for patient populations such as the Disability Assessment for Dementia scale (Gelinas et al., 1999). Assessment of ADLs can be challenging as this requires knowledge about the individual's expected level of function in their usual environment at the current stage of their life. It may also be difficult to judge between decline in physical functioning that is age related or related to coexisting medical problems and that which is related to cognitive impairment. Given that any degree of cognitive impairment will have an effect on certain activities, a differentiation between complex and basic ADLs has been proposed by some authors (e.g. Perneczky et al., 2006). Basic ADLs refer to day-to-day core abilities, such as eating, washing, walking and dressing. Complex or instrumental ADLs are defined by their higher level of complexity, incorporating tasks such as managing finances and medication and meal preparation (Table 4.4).

## 4.4 COGNITIVE CHANGE WITH AGEING

In order to draw useful conclusions about the effect of interventions, we will briefly survey evidence of the cognitive changes typical in healthy ageing. There are two broad categories of cognitive change that occur with age. One is an increase in general knowledge and know-how, for example, vocabulary and other acquired knowledge, referred to as crystallized abilities (Christensen, 2001). The other is a decline in cognitive performance, in particular, deterioration in memory, spatial abilities, reasoning and mental speed (Salthouse, 2010). Bäckman et al. (2004) describe a pattern of cognitive ageing whereby those tasks which are highly automated, have

---

**TABLE 4.4**
**Summary of Section 4.3**

**Practical Guide to Cognitive Assessment**

Consider gathering data from variable sources to look for consistencies in cognitive performance.

Sensitive cognitive screening tools are also needed to identify patients for enrolment into studies of potential nutritional interventions and offer direction as to the cognitive domains that need to be specifically addressed with more detailed neuropsychological assessment, imaging and other investigations.

Detailed cognitive assessment should assess memory, language, attention and visuospatial skills.

Interviewing a family member or caregiver may add valuable perspective to any change in cognition.

Assessing activities of daily living (ADLs) can be used to estimate the *real-world* impact of an intervention.

---

limited speed demands or depend on prior experience remain stable. Conversely, tasks that require new learning, speed and mental flexibility, sometimes referred to as *fluid intelligence*, are greatly affected. Importantly, the course of cognitive decline follows a similar pattern whether it occurs as a result of normal ageing or due to pathological processes (Bäckman et al., 2004). It can therefore be difficult to discriminate early pathological decline from normal ageing, purely on the basis of cognitive testing.

Research supports the notion that knowledge increases with age and experience. For example, data from the Betula project, a large longitudinal study of cognition throughout adulthood, indicated there was an increase in semantic memory (vocabulary and general knowledge) from middle adulthood up until early old age (55–65 years) although it decreased in older old age (70–80 years) (Nyberg et al., 2003). Similarly, another study observed that semantic representation (in this case, knowledge about the categories or attributes of items) was preserved in old age, despite slower responses (Eustache et al., 1998). In the Canberra Longitudinal Study, crystallized abilities, as measured by the NART, remained stable after 7 years of follow-up in elderly participants (Christensen, 2001).

Interestingly, forgetting rates are stable across the lifespan (Fjell et al., 2005). Although less information is encoded overall, it is retained in older people in the same proportion as it is in younger people (Salthouse, 1992). This suggests that memory loss is due to processes involved with encoding memories, rather than retrieving them.

### 4.4.1 Cognitive Decline

Although some functions do improve, other mental faculties show clear decline with age. Specifically, impairments in performance occur in cognitive speed, memory, executive function and spatial abilities, among others. There is still some debate regarding the nature of the impairments. Some authors argue that there is evidence of a single general factor underlying cognitive decline (Malec et al., 1991; Salthouse, 2010). This is proposed to be processing speed, that is, a general slowing in cognitive ability which affects performance in all other cognitive domains (Salthouse, 1996). However, other research has shown decrements in specific areas in addition to processing speed. Research has demonstrated that different cognitive functions decline at different rates, with the greatest decline observed in tasks assessing spatial working memory and contextual memory (Ahmed et al., 2008b; Pipingas et al., 2010). Test performance in a community cohort of older people was significantly different in all tests for episodic and semantic memory, but not in tests for working memory, processing speed and language in a study by de Jager et al. (2002). Processing speed partialled out the age effect on memory performance for the whole cohort, but for the subgroup with poor episodic memory, memory performance was not associated with age or processing speed. This indicated that memory decline was greater than that expected for age in this cohort.

Cognitive decline becomes most apparent in older age; however, a reduction in performance can be observed from early adulthood (Pipingas et al., 2010; Salthouse, 2009). In cross-sectional studies, decline is observed to be linear and mild throughout adulthood, becoming steeper after 70 years of age (Rabbitt et al., 2001). In longitudinal studies, the decline does not appear to be as steep, but this might be due in part to practice effects (Salthouse, 2010).

### 4.4.2 Effect of Slowing on Other Cognitive Domains

A general reduction in mental processing speed may manifest as poorer performance in tasks which are more complex than those described earlier, affecting performance in accuracy as well as response time. The processing speed theory was comprehensively addressed by Salthouse (1996) where he contended that processing speed manifests as a simple slowing and that it affects other cognitive functions as well, such as memory and executive function.

Some research supports the processing speed theory. For example, in a large study in twins, it was determined that processing speed could account for most of the variation in cognitive performance as well as the acceleration of cognitive decline in later years (Finkel et al., 2005). The study also noted that a significant proportion of the genetic influences on cognitive ability were mediated by genetic factors that affected processing speed. In a further study, this group reported that processing speed was the best indicator of age-related changes in spatial function and memory, although not verbal ability (Finkel et al., 2007). Contrarily, it has been argued that the reverse might be true, since many other functions underpin performance on a processing speed task (Eckert, 2011). The trail making task was used as an example. Performance of this task requires many cognitive processes, including perception, attention, working memory, decision making, motor planning and praxis and performance evaluation. This requires the coordination of several neural systems which may themselves be affected with age, and these can have additive effects on the speed at which the task is performed.

Language is a domain that in general is unaffected with ageing and, in fact, can improve with improved vocabulary, life experience and ongoing education. However, word-finding difficulty and the tip-of-the-tongue phenomenon may be affected by neural plasticity or by circuits that need to bypass areas of neural damage or atrophy (Lesk & Womble, 2004). Early life language ability for idea density and grammatical complexity has been shown to be protective against Alzheimer's disease (Ahmed et al., 2013; Snowden et al., 1996) (Table 4.5).

---

### TABLE 4.5
### Summary of Section 4.4

**Cognitive Change with Ageing**

Research shows that there are two broad categories of cognitive change that occur with age.

One is an increase in general knowledge, for example, in vocabulary and other acquired knowledge. These are referred to as crystallized abilities.

The second is a decline in performance in selected cognitive domains, particularly in memory, spatial abilities, reasoning and mental speed.

---

## 4.5 CONCLUDING SUMMARY

Cognitive assessment provides a scientific method to describe and quantify cognitive abilities. The goal in using cognitive assessment in nutrition intervention studies is to provide objective measures of the utility of a nutritional supplement or diet for improving cognition. More scientific data regarding the utility of particular cognitive assessments for this task are now emerging. This chapter has outlined some key guidelines for researchers planning such studies. The measurement of cognitive function requires careful planning taking into account the methodology of the tests being considered, but also the assessment procedures and those being assessed. Keeping in mind these methodological guidelines will ensure that well-designed and reliable trials will continue to contribute to our knowledge of the effects of food and nutrients on cognition.

### TOP 4 SUMMARY POINTS FROM CHAPTER

- Methodological principles are the foundation of a good cognitive test. The psychometric properties of each test to be used must be well considered.
- Once methodological principles have been established, characteristics of the population being assessed are the next key consideration.
- Tailor assessment to the population being examined in order to extract the most accurate evaluation of the effect of a nutritional intervention.
- Comprehensive cognitive assessment will include a cognitive screen, detailed cognitive evaluation, functional assessment and information from an informant.

## REFERENCES

Ahmed, S., Mitchell, J., Arnold, R., Dawson, K., Nestor, P. J., & Hodges, J. R. (2008). Memory complaints in mild cognitive impairment, worried well, and semantic dementia patients. *Alzheimer Disease and Associated Disorders, 22*(3), 227–235. doi: 10.1097/WAD.0b013e31816bbd27. PubMed PMID: 18580592.

Ahmed, S., Arnold, R., Thompson, S. A., Graham, K. S., & Hodges, J. R. (2008). Naming of objects, faces and buildings in mild cognitive impairment. *Cortex, 44*(6), 746–752. doi: 10.1016/j.cortex.2007.02.002. Epub 2007 Dec 23. PubMed PMID: 18472044.

Ahmed, S., Mitchell, J., Arnold, R., Nestor, P. J., & Hodges, J. R. (2008). Predicting rapid clinical progression in amnestic mild cognitive impairment. *Dementia and Geriatric Cognitive Disorders, 25*(2), 170–177. doi: 10.1159/000113014. Epub 2008, January 22. PubMed PMID: 18212499.

Ahmed, S., de Jager, C., & Wilcock, G. (2012). A comparison of screening tools for the assessment of mild cognitive impairment: Preliminary findings. *Neurocase, 18*(4), 336–351. doi:10.1080/13554794.2011.608365

Ahmed, S., Haigh, A. M., de Jager, C. A., & Garrard, P. (2013) Connected speech as a marker of disease progression in autopsy-proven Alzheimer's disease. *Brain, 136*(12), 3727–3737.

Anastasi, A. (1968). *Psychological testing*. New York: MacMillan Publishing Co Inc.

Bäckman, L., Jones, S., Berger, A. K., Laukka, E. J., & Small, B. J. (2004). Multiple cognitive deficits during the transition to Alzheimer's disease. *Journal of Internal Medicine, 256*(3), 195–204. Review. PubMed PMID: 15324363.

Basso, M., Bornstein, R., & Lang, J. (1999). Practice effects on commonly used measures of executive function across 12 months. *The Clinical Neuropsychologist, 13*, 283–292.

Bright, P., Jaldow, E., & Kopelman, M. D. (2002). The National Adult Reading Test as a measure of premorbid intelligence: A comparison with estimates derived from demographic variables. *Journal of the International Neuropsychological Society, 8*(6), 847–854.

Bryan, J., Calvaresi, E., & Hughes, D. (2002). Short-term folate, vitamin B-12 or vitamin B-6 supplementation slightly affects memory performance but not mood in women of various ages. *Journal of Nutrition, 132*(6), 1345–1356.

Casini, M. L., Marelli, G., Papaleo, E., Ferrari, A., D'Ambrosio, F., & Unfer, V. (2006). Psychological assessment of the effects of treatment with phytoestrogens on postmenopausal women: A randomized, double-blind, crossover, placebo-controlled study. *Fertility and Sterility, 85*(4), 972–978. doi:10.1016/j.fertnstert.2005.09.048

Christensen, H. (2001). What cognitive changes can be expected with normal ageing? *Australian and New Zealand Journal of Psychiatry, 35*(6), 768–775.

Crews, W. D., Jr., Harrison, D. W., & Wright, J. W. (2008). A double-blind, placebo-controlled, randomized trial of the effects of dark chocolate and cocoa on variables associated with neuropsychological functioning and cardiovascular health: Clinical findings from a sample of healthy, cognitively intact older adults. *American Journal of Clinical Nutrition, 87*(4), 872–880.

Cullen, B., O'Neill, B., Evans, J. J., Coen, R. F., & Lawlor, B. A. (2007). A review of screening tests for cognitive impairment. *Journal of Neurology, Neurosurgery, and Psychiatry, 78*(8), 790–799. doi:10.1136/jnnp.2006.095414

de Jager, C. A., Milwain, E., & Budge, M. (2002). Early detection of isolated memory deficits in the elderly: The need for more sensitive neuropsychological tests. *Psychological Medicine, 32*(3), 483–91.

de Jager, C. A., Oulhaj, A., Jacoby, R., Refsum, H., & Smith, A. D. (2012). Cognitive and clinical outcomes of homocysteine-lowering B-vitamin treatment in mild cognitive impairment: A randomized controlled trial. *International Journal of Geriatric Psychiatry, 27*(6), 592–600. doi:10.1002/gps.2758

de Jager, C. A., Dye, L., de Bruin, E. A., Butler, L., Fletcher, J., Lamport, D. J., Latulippe, M. E., Spencer, J. P., & Wesnes, K. (2014). Criteria for validation and selection of cognitive tests for investigating the effects of foods and nutrients. *Nutrition Reviews, 72*(3), 162–79. Review.

Deijen, J. B., van der Beek, E. J., Orlebeke, J. F., & van den Berg, H. (1992). Vitamin B-6 supplementation in elderly men: Effects on mood, memory, performance and mental effort. *Psychopharmacology (Berlin), 109*(4), 489–496.

Duffy, R., Wiseman, H., & File, S. E. (2003). Improved cognitive function in postmenopausal women after 12 weeks of consumption of a soya extract containing isoflavones. *Pharmacology Biochemistry and Behavior, 75*(3), 721–729.

Eckert, M. A. (2011). Slowing down: Age-related neurobiological predictors of processing speed. *Frontiers in Neuroscience, 5*, 25.

Eustache, F., Desgranges, B., Jacques, V., Platel, H. (1998). Preservation of the attribute knowledge of concepts in normal aging groups. *Perceptual and Motor Skills, 87*(3 Part 2), 1155–1162.

Field, D. T., Williams, C. M., & Butler, L. T. (2011). Consumption of cocoa flavanols results in an acute improvement in visual and cognitive functions. *Physiology & Behavior, 103*(3–4), 255–260. doi:10.1016/j.physbeh.2011.02.013

Fjell, A. M., Walhovd, K. B., Reinvang, I., Lundervold, A., Dale, A. M., Quinn, B. T.,& Fischl, B.(2005). Age does not increase rate of forgetting over weeks - Neuroanatomical volumes and visual memory across the adult life-span. *Journal of the International Neuropsychological Society , 11*(1), 2–15.

File, S. E., Hartley, D. E., Elsabagh, S., Duffy, R., & Wiseman, H. (2005). Cognitive improvement after 6 weeks of soy supplements in postmenopausal women is limited to frontal lobe function. *Menopause, 12*(2), 193–201.

File, S. E., Jarrett, N., Fluck, E., Duffy, R., Casey, K., & Wiseman, H. (2001). Eating soya improves human memory. *Psychopharmacology (Berlin), 157*(4), 430–436. doi:10.1007/s002130100845

Finkel, D., Reynolds, C. A., McArdle, J. J., & Pedersen, N. L. (2005). The longitudinal relationship between processing speed and cognitive ability: Genetic and environmental influences. *Behavior Genetics, 35*(5), 535–549.

Finkel, D., Reynolds, C. A., McArdle, J. J., & Pedersen, N. L. (2007). Age changes in processing speed as a leading indicator of cognitive aging. *Psychology and Aging , 22*(3), 558–568.

Fioravanti, M., Ferrario, E., Massaia, M., Cappa, G., Rivolta, G., Grossi, E., & Buckley, A. E. (1998). Low folate levels in the cognitive decline of elderly patients and the efficacy of folate as a treatment for improving memory deficits. *Archives of Gerontology and Geriatrics, 26*(1), 1–13.

Folstein, M. F., Folstein, S. E., & McHugh, P. R. (1975). "Mini-mental state". A practical method for grading the cognitive state of patients for the clinician. *Journal of Psychiatric Research, 12*(3), 189–198.

Franzen, M. (2000). *Reliability and validity in neuropsychological testing* (2nd ed.). New York: Kluwer Academic/Plenum Publishers.

Gelinas, I., Gauthier, L., McIntyre, M., & Gauthier, S. (1999). Development of a functional measure for persons with Alzheimer's disease: The disability assessment for dementia. *The American Journal of Occupational Therapy, 53*(5), 471–481.

Gleason, C. E., Carlsson, C. M., Barnet, J. H., Meade, S. A., Setchell, K. D., Atwood, C. S., … Asthana, S. (2009). A preliminary study of the safety, feasibility and cognitive efficacy of soy isoflavone supplements in older men and women. *Age and Ageing, 38*(1), 86–93. doi:10.1093/ageing/afn227

Hsieh, S., McGrory, S., Leslie, F., Dawson, K., Ahmed, S., Butler, C., … Hodges, J. (2015). The mini-Addenbrooke's cognitive examination: A new assessment tool for dementia. *Dementia and Geriatric Cognitive Disorders, 39*, 1–11.

Ivnik, R. J., Smith, G. E., Lucas, J. A., Petersen, R. C., Boeve, B. F., Kokmen, E., & Tangalos, E. G. (1999). Testing normal older people three or four times at 1- to 2-year intervals: Defining normal variance. *Neuropsychology, 13*(1), 121–127.

Jorm, A. F. (2004). The informant questionnaire on cognitive decline in the elderly (IQCODE): A review. *International Psychogeriatrics, 16*(3), 275–293.

Karr, J. E., Grindstaff, T. R., & Alexander, J. E. (2012). Omega-3 polyunsaturated fatty acids and cognition in a college-aged population. *Experimental and Clinical Psychopharmacology, 20*(3), 236–242. doi:10.1037/a0026945

Krikorian, R., Shidler, M. D., Nash, T. A., Kalt, W., Vinqvist-Tymchuk, M. R., Shukitt-Hale, B., & Joseph, J. A. (2010). Blueberry supplementation improves memory in older adults. *Journal of Agricultural and Food Chemistry, 58*(7), 3996–4000. doi:10.1021/jf9029332

Kritz-Silverstein, D., Von Muhlen, D., Barrett-Connor, E., & Bressel, M. A. (2003). Isoflavones and cognitive function in older women: The SOy and postmenopausal health in aging (SOPHIA) study. *Menopause, 10*(3), 196–202.

Lee, L. K., Shahar, S., Chin, A. V., & Yusoff, N. A. (2013). Docosahexaenoic acid-concentrated fish oil supplementation in subjects with mild cognitive impairment (MCI): A 12-month randomised, double-blind, placebo-controlled trial. *Psychopharmacology (Berlin), 225*(3), 605–612. doi:10.1007/s00213-012-2848-0

Lesk, V. E., & Womble, S. P. (2004). Caffeine, priming, and tip of the tongue: Evidence for plasticity in the phonological system. *Behavioral Neuroscience, 118*(3), 453–61.

Lewerin, C., Matousek, M., Steen, G., Johansson, B., Steen, B., & Nilsson-Ehle, H. (2005). Significant correlations of plasma homocysteine and serum methylmalonic acid with movement and cognitive performance in elderly subjects but no improvement from short-term vitamin therapy: A placebo-controlled randomized study. *The American Journal of Clinical Nutrition, 81*(5), 1155–1162.

Malec, J. F., Ivnik, R. J., & Hinkeldey, N. S. (1991). Visual spatial learning test. *Psychological Assessment, 3*(1), 82–88.

McCaffrey, R. J. & Westervelt, H. J. (1995). Issues associated with repeated neuropsychological assessments. *Neuropsychology Review, 5*(3), 203–221.

Mitrushina, M., Boone, K., Razani, L., & D'Elia, L. (2005). *Handbook of normative data for neuropsychological assessment* (2nd ed.). New York: OUP.

Nasreddine, Z. S., Phillips, N. A., Bedirian, V., Charbonneau, S., Whitehead, V., Collin, I., ... Chertkow, H. (2005). The Montreal Cognitive Assessment, MoCA: A brief screening tool for mild cognitive impairment. *Journal of the American Geriatrics Society, 53*(4), 695–699. doi:10.1111/j.1532-5415.2005.53221.x

Nyberg, L., Rönnlund, M., Dixon, R. A., Maitland, S. B., Bäckman, L., Wahlin, Å.,& Nilsson, L. G. (2003). Selective adult age differences in an age-invariant multifactor model of declarative memory. *Psychology and Aging, 18*(1), 149–160.

Perneczky, R., Pohl, C., Sorg, C., Hartmann, J., Komossa, K., Alexopoulos, P., ... Kurz, A. (2006). Complex activities of daily living in mild cognitive impairment: Conceptual and diagnostic issues. *Age and Ageing, 35*(3), 240–245. doi:10.1093/ageing/afj054

Pipingas, A., Silberstein, R. B., Vitetta, L., Rooy, C. V., Harris, E. V., Young, J. M., ... Nastasi, J. (2008). Improved cognitive performance after dietary supplementation with a *Pinus radiata* bark extract formulation. *Phytotherapy Research, 22*(9), 1168–1174. doi:10.1002/ptr.2388

Pipingas, A., Harris, E., Tournier, E., King, R., Kras, M., & Stough, C. (2010). Assessing the efficacy of nutraceutical interventions on cognitive functioning in the elderly. *Current Topics in Nutraceutical Research, 8*(2–3), 79–87.

Rabbitt, P., Diggle, P., Smith, D., Holland, F., & Mc Innes, L. (2001). Identifying and separating the effects of practice and of cognitive ageing during a large longitudinal study of elderly community residents. *Neuropsychologia, 39*(5), 532–543.

Roth, M., Tym, E., Mountjoy, C. Q., Huppert, F. A., Hendrie, H., Verma, S., & Goddard, R. (1986). CAMDEX. A standardised instrument for the diagnosis of mental disorder in the elderly with special reference to the early detection of dementia. *The British Journal of Psychiatry, 149*, 698–709.

Ryan, J., Croft, K., Mori, T., Wesnes, K., Spong, J., Downey, L., ... Stough, C. (2008). An examination of the effects of the antioxidant Pycnogenol on cognitive performance, serum lipid profile, endocrinological and oxidative stress biomarkers in an elderly population. *Journal of Psychopharmacology, 22*(5), 553–562. doi:10.1177/0269881108091584

Saka, E., Mihci, E., Topcuoglu, M. A., & Balkan, S. (2006). Enhanced cued recall has a high utility as a screening test in the diagnosis of Alzheimer's disease and mild cognitive impairment in Turkish people. *Archives of Clinical Neuropsychology, 21*(7), 745–751. doi:10.1016/j.acn.2006.08.007

Salthouse, T. A. (1992). Influence of processing speed on adult age differences in working memory. *Acta Psychologica, 79*(2), 155–170.

Salthouse, T. A. (1996). The processing-speed theory of adult age differences in cognition. *Psychological Review, 103*(3), 403–428.

Salthouse, T. A. (2009). When does age-related cognitive decline begin? *Neurobiology of Aging, 30*(4), 507–514.

Salthouse, T. A. (2010). Selective review of cognitive aging. *Journal of the International Neuropsychological Society, 16*(5), 754–760.

Scholey, A. B., French, S. J., Morris, P. J., Kennedy, D. O., Milne, A. L., & Haskell, C. F. (2010). Consumption of cocoa flavanols results in acute improvements in mood and cognitive performance during sustained mental effort. *Journal of Psychopharmacology, 24*(10), 1505–1514. doi:10.1177/0269881109106923

Shulman, K. I., Herrmann, N., Brodaty, H., Chiu, H., Lawlor, B., Ritchie, K., & Scanlan, J. M. (2006). IPA survey of brief cognitive screening instruments. *International Psychogeriatrics, 18*(2), 281–294. doi:10.1017/S1041610205002693

Slavin, M. J., Sandstrom, C. K., Tran, T. T., Doraiswamy, P. M., & Petrella, J. R. (2007). Hippocampal volume and the mini-mental state examination in the diagnosis of amnestic mild cognitive impairment. *AJR: American Journal of Roentgenology, 188*(5), 1404–1410. doi:10.2214/AJR.06.1052

Stott, D. J., MacIntosh, G., Lowe, G. D., Rumley, A., McMahon, A. D., Langhorne, P., … Westendorp, R. G. (2005). Randomized controlled trial of homocysteine-lowering vitamin treatment in elderly patients with vascular disease. *The American Journal of Clinical Nutrition, 82*(6), 1320–1326.

Thorp, A. A., Sinn, N., Buckley, J. D., Coates, A. M., & Howe, P. R. (2009). Soya isoflavone supplementation enhances spatial working memory in men. *The British Journal of Nutrition, 102*(9), 1348–1354. doi:10.1017/S0007114509990201

van Asselt, D. Z., Pasman, J. W., van Lier, H. J., Vingerhoets, D. M., Poels, P. J., Kuin, Y., … Hoefnagels, W. H. (2001). Cobalamin supplementation improves cognitive and cerebral function in older, cobalamin-deficient persons. *The Journals of Gerontology. Series A, Biological Sciences and Medical Sciences, 56*(12), M775–M779.

Walker, J. G., Batterham, P. J., Mackinnon, A. J., Jorm, A. F., Hickie, I., Fenech, M., … Christensen, H. (2012). Oral folic acid and vitamin B-12 supplementation to prevent cognitive decline in community-dwelling older adults with depressive symptoms – the Beyond Ageing Project: A randomized controlled trial. *The American Journal of Clinical Nutrition, 95*(1), 194–203. doi:10.3945/ajcn.110.007799

Wedderburn, C., Wear, H., Brown, J., Mason, S. J., Barker, R. A., Hodges, J., & Williams-Gray, C. (2008). The utility of the Cambridge Behavioural Inventory in neurodegenerative disease. *Journal of Neurology, Neurosurgery, and Psychiatry, 79*(5), 500–503. doi:10.1136/jnnp.2007.122028

Wilson, B. A., Watson, P. C., Baddeley, A. D., Emslie, H., & Evans, J. J. (2000). Improvement or simply practice? The effects of twenty repeated assessments on people with and without brain injury. *Journal of the International Neuropsychological Society, 6*(4), 469–479.

Yurko-Mauro, K., McCarthy, D., Rom, D., Nelson, E. B., Ryan, A. S., Blackwell, A., … Investigators, M. (2010). Beneficial effects of docosahexaenoic acid on cognition in age-related cognitive decline. *Alzheimer's Dement, 6*(6), 456–464. doi:10.1016/j.jalz.2010.01.013

# 5 Measuring Mood
## Considerations and Innovations for Nutrition Science

*Maria A. Polak, Aimee C. Richardson, Jayde A. M. Flett, Kate L. Brookie and Tamlin S. Conner*

## CONTENTS

## SUMMARY

There is growing evidence that nutritional factors such as macro- and micronutrients, fruits and vegetables, dietary patterns and supplements are implicated in mood. The goal of this chapter is to review a range of traditional and innovative tools for assessing mood in relation to nutrition. We start by defining mood as a positive or negative emotional state of varying intensity that changes in response to life's circumstances and then discuss psychometrically validated questionnaires that measure singular moods (e.g. depression) and multiple types of moods (e.g. sadness, anxiety, anger, vitality). We review questionnaires that also measure positive mood (e.g. calmness, happiness, vitality) and suggest that researchers expand their toolkit to include a broader range of well-being measures (happiness, life satisfaction and eudaemonia – positive mood associated with purpose, engagement and meaning).

We review innovative methodological and technological components of real-time measures of moods using daily diaries and experience sampling methods (ESMs) and ecological momentary assessment (EMA) which measure moods as they occur on a moment-by-moment or day-by-day basis, for example, through the use of smart-phones. We end by a recommendation to integrate more technologically advanced platforms and an emphasis on incorporating a range of ambulatory methods and sampling strategies. These real-time approaches mitigate memory biases that can occur when people reflect on their mood over the last week or *in general* as with standard questionnaire time frames. As technology develops, real-time assessment will continue to offer an ecologically valid way of assessing the food and mood connection as it occurs in daily life, giving us new perspectives.

## 5.1  MEASURING MOOD: CONSIDERATIONS AND INNOVATIONS FOR NUTRITION SCIENCE

There is growing research on the role of nutritional factors in mental health and, in particular, the effect of diet on mood. A range of dietary factors have been linked to poorer mood including traditional Western diets, sodas, snacks, chocolate, lower fruit and vegetable (FV) consumption (e.g. Jacka et al., 2010; Rahe et al., 2014) and certain micronutrient deficits (e.g. Colangelo et al., 2014; Polak et al., 2014; Yi et al., 2011; also see Rucklidge & Kaplan, 2013 for a review). But what is mood exactly? And how can nutrition researchers measure it in a psychologically sophis-ticated way using validated questionnaires? In this chapter, we define mood and review a range of tools for measuring mood in nutrition research. We cover well-used self-report questionnaires such as the Center for Epidemiologic Studies Depression (CES-D) Scale (Radloff, 1977) and the Profile of Mood States (POMS) question-naire (McNair et al., 1971) and other tools commonly used in the nutrition literature (e.g. 12-Item General Health Questionnaire [GHQ-12], Goldberg & Williams, 1991; Positive and Negative Activation Schedule [PANAS], Watson et al., 1988). We dis-cuss the strengths and weaknesses of these well-used measures from a psychological perspective and suggest additional tools to measure positive states of well-being, such as the Psychological Well-Being (PWB) Scale (Ryff & Keyes, 1995), which are relatively underutilised in nutrition research. We then introduce novel ways of tracking mood in real time using EMA or ESMs on mobile phones and via Internet surveys. Our goal is to provide practical guidelines for choosing the right mood mea-sure for the research question to be addressed.

### 5.1.1  DEFINING MOOD

In the field of psychology, mood refers to a positive or negative emotional state of varying intensity that changes in response to life's circumstances. Moods are often undifferentiated, slower to change and *object-less* in that people may not know the cause or source of the mood (Russell, 2003). For example, a person may feel *down* or *blue*, which could last for days or even weeks in the case of depression, and a person may not know why he or she feels this way. By contrast, emotion refers to an

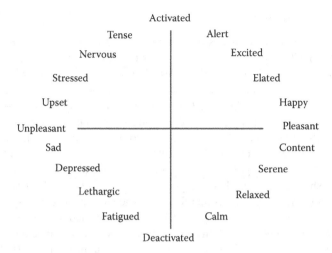

**FIGURE 5.1** A circumplex model of mood reflecting differences in valence (positivity/negativity) and activation (high energy/low energy). (Adapted from Barrett, L.F. and Russell, J.A., *Curr. Dir. Psychol. Sci.*, 8, 10, 1999.)

acute, specific feeling state felt in response to an event (Russell, 2003). For example, a person might feel the rush of anger in response to a challenging situation, but this feeling dissipates. Whereas emotion refers to prototypical reactionary states such as anger, sadness, fear, disgust, happiness or surprise, moods often reflect feelings of valence (feeling good/bad) and activation (feeling sleepy/awake) (Barrett & Russell, 1999). These two dimensions have been discovered through principal component analysis of multiple mood reports, which have yielded a *circumplex* reflecting four broad types of moods: positive high activation (enthusiastic, excited and cheerful), positive low activation (calm, relaxed and peaceful), negative high activation (anxious, hostile and stressed) and negative low activation (sad, depressed and dejected) as shown in Figure 5.1 (Barrett & Russell, 1999).

A good way to think about mood measures is to understand which parts of the circumplex they are capturing. Some questionnaires target specific quadrants in the circumplex such as depression (representing a low activation negative mood) or vitality (a high activation positive mood), whereas others target the broader dimensions of positive and negative affect (PA/NA).

## 5.2 COMMON TOOLS FOR MEASURING MOOD IN NUTRITION SCIENCE

In this section, we review several common mood measures used in nutrition research, focusing on questionnaire measures of depression, anxiety and multiple moods. We also introduce measures of positive mood and PWB that may provide good counterpoint to the nearly exclusive focus on negative mood in nutrition research. For each section, we give recommendations for the use of these measures.

### 5.2.1 Measuring Depression

One of the most popular measures of depressed mood is the 20-item CES-D Scale (Radloff, 1977). CES-D is made up of 20 items that are answered on a Likert scale from zero (*rarely or none of the time*, i.e. less than 1 day) to three (*most or all of the time*, i.e. 5–7 days). Items are answered with reference to the past week. Example items include *I thought my life had been a failure* and *I had crying spells*. After reverse scoring of four items (items 8, 12, 16 and 20), all items are summed to give a total score within the range of 0–60. A cut-off score of ≥16 is recommended to indicate those who are at risk of depression, although higher cut-off scores of ≥19 (e.g. Yi et al., 2011) and ≥27 (e.g. Colangelo et al., 2014) have also been used. However, this measure should not be used as a diagnostic tool per se. The CES-D was designed for use in community populations and focuses largely on the affective symptoms of depression. Nutrition research using the CES-D has reported associations between higher depressive symptoms and higher selenium exposure (Colangelo et al., 2014), lower serum ferritin levels (Yi et al., 2011) and lower vitamin D levels (Polak et al., 2014) and associations between lower depressive symptoms and consumption of whole foods (Akbaraly et al., 2009) and higher intake of fruit, vegetables and fibre and lower intake of *trans* fat (Akbaraly et al., 2013). Furthermore, it has been found that micronutrient supplementation (containing folic acid, iron, vitamin B12 and zinc) for 12 weeks results in decreases on the total CES-D score (Nguyen et al., 2009; see Rucklidge & Kaplan, 2013, for a review).

The Beck Depression Inventory (BDI), on the other hand, was designed for use in clinical populations to assess the severity of depression (original, version II and fast screen for medical patients, Beck et al., 1961; Beck et al., 1996; see also Richter et al., 1998, for a review of its validity). The BDI-II (1996) is the most recent version of this measure; it contains 21 items based on the *Diagnostic and Statistical Manual of Mental Disorders* criteria of major depressive disorder, 4th ed. (DSM-IV; American Psychiatric Association, 1994) although there were no changes to the symptomatology of major depressive disorder from DSM-IV to DSM-5 (American Psychiatric Association, 2013). The BDI-II is completed with reference to the past 2 weeks. Items are answered on a Likert scale from zero to three. Example items include *self-criticalness* (0 = I don't criticise or blame myself more than usual; 3 = I blame myself for everything bad that happens) and *worthlessness* (0 = I do not feel worthless; 3 = I feel utterly worthless). Items are summed to give a total score, which is interpreted as minimal depression (0–13), mild depression (14–19), moderate depression (20–28) or severe depression (29–63). The BDI-II emphasises the cognitive symptoms of depression, unlike the CES-D which emphasises more affective symptoms. Studies using various versions of the BDI have reported associations between more depressive symptoms and lower serum ferritin levels (Vahdat Shariatpanaahi et al., 2007) and infrequent fish consumption (Tanskanen et al., 2001).

For research in specific populations such as the elderly or pregnant women, the Geriatric Depression Scale (GDS) and the Edinburgh Postnatal Depression Scale (EPDS) have been used, respectively. The GDS (Yesavage et al., 1983) contains 30 items and is answered on a yes/no scale. Items include *Do you feel pretty worthless the way you are now? Do you feel that your life is empty?* Responses are summed and the total score is then used to indicate likely depression; a cut-off score of ≥11 is recommended. The GDS has been used to examine links between increased depressive symptoms and lower selenium exposure (Gao et al., 2012; Johnson et al., 2013) and lower dietary intake of vitamin A, riboflavin, vegetables and fibre (Woo et al., 2006).

The EPDS (Cox et al., 1987) contains 10 items and is designed to screen for postpartum depression in women who have recently given birth. As a screen for postpartum depression, the EPDS should be administered within 8 weeks of giving birth, although it has also been validated as a major depression screening tool during pregnancy (Murray & Cox, 1990). Items are answered with respect to the past week; examples of the items include *I have blamed myself unnecessarily when things went wrong* and *I have felt sad or miserable*. Responses are scored zero to three and scores are then summed. However, the utility of the EPDS as a screening tool has been criticised due to the wide variation in sensitivity and specificity (Gibson et al., 2009). A cut-off score of 13 or more is recommended as indicating probable postpartum depression (Cox et al., 1987; Matthey et al., 2006), whereas a cut-off score of 15 or more is recommended as indicating probable antepartum depression (Murray & Cox, 1990). Researchers using the EPDS have reported that selenium supplementation (Mokhber et al., 2011) and iron supplementation (Beard et al., 2005) significantly reduced postpartum depression levels.

The Hospital Anxiety and Depression Scale (HADS) (Zigmond & Snaith, 1983) was designed as a screening tool for anxiety and depression in general medical outpatients. Given that the measure was designed for those who are likely to have physical health complaints, the authors tried to include items that did not assess somatic symptoms of anxiety or depression. This measure contains 14 items that are answered on a Likert scale from zero to three. Seven items assess depression and seven items assess anxiety. Example depression items include *I felt cheerful* and *I look forward with enjoyment to things* (both reverse scored). A cut-off score of eight on each subscale is recommended to indicate potential cases of depression and anxiety (Bjelland et al., 2002). Nutrition research using the HADS has reported associations between higher depression symptoms and lower magnesium intake (Jacka et al., 2009) and associations between lower depression levels and a more healthful diet (vegetables, fruits, cereals, non-processed meats, etc.; Jacka et al., 2011). HADS scores have also been shown to reduce significantly following micronutrient supplementation (containing selenium, vitamin C and folate) for 8 weeks (Gosney et al., 2008; also see Rucklidge & Kaplan, 2013 for a review).

*Recommendation*: Overall, for use in the general population, the CES-D or the HADS is recommended. These measures were designed for use in non-clinical populations and there is a large body of evidence supporting their use. Reviews of the observational studies of dietary intake and depressive symptoms indicate that the CES-D appears to be the most commonly used measure (Lai et al., 2014; Murakami & Sasaki, 2010). For clinical populations, the BDI-II is recommended. The BDI-II allows for comparison of groups according to depression severity (minimal, mild, moderate and severe). However, the CES-D and the BDI-II all contain items assessing appetite, concentration and sleep difficulties. In populations where physical health conditions are common, or where nutritional deficiency is likely to produce physical symptoms, the HADS is recommended as this scale contains less somatically laden items than the CES-D and the BDI-II. In elderly populations, the GDS is recommended as the language is more straightforward and the response format is simpler than other depression measures (yes/no), although like the CES-D and the BDI-II, this measure contains items assessing the somatic symptoms of depression (sleep, concentration and memory difficulties). For women who have recently given birth, the EPDS should be used as it is specifically designed for this population (women within 8 weeks of birth). The EPDS is also validated as a screening tool for depression in pregnant women.

### 5.2.2 MEASURING ANXIETY

The role of food in anxiety-related mood is less established than the research on depressed mood. However, anxiety has been measured in several nutrition-related research areas, from experimental supplementation studies to cross-sectional population diet studies. The most common anxiety-specific mood measure is the State–Trait Anxiety Inventory (STAI: Form Y) (Spielberger, 1983). The STAI is a 40-item self-report scale that measures both state (current feelings at this moment) and trait (general feelings of anxiety) factors of anxiety. Example items from the state anxiety scale include *I am tense* or *I am worried*, whereas the trait anxiety subscale includes items such as *I worry too much over something that really doesn't matter* or reverse-scored items such as *I am a steady person*. This measure is well established in diagnostic and clinical settings, as well as medical and research domains. Sound psychometric properties are reported including internal consistency coefficients ranging between 0.86 and 0.95 (Spielberger et al., 1983). The STAI has been used in nutritional and herbal supplementation research including a study that showed a reduction in anxiety in perimenopausal women with kava supplementation (Cagnacci et al., 2003) and a reduction in state anxiety in individuals following an essential amino acid – L-lysine and L-arginine supplement (Jezova et al., 2005). The STAI was also used in an observational study of eating behaviours among high school students in an urban setting (Pastore et al., 1996). Although no differences in state or trait anxiety were found between normal and overweight individuals, increased anxiety was associated with eating attitudes such as dieting and food preoccupation (Pastore et al., 1996). The STAI state anxiety measure has also been used to assess current levels of anxiety, concluding that the consumption of sweets and meat was associated with higher current feelings of anxiety (Yannakoulia et al., 2008).

The Hamilton Anxiety Rating Scale (HAM-A) (Hamilton, 1959) is a clinician-rated instrument that is widely used in both clinical and research settings. This scale consists of 14 items measuring the severity of both psychological (mental agitation and psychological distress) and somatic anxiety symptoms (physical anxiety complaints) (Hamilton, 1959). This scale includes domains such as tension and worry, and clinicians make observations rated on a scale of 0 (not present) to 4 (severe).

Scores between 18 and 24 indicate mild to moderate severity, whereas 25–30 indicate moderate to severe anxiety symptoms (Hamilton, 1959). A reduction in anxiety as indicated by the HAM-A has been shown in a number of plant-based supplement studies including a 4-week supplementation of *Ginkgo biloba*, an 8-week supplementation of chamomile and a number of kava supplementation trials (for review, see Sarris et al., 2013). Whilst still commonly used, the HAM-A has been criticised in terms of its ability to distinguish between depressant and anxiolytic symptoms (Maier et al., 1988), preventing it from being a measure of choice when trying to compare anxiety and depression. Furthermore, it has found to be only moderately associated with other strong predictors of anxiety such as the Beck Anxiety Inventory (BAI) (Beck & Steer, 1993). The BAI is a 21-item self-report inventory which shows high internal consistency and test–retest reliability for measuring the severity of anxiety in psychiatric populations. The BAI discriminates anxious diagnostic groups well from non-anxious diagnostic groups (Beck et al., 1988), but has not been used in nutrition research due to its focus on clinical populations.

Anxiety can also be measured with the HADS (Zigmond & Snaith, 1983). As outlined in the previous section, the HADS is a well-established 14-item scale that has been widely used in medical outpatient and epidemiological research studies. In addition to the seven items that assess depression, seven items assess anxiety, for example, *I feel tense or wound up* and *I get sudden feelings of panic* (Zigmond & Snaith, 1983). The responses are recorded on a Likert scale from zero to three. A cut-off score of 8 for anxiety provides specificity of 0.78 and sensitivity of 0.9 (Bjelland et al., 2002). In a cross-sectional study of middle age and elderly adults, a diet characterised largely by FVs, whole grains, fish and non-processed meat (a *traditional* diet) was associated with reduced likelihood of HADS anxiety scores in Norwegian women (Jacka et al., 2011). Conversely, a diet characterised by unhealthy and processed foods (a *Western* diet) was associated with a greater risk of anxiety for both men and women, as indicated by increased scores on the HADS (Jacka et al., 2011). In a study of adherence to a gluten-free diet in a sample of individuals with coeliac disease (CD), a greater difficulty of adherence was associated with greater anxiety as measured by the HADS (Barrat et al., 2011). Supplementation using a multivitamin (magnesium, zinc and calcium) showed a reduction in anxiety as measured by the HADS after 28-day supplementation treatment (Carroll et al., 2000). The HADS appears to be a reliable measure, efficient for use in research simultaneously measuring anxiety and depression symptomatology.

The GHQ-12 (Goldberg & Williams, 1991) is a common, brief self-report screening instrument for common mental disorders, which is widely used within general medical practice (Kalliath et al., 2004). It is comprised of common mental health domains of depression, anxiety, somatic symptoms and social withdrawal. The anxiety subscale includes items such as *Have you been getting scared and panicky for no good reason?* And individuals respond using a Likert scale ranging from zero to three (Goldberg & Williams, 1991). This measure has been translated into over 38 different languages and its reliability coefficients have been reported between 0.78 and 0.95 (Jackson, 2007). Whilst the GHQ-12 should not be used for predictive or diagnostic purposes (Jackson, 2007), it provides adequate screening of those identified as *at risk* of developing psychological distress. In the current literature, the

GHQ-12 has mainly been used in cross-sectional studies of diet quality. It was found that consumption of unhealthy Western diet patterns was generally associated with higher GHQ-12 scores, whereas the consumption of a traditional diet was generally associated with lower GHQ-12 scores (Jacka et al., 2010). Furthermore, reduced GHQ-12 scores were found in a study of the relationship between anxiety and polyunsaturated fatty acid (PUFA) intake and fish consumption (Jacka et al., 2012b), as well as decreased red meat consumption (Jacka et al., 2012a). However, these studies used the GHQ-12 to assess common mental disorders (anxiety and depression), reflecting an overall reduction in psychological distress, rather than anxiety specifically. The studies mentioned previously used the GHQ-12 in conjunction with a *gold standard* diagnostic interview to assess for specific anxiety-related disorders. It is not recommended that the GHQ-12 be used in isolation to assess for anxiety in nutrition research, due to its brevity and broad approach to general mental health.

Lastly, the Structured Clinical Interview for DSM-IV (text revised), non-patient edition (SCID-I/NP) (First et al., 2002), is a semi-structured diagnostic interview, considered a *gold standard* assessment tool for anxiety (Sarris et al., 2013). It is the primary diagnostic instrument in assessing for anxiety-related disorders including panic, agoraphobia, social, specific, OCD, GAD and anxiety due to substance or other medical disorder (First et al., 2002). For these diagnoses, symptoms are identified as *present, sub-threshold* or *absent*. This instrument is reasonably time consuming and is designed to be administered by a clinician or trained mental health specialist. However, it provides an indication of specific anxiety diagnoses rather than the presence of general anxiety symptomatology, making it a clinically relevant tool. The Structured Clinical Interview for DSM-5 is currently in the final stages of publication. A number of studies have found that a Western diet, characterised by unhealthy and processed food (Jacka et al., 2010, 2011, 2012b) and decreased red meat consumption in women (Jacka et al., 2012a), is associated with a higher prevalence of diagnosed anxiety disorders.

A number of physiological measures of anxiety have been used in nutritional research. Although these are not widely researched, they offer a promising route of objective anxiety indicators. For example, a significant improvement in vagal heart rate control was seen after a 4-week randomised controlled trial (RCT) of kava (Watkins et al., 2001). Similarly, an RCT in healthy adults found that L-lysine supplementation over 1 week was associated with decreased hormonal stress response, as indicated by lower levels of salivary cortisol (Smriga et al., 2007).

*Recommendation*: Overall, for use in the general population, the STAI offers a sound anxiety measure when looking at anxiety in isolation. This measure has been well used in micronutrient supplement studies (Lakhan & Vieira, 2010; Sarris et al., 2013). This measure may be more useful for pre- and post-intervention comparison but holds little predictive power in terms of diagnostic value. When research aims are clinically based, the SCI-DSM-IV is considered the *gold standard* for diagnosis and provides not only an indication of anxiety-related symptomatology but can differentiate between types of anxiety disorders. It does not provide a score which can be statistically compared pre- and post-intervention; however, it can be used in research in combination with the STAI.

## 5.3 MEASURING MULTIPLE ASPECTS OF MOOD

Other questionnaires target multiple types of mood within the same questionnaire. For example, the POMS (McNair et al., 1971) is a 65-item rating scale that yields a total mood index, plus a single index of positive mood (vigour/activity) and five indices of negative mood (tension/anxiety, depression/dejection, anger/hostility, fatigue/inertia and confusion/bewilderment). Respondents use a unipolar scale to rate the extent to which they are experiencing or have experienced 65 affect states in the past week (e.g. *sad, tense, angry, energetic, weary, confused*) using a 5-point scale (0 = *not at all*, 4 = *extremely*). There are several other versions of the POMS including the revised POMS 2 that adds an additional scale (friendliness) (Heuchert & McNair, 2004), the youth version for adolescents ages 13–17 (POMS 2-Y) and also several shortened versions. The POMS, POMS 2 and their shortened variants are good measures because they capture a range of different negative moods, and they include a measure of positive mood through the vigour subscale (vigour items: lively, active, energetic, cheerful, alert, full of pep, carefree and vigorous). However, the vigour subscale only measures higher activation positive mood, not lower activation positive mood, which would be limiting if a nutritional intervention was designed to promote calmness. Nevertheless, growing evidence suggests that good nutrition may be associated with high activation positive mood states. Recent intervention studies have shown that fruit consumption and iron consumption increased scores on the vigour subscale of the POMS (fruit, Carr et al., 2013; iron, McClung et al., 2009). Research using the POMS-Bipolar form (POMS-BI) has reported that selenium supplementation resulted in increased mood scores on four of the six subscales (Benton & Cook, 1991).

Another popular mood measure is the PANAS (previously called the Positive and Negative Affect Schedule) (Watson et al., 1988). The PANAS is a 20-item scale that is commonly used to obtain separate measures of PA and NA; however, in truth, this questionnaire yields measures of high positive activation and negative activation because all of the items capture high activation states, for example, *attentive, interested, alert, enthusiastic, excited, inspired, proud, determined, strong and active* for PA and *distressed, upset, hostile, irritable, scared, afraid, ashamed, guilty, nervous and jittery* for NA. There is also a shortened 10-item version of the PANAS that contains five items for PA and five items for NA (Mackinnon et al., 1999). Although this measure is very popular, researchers should be cautious when using it because neither the 20-item nor 10-item PANAS captures lower activation feelings of calmness, happiness or sadness. An extended version, the PANAS-X, is a 60-item scale available to measure more discrete feelings including some, but not all, lower level activation states (sadness, serenity and fatigue) in addition to the broader positive and negative activation states (Watson & Clark, 1994). The 20-item version of the PANAS has been used to examine links between mood and folate status (Williams et al., 2008) and zinc status (McConville et al., 2005). The 10-item version of the PANAS has been used in research to demonstrate a link between a diet rich in Mediterranean foods (e.g. fruit, vegetables, whole grains) and higher PA and lower NA (Ford et al., 2013).

Another approach to measuring mood is to use items reflecting all the combinations of valence and activation. For example, Polak and colleagues used an 18-item scale to measure PA and NA across three levels of activation (Polak et al., in preparation). The scale is based on the affective circumplex (Barrett & Russell, 1999; Tugade et al., 2007) and includes a 9-item measure of PA (high activation, *energetic, enthusiastic, excited*; medium activation, *happy, cheerful, pleasant*; low activation, *calm, content, relaxed*) and a 9-item measure of NA (high activation, *hostile, angry, irritable*; medium activation, *nervous, anxious, tense*; low activation, *dejected, sad, unhappy*). This measure can be adapted to capture trait affect (*Typically, how happy do you feel?*) or state affect (*How happy do you feel today/ right now?*). Questions are usually answered on a 5-point scale from 1 (not at all) to 5 (extremely) or from 0 (not at all) to 4 (extremely). This affective circumplex measure has not been validated, although it does show adequate internal consistency within the separate 9-item PA and NA scales (White et al., 2013). Because there are no norms, researchers might have difficulty linking this scale to previous research. However, we recommend a circumplex approach if there is a need to explicitly differentiate between high, medium and low activation positive and negative mood states.

Verbal and visual analogue measures of mood are also used in nutrient intervention studies. As a recent example, the effects of multivitamin supplementation on mood and well-being were assessed using several measures, including the 16-item Bond–Lader visual analogue scale (VAS) (Pipingas et al., 2013). This scale comprises 16, 100 mm lines, anchored at both ends with adjective pairs such as happy–sad. Participants mark their degree of agreement between the adjectives based on their current subjective state, allowing fine discrimination along the 100 mm scale (Bond & Lader, 1974). Scoring is calculated as the distance from the negative anchor. Analogue scales have been successfully used in appetite control studies (e.g. Parker et al., 2004); they show high reproducibility, power and validity in appetite assessment in single meal studies (Flint et al., 2000), as well as good validity and reliability in mood disorders (Ahearn, 1997). VASs may be particularly good to use with children because the questions are answered on a linear pictorial rather than a verbal scale (Miller & Ferris, 1993).

*Recommendation*: We recommend the POMS, POMS 2 and its variants to measure multiple mood states. The PANAS should only be used to measure high activation states. Otherwise, the PANAS-X or POMS would be the better choice. An underutilised option is the mood circumplex that captures both valence (negative–positive) and activation (high–medium–low) of mood states.

## 5.4   BEYOND NEGATIVE MOOD: MEASURING POSITIVE MOOD AND PSYCHOLOGICAL WELL-BEING

Measures of negative mood, depression and anxiety are much more common in nutrition research than measures of happiness and life satisfaction. Yet there is emerging evidence that dietary factors may also play a role in these states of positive well-being. A recent study of over 80,000 British people found a strong link between consumption of FVs and greater life satisfaction that was not accounted for by demographic or health factors (Blanchflower et al., 2013). Contrary to common assumptions, these negative states of ill-being and positive states of well-being are not two sides of the same coin. Well-being reflects an optimal level of emotional experience and functioning, not simply the absence of depression or anxiety (Deci & Ryan, 2008). It is an empirical question whether good nutrition increases well-being over and above any neutralising effect on ill-being.

There are several psychometrically validated measures of well-being that we recommend. Some measures target hedonic well-being, that is, whether people feel happy and are satisfied with their lives (Veenhoven, 2003). Measures of happiness include the first item in the Fordyce Happiness Measures (Fordyce, 1988), which asks people to answer *In general, how happy or unhappy do you usually feel?* on a scale from 0 (extremely unhappy) to 10 (extremely happy), and the 4-item Subjective Happiness Scale (SHS) (Lyubomirsky & Lepper, 1999). Measures of life satisfaction include the OECD's single-item question of *Overall, how satisfied are you with your life as a whole these days?*, answered from 0 *not at all satisfied* to 10 *completely satisfied* (OECD, 2013); the 1-item Cantril scale (Cantril, 1965), which asks people to place themselves on a ladder where the bottom step (0) represents the *worst possible life for you* and the top step (10) is *the best possible life for you* (scores 7+ indicate thriving; scores ≤ 4 indicate suffering); and the 5-item Satisfaction with Life Scale (Pavot & Diener, 1993).

Other measures target eudaemonic well-being, that is, whether people are engaged in life's activities and experience greater vitality, purpose and meaning in life (McKnight & Kashdan, 2009; Ryan et al., 2008). It could be argued that the POMS vigour/activity subscale measures a rudimentary form of eudaemonia by capturing differences in vitality (lively, active, energetic, cheerful, alert, full of pep, carefree and vigorous); however, it was not intended to measure eudaemonia. Established measures of eudaemonic well-being include the PWB Scale, which covers six dimensions of eudaemonic well-being: autonomy, environmental mastery, personal growth, positive relations with others, purpose in life and self-acceptance (Ryff & Keyes, 1995), the Flourishing Scale (Diener et al., 2010) and the Warwick-Edinburgh Mental Well-being Scale (Tennant et al., 2007). The PWB Scale covers six dimensions of eudaemonic well-being: autonomy, environmental mastery, personal growth, positive relations with others, purpose in life and self-acceptance (Ryff & Keyes, 1995). There are two versions – a 42-item format and a shorter 18-item version – that are both suitable for investigating eudaemonic well-being. It includes items like *In general, I feel I am in charge of the situation in which I live (environmental mastery)* and *Some people wander aimlessly through life, but I am not one of them (purpose in life)*. Other shorter options include the 8-item Flourishing Scale (Diener et al., 2010) with items like *I lead a purposeful and meaningful life* or *I am optimistic about my future* that capture important aspects of a successful life where participants rate their answers on a scale from 1 (strongly disagree) to 7 (strongly agree). The total score ranges from 8 to 56, with a higher score reflecting greater flourishing (for an example, see Conner et al., 2014). The 14-item Warwick-Edinburgh Mental Well-being Scale provides another useful tool to examine positive mental well-being (Tennant et al., 2007). This scale includes both hedonic and eudaemonic perspectives and focuses on the positive psychological outcomes only. The scale has been applied in research on FV consumption and showed that highest well-being was associated with about seven servings per day (Blanchflower et al., 2013).

*Recommendation*: Positive psychological states are not simply the reverse of ill-being. For this reason, we recommend incorporating positive well-being measures into nutrition research to open up novel scientific discoveries. Large-scale nutrition surveys could benefit from including the single-item happiness measure and either the OECD life satisfaction measure or the Cantril scale, which are roughly interchangeable. We also recommend the Warwick-Edinburgh Mental Well-being Scale for measuring both hedonic and eudaemonic well-being in a short questionnaire. Researchers interested specifically in eudaemonic well-being should administer the PWB Scale or the Flourishing Scale.

## 5.5  INNOVATIVE REAL-TIME MOOD MEASUREMENT

One of the exciting recent developments for nutritional research is to use *real-time* or *near to real-time* measures of mood. Most research asks people to report their mood in general trait terms (how people feel typically), retrospectively over the past week(s) or prospectively at a given time of day usually relative to the time of ingestion of a food or supplement. Real-time measures of mood enable researchers to track mood on a daily or momentary basis over a period of time (usually 1–4 weeks) using technology such as Internet diaries and smartphones. This latter point is important to nutrition research. Micronutrient treatment or dietary interventions should show stronger or earlier effects on mood reported in near to real time compared to mood reported over a 1-week recall time frame or longer (see Lenderking et al., 2008, for an example in pharmacology; see also Pipingas et al., 2013). The reason is that micronutrients or dietary changes are thought to affect underlying neurotransmitter processes (Rooney et al., 2013) which are more closely tied to actual/immediate mood responses compared to delayed reflections on mood (Conner & Barrett, 2012). Tracking mood over time can also reveal the pattern in how mood changes following the intervention – whether it is a gradual change, a sharp change, a delayed change, etc. This temporal resolution is not possible with traditional pre-/post-test forms of mood measurement.

Collectively, these real-time methods of assessing behaviour, physiology, affect and cognition, repeatedly over a period of time in naturalistic or unconstrained settings, are often referred to as ESMs, EMA (Hamer et al., 2014; Shiffman et al., 2008) or ambulatory assessment (Fahrenberg & Myrtek, 1996). These are a range of real-time methods that can be used in nutrition research. These approaches include daily diaries, experience sampling, behavioural observations, self-monitoring systems, ambulatory monitoring of physiological functions, physical activity and/or movement and the technological tools and hardware used to measure these features. Tables 5.1 and 5.2 present a breakdown of these methods.

## TABLE 5.1

## Measures and Sampling Techniques Suitable for Studies on the Relationship between Nutrition and Mood

| Measure | Author | Description |
|---|---|---|
| CES-D Scale | Radloff (1977) | A measure of depressed mood, suitable for use in a community sample. |
| BDI and BDI-II | Beck et al. (1961, 1996) | A measure of depression severity, designed for use in clinical population. Researchers must consider the crossover between somatic depression symptoms and the physical symptoms of nutritional deficiency. |
| GDS | Yesavage et al. (1983) | A measure of depression, specifically for use in elderly population. |
| EPDS | Cox et al. (1987) | A measure of depression, specifically for use of postpartum women (within 8 weeks of giving birth). |
| HADS | Zigmond & Snaith (1983) | A screening tool for indications of anxiety and depression. This tool is considered efficient to measure depression and anxiety symptoms simultaneously – a recommended tool for nutritional research. |
| STAI | Spielberger (1983) | A self-report measure of both current and general feelings of anxiety. This measure is commonly used in supplement studies. |
| HAM-A | Hamilton (1959) | A clinician-rated measure of anxiety severity. Researchers must consider the potential crossover between somatic anxiety symptoms and physical symptoms of nutritional deficiency. This measure has also shown to have crossover with depressive symptomatology. |
| BAI | Beck & Steer (1993) | Includes both cognitive and somatic components of anxiety and is suitable for clinical populations. |
| GHQ-12 | Goldberg & Williams (1991) | A brief self-report screening tool for common mental health disorders, with subscales including depression, anxiety, somatic symptoms and social withdrawal. This measure provides an indication of general psychological distress, rather than measurement of particular mood states. |
| SCID-I/NP | First et al. (2002) | A semi-structured diagnostic interview, which indicates the presence and severity of DSM-IV diagnoses. Whilst being the *gold standard* instrument to indicate the presence of a mental illness, it requires extensive training to administer. |

*(Continued)*

**TABLE 5.1 (*Continued*)**
**Measures and Sampling Techniques Suitable for Studies on the Relationship between Nutrition and Mood**

| Measure | Author | Description |
|---|---|---|
| POMS and POMS2 | McNair et al. (1971) and Heuchert & McNair (2004) | A total mood measure, which incorporates a range of different negative moods and a measure of positive mood. The inclusion of *vigour* is important given the relationship between healthy eating and feelings of energy. There are several shortened versions. |
| PANAS | Watson et al. (1988) | A mood measure which yields separate measures of positive and negative activation states. This measure is limited to high activation states, rather than lower-level activation (e.g. fatigue). There is also a shortened version available. |
| VAS | Bond & Lader (1974) | A measure of various moods using a continuum, in which individuals indicate their position along a continuous line between two points (e.g. happy–sad). VAS may provide a good option for the measurement of mood in children. |
| Affective circumplex | Barrett & Russell (1999) | A self-report measure encompassing both positive and negative affect. This measure also reflects high, medium and low levels of activation and differentiates between state and trait affect. |
| Fordyce Happiness Measure | Fordyce (1988) | A remarkably quick single-item instrument to measure happiness with good reliability and stability. |
| SHS | Lyubomirsky & Lepper (1999) | A quick 4-item measure of happiness in general and in comparison to peers. |
| OECD life satisfaction measure | OECD (2013) | Measure of life satisfaction used in OECD country surveys, suitable for nutrition research. |
| Cantril scale | Cantril (1965) | Quick single-item measure of life satisfaction, where respondents rate their life from worst possible to best possible. |
| Satisfaction with Life Scale | Pavot & Diener (1993) | This 5-item questionnaire measures global cognitive judgments on satisfaction with life. |
| PWB Scale | Ryff & Keyes (1995) | A self-report measure of various dimensions of eudaemonic well-being. |
| Flourishing Scale | Diener et al. (2010) | A measure of flourishing, capturing aspects of what is considered a *successful* life. |
| Warwick-Edinburgh Mental Well-being Scale | Tennant et al. (2007) | A measure of hedonic and eudaemonic well-being, with a specific focus on positive psychological outcomes. |

## TABLE 5.2
## Sampling Strategies Suitable for Studies on the Relationship between Nutrition and Mood

| Sampling Strategy | Example | Description |
|---|---|---|
| Daily diary method | Conner & Lehman (2012) and White et al. (2013) | A method that requires individuals to complete a survey each day, typically at the end of each day. This diary can be tailored to include measures of mood, daily nutritional intake and other aspects of experience that vary on a daily basis. Daily diaries are useful for testing covariation between food and mood and for detecting mood changes in intervention/supplementation trials. Diary surveys can also be delivered through smartphones, which can enable large-scale delivery. |
| ESM/EMA | Conner & Lehman (2012), Macht et al. (2005), and Lathia et al. (2013) | A method that utilises pagers, text messaging or mobile phone *apps* to signal self-report measurements multiple times per day, typically on a semi-random schedule. ESM is used to measure current mood or other experiences (e.g. stress, pain) that are variable and ongoing across a short period of time in naturalistic free-range (ambulatory) settings. Smartphone usage will increase feasibility of this method in the near future. |
| Event contingent experience sampling | Lowe & Fisher (1983) | A method in which mood and other experiences are measured followed a specified event. This method is commonly used to tap mood that follows infrequent events (e.g. following binges). |
| Continuous sampling/ adaptive sensor sampling | Rachuri (2012) | A method in which psychological and physiological experiences are measured using various technologies including GPS, voice recorder, microphone, text messaging and call logs. Whilst not yet utilised in the field of nutrition, this continuous sampling method offers insight into routines and habits as individuals navigate their daily life. |

### 5.5.1 DAILY DIARY METHODS

Daily diary methods are an example of *interval contingent sampling* and involve completing a survey (called a diary) after a specified interval of time, often once a day in the evening before going to bed. People answer questions about their experiences that occurred that day – for example, what they ate, their mood and other experiences. Daily diaries are subject to mental averaging of the day's experience and are more subject to memory biases than prospectively administered VAS or other scales hourly in the lab or in free-living situations (Hamer et al., 2014); however, tests of end-of-day reports compared to averaged hourly reports during the same day show good correspondence (Parkinson et al., 1995). The typical daily diary study lasts from 1 to 3 weeks; however, the quality of data may decline after approximately 2–4 weeks of data collection possibly due to participant burden (Stone et al., 1991). If a longer time period is required, researchers can adopt a measurement burst design by surveying a few days to 1 week every month. Daily diaries are popular with researchers because of their ease of administration (through Internet surveys), low-frequency sampling and option to include many items. However, daily diaries are not suitable for projects requiring a more fine-grained temporal resolution across the day.

In nutrition research, daily diaries are well-suited for measuring both moods and foods together to investigate, for instance, how mood states change in response to, or in advance of, daily eating habits. For example, White et al. (2013) investigated the bidirectional relationships between daily negative and positive mood and food consumption in 281 healthy young adults using an Internet-based daily diary for 21 consecutive days. Self-reported daily servings of fruit, vegetables and several unhealthy foods were reported each day along with the 18-item circumplex mood measure (described earlier) adapted for a daily format (how they felt *today*). Using multilevel linear modelling, within-person associations revealed that on days when individuals reported eating more servings of FVs, they experienced greater positive mood. Next-day lagged analysis showed that FV consumption predicted improvements in positive mood the following day and not vice versa, suggesting that the FV consumption was antecedent to changes in positive mood. By utilising a daily diary method, the authors were able to show how FV consumption was tightly yoked to changes in positive mood within the same person over time. This finding at the within-person level complements cross-sectional evidence at the between-person level that FV consumption is correlated positively with greater happiness and life satisfaction (Blanchflower et al., 2013).

In another study utilising a daily diary method, Newman et al. (2007) examined the relationship between cortisol reactivity and snacking behaviours in response to stressors. Fifty pre-menopausal women completed reports of daily hassles and snack intake diaries for 14 consecutive days. Previous to this, they completed a social stress test in the lab and cortisol reactivity was measured to determine their reactivity status (high/low). Using hierarchical multivariate linear modelling, they found significant within-person associations between daily hassles and snack intake for the overall sample, where an increased number of hassles were associated with increased snack intake. Additionally, those with higher cortisol reactivity to stressors from a laboratory task were more likely to snack in response to stress than low reactors. This finding suggests that stress reactivity may play a moderating role of eating style on stress-induced eating in daily life.

Daily diary methods may be particularly useful for intervention research. For example, a recent study by Pipingas et al. (2013) found no effect of multivitamin supplementation on standard measures of mood like the POMS administered at baseline, 8 and 16 weeks following daily supplementation with a high-potency multivitamin. However, participants in the active ingredient group did report lower stress, anxiety and fatigue when they reported their mood using mobile phones at home, suggesting that the temporal proximity of real-time measures may be more sensitive to mood changes than chronic measures (Pipingas et al., 2013). However, as the authors note, these patterns could be due to mobile phone reports being made soon after participants took their daily multivitamin supplement, whereas participants refrained from taking their daily supplement at their 8- and 16-week testing settings.

Many of the shorter trait measures of mood and PWB can be adapted to a daily diary format by changing the wording from *in general* to *today*. This is common practice in daily diary research. However, shorter measures (<10 items) are better suited to daily diary formats. Reliability estimates of daily diary measures cannot be computed using standard Cronbach's alphas because the data are *nested* (multiple observations over time nested within participants), which violates assumptions of independence. Reliability should be computed taking into account the nested nature of the data – see Nezlek (2012) or Shrout and Lane (2012).

### 5.5.2 EXPERIENCE SAMPLING METHODS

The term *experience sampling* is used to refer to *signal contingent sampling* that involves more frequent reports combined with periodic signalling in natural settings (Csikszentmihalyi & Larson, 1987). Unlike a daily diary that is done once per day, with an ESM, people are signalled semi-randomly between 6 and 10 times per day, usually over the course of several days to weeks. At each signal, participants answer questions about their experiences at that moment. This style of sampling is suited to recording momentary experiences that are ongoing and variable (e.g. quicker changes in emotional states) and most susceptible to memory biases (e.g. pain). Although the number of items in experience sampling is usually quite small, which limits the breadth of questioning, reliability can be constructed by aggregating single items over time (Csikszentmihalyi & Larson, 1987). Researchers usually try to choose items and questions with good face validity. For example, researchers might ask people to rate how pleasant and unpleasant they currently feel (each item rated on 0, not at all, and 9, extremely) to capture valence, or they may try to target different levels of valence and activation (energetic, relaxed, tense and sad).

In most experience sampling studies, participants are prompted by a randomly timed signal, which is now usually accomplished using either a text message or audible signal from a smartphone application (*app*; for a review of current options, see Conner & Lehman, 2012, and the website for the Society of Ambulatory Assessment, http://www.ambulatory-assessment.org/an international society for researchers interested in mobile assessment of behaviour). Following this signal, participants respond to survey questions by either replying back to the text message, clicking through to a web survey delivered by text to their smartphone, responding directly into a survey app or completing a paper questionnaire (although paper questionnaires are becoming less common). Macht et al. (2005) used the ESM approach to investigate changes in eating in response to the stress of studying for exams in college students. Participants reported their emotional state, motivations to eat and perceived functions of eating 10 times a day on 2 successive days during baseline

(3–4 weeks before exams) and during the *stress* period (3–4 days before exams). Control participants did not have an exam. A cellular pager was used to randomly signal participants as a prompt to perform the ratings on supplied questionnaires. Students were screened to exclude any participants who reported pathological eating patterns. In the lead up to an exam, students experienced increased fear, tension and emotional stress. They also reported a higher tendency to eat in order to distract from stress but did not eat in order to relax or feel better.

In another study, Tomiyama et al. (2009) investigated the eating behaviour motivations of restrained eaters in their daily lives. In this study, 137 female participants used a personal digital assistant (PDA) (also known as a palmtop computer) to report approximately every hour (±10 min, disregarding sleeping hours) for 2 days about their positive and negative mood, levels of perceived anxiety and distraction, level of hunger and whether food had been consumed since the previous response. Contrary to findings from laboratory settings, in real-life settings, restrained eaters did not overeat in response to anxiety and ate more in response to hunger (Tomiyama et al., 2009).

### 5.5.3  EVENT SAMPLING

Another useful approach is *event contingent sampling*, which refers to data collection initiated by the participant following a specified event. This sampling style is well utilised in nutritional and craving research. For example, Lowe and Fisher (1983) found that when obese female college students recorded their food intake and mood using a Food and Mood Self-Monitoring (FMSM) form just prior to eating, they were more emotionally reactive and more likely to engage in emotional snacking than their *normal weight* comparisons.

In another example, Sayegh et al. (1995) used a computerised telephone system to have their participants report mood and appetite. Twenty-four women with premenstrual syndrome (PMS) were enrolled in a double-blind study to test the efficacy of specific beverages on PMS symptoms. Participants used the number pad of their telephone to quantify responses to mood and appetite questions before and 30, 90 and 180 min after consumption of the beverages. Cognitive tests were also administered by phone interview. Results show that consuming a specially formulated carbohydrate-rich beverage known to increase serum tryptophan levels during the late luteal phase of the menstrual cycle was associated with a significant decrease in self-reported depression, anger, confusion and carbohydrate craving 90–180 min after initial intake.

Event contingent sampling methods have also been used to challenge common assumptions in nutrition. For example, Stein et al. (2007) used palmtop computers to investigate the relationship between NA and binge eating in a sample of overweight women with binge eating disorder. They found that, contrary to prior research, NA did not decrease significantly following a binge. In addition, contrary to the popular restraint theory was the finding that the breaking of a *food rule* was not a primary cause for binge eating. This study underscores the important role of testing the contingencies of health behaviours and mood in real-world contexts.

### 5.5.4 SENSOR SAMPLING: A NEW FRONTIER

One of the newest real-time methods is the use of sensor sampling to infer moods and other psychological states over time in daily life. In *continuous sensor sampling*, activities and physiological measures are recorded continuously over a designated time period using voice or audio recorders (e.g. EAR, Mehl et al., 2001; cellular microphone), pedometers, GPS, enhanced pedometers (e.g. FitBit®) and more recently from the built-in sensors in off-the-shelf smartphones. Data from continuous recording (e.g. movement or heart rate) are often useful in conjunction with self-reports of experience (Rachuri et al., 2011). Similarly, *adaptive sensor sampling* refers to an adjusted sampling rate of these sensors to conserve energy and reduce local memory use and processing power (Rachuri et al., 2011).

The trend towards real-time ambulatory measures opens up other interesting tools in nutrition science. For example, heart rate monitor phone *apps* and self-assessed salivary cortisol levels may provide real-time anxiety data (see Schlotz, 2011). Similarly, continuous interstitial ambulatory glucose-monitoring devices (AGDs; such as the Glucoday®, see Dye et al., 2010) can allow for a more comprehensive view of an individual's glucose levels in relation to diet, exercise and mood when combined with experience sampling strategies. Meanwhile, other *apps* utilising built-in sensors in smartphones can be used to detect stress (Lu et al, 2012), infer mood (LiKamWa et al., 2011) or develop a pattern of a person's habits, activities, routines and emotions (Lathia et al., 2013).

Many off-the-shelf smartphones have built-in sensors such as the accelerometer (which can be used for activity recognition), microphone (speaker, conversation detection) and GPS (location). By extracting features from the sensor data, it is possible to draw inferences about physical activities such as running, cycling and walking, using the accelerometer sensor and movement speed using readings from the GPS sensor (Park et al., 2012). Classification tasks such as speech recognition (e.g. Siri on the iPhone 4S6) can also be enhanced by accessing dictionaries available in alternative servers (Rachuri, 2012). Although these sensors were initially incorporated to improve user experience of the smartphones, utilising these built-in sensors can enhance the accurate observation of spontaneous behaviour and speech and they are especially useful when the social sensing is performed passively (Rachuri et al., 2011). For example, StressSense (Lu et al., 2012) is a mobile sensing system that uses audio recorded through the microphone sensor to detect stress in the user's voice by classifying the standard deviation of pitch, perturbation and speaking rate. Likewise, the MoodSense system can be used to infer the user's mood from information already available in smartphones by analysing communication history and application usage patterns. For example, the MoodSense system inferred users' daily mood average with a 93% accuracy rate and sudden mood change with an accuracy rate of 74% (LiKamWa et al., 2011). Similarly, University of Cambridge's EmotionSense system combines self-reports of mood and data recorded using the phone's built-in GPS, accelerometer and microphone, to develop a pattern of that person's habits, daily activities, social interactions and emotions (Rachuri, 2012). EmotionSense achieves greater than 90% accuracy for speaker identification and greater than 70% accuracy for broad emotion recognition (Lathia et al., 2013).

By combining the data from built-in sensors with a log of the user's calling and texting patterns, a study of a person's smartphone can offer nutrition researchers a very useful record of their participants' natural habits, activities and routines. In addition, these software applications are becoming readily available for external researchers to utilise and modify to suit their researching needs. For nutrition researchers, this could include the incorporation of food intake recording methodologies. For example, My Meal Mate is a free smartphone application developed at the University of Leeds which utilises goal setting, progress feedback and self-monitoring of diet, physical activity and weight to promote user weight loss (Carter et al., 2013). Another example of utilising built-in smartphone features for nutrition research is the Remote Food Photography Method (RFPM) in which users capture images of food selection and plate waste. This method enhances individuals' food and energy intake estimation by reducing retrospective recall-based error when compared to 24 h food recall and pen-and-paper food records (Martin et al., 2009). Consistent with standard ESM protocols, customised prompts (delivered at personalised meal times) are sent to the participants to remind them to capture food images. Energy intake in a customised prompt condition was compared against doubly labelled water (DLW), considered the gold standard metabolic measure used to assess free-living energy expenditure. When customised prompts were utilised, energy intake estimated by the RFPM did not significantly differ from the energy intake measured by the more labour-intensive, and expensive, DLW method. The authors reported that RFPM underestimated energy intake by 3.7%, which represented an improvement over alternative self-report methods (food records and 24 h recall which underestimate energy intake and micronutrient intake, respectively; Poslusna et al., 2009). If RFPM was combined with a passive sensing system such as StressSense (Lu et al., 2012), MoodSense system (LiKamWa et al., 2011) or EmotionSense (Rachuri, 2012), it would be plausible to deploy large-scale studies with reduced logistical and financial constraints whilst achieving accurate nutrition, mood and physical activity data.

Whilst these applications are relatively recent, they demonstrate the potential of utilising off-the-shelf smartphones to combine passive sensor data collection and machine learning to provide continuous monitoring of participants' emotional states, interactions and mobility (Lathia et al., 2013). Researchers can utilise these systems to facilitate the collection of data by automatically capturing and classifying data to enhance their understanding of social interactions, nutrition and physiological responses, on emotions, mood and behaviour.

*Recommendation*: Whilst it is clear that good research design and careful selection of measures are of the utmost importance, nutrition researchers should aim to take advantage of real-time mood measures and advances in technology. In the near future, it will be less acceptable to rely solely upon pre- and post-test measures of mood when there are such rich data points to be measured in between assessment periods. Internet or app-based daily diaries should be used more frequently in nutrition science to track a range of daily measures of food and mood. Of course, technology cannot replace careful design of existing measures, which suggests that a multi-method approach is valuable. We also urge researchers to avoid paper-and-pen diaries or paper ESM booklets given the near ubiquitous access to the Internet and mobile phones. For a review of technology and ESM-capable software, see www. ambulatory-assessment.org.

## 5.6   CONCLUSION

Multiple options are available for measuring mood in nutrition research. Some of these involve more traditional approaches of examining trait and state moods using a paper-and-pen questionnaire. However, more recent technological advances and multimodal research approaches now allow us to capture new facets of the relationship between nutritional factors and moods. Whilst trait reports of global or longer-term retrospective well-being are still the method of choice for cross-sectional studies to establish links between typical eating patterns and macro-level moods, real-time approaches can be extremely useful for intervention research where real-time measures of mood can potentially show earlier changes in mood than traditional measures. These approaches could also help nutrition researchers illustrate micro-level changes in mood as a function of nutrition intake, offering a finer-grained resolution of temporal sequencing that cannot be achieved with pre- and post-test reports. However, the method utilised for measuring mood in nutrition research in any specific project needs to be suitable for the aims of the research and the study population. Most importantly, the growing development in the fascinating new area of the nutrition–mood link research requires understanding of the range of mood measures available to researchers.

### CURRENT TRENDS

- A trend towards including measures that assess both negative and positive mood states is warranted.
- New trends in ambulatory research may give rise to the use of subjective state measures as well as real-time, objective physiological measures.
- Real-time data capture approaches are beginning to integrate more technologically advanced platforms for research such as SMS-based, smartphone app–based and Internet-based experience sampling with an emphasis on incorporating a range of ambulatory methods. These methods often necessitate advanced forms of statistics such as multilevel modelling.

## REFERENCES

Ahearn, E. P. (1997). The use of visual analog scales in mood disorders: A critical review. *Journal of Psychiatric Research, 31*, 569–579.

Akbaraly, T., Sabia, S., Shipley, M. J., Batty, G. D., & Kivimaki, M. (2013). Adherence to healthy dietary guidelines and future depressive symptoms: Evidence for sex differentials in the Whitehall II study. *The American Journal of Clinical Nutrition, 97*, 419–427.

Akbaraly, T. N., Brunner, E. J., Ferrie, J. E., Marmot, M. G., Kivimaki, M., & Singh-Manoux, A. (2009). Dietary pattern and depressive symptoms in middle age. *The British Journal of Psychiatry, 195*, 408–413.

American Psychiatric Association. (1994). *Diagnostic and statistical manual of mental disorders* (4th ed.). Washington, DC: American Psychiatric Association.

American Psychiatric Association. (2013). *Diagnostic and statistical manual of mental disorders* (5th ed.). Arlington, VA: American Psychiatric Publishing.

Barratt, S. M., Leeds, J. S., & Sanders, D. S. (2011). Quality of life in Coeliac Disease is determined by perceived degree of difficulty adhering to a gluten-free diet, not the level of dietary adherence ultimately achieved. *Journal of Gastrointestinal & Liver Diseases, 20*, 241–245.

Barrett, L. F., and Russell, J. A. (1999). Structure of current affect. *Current Directions in Psychological Science, 8*, 10–14.

Beard, J. L., Hendricks, M. K., Perez, E. M., Murray-Kolb, L. E., Berg, A., Vernon-Feagans, L., & Tomlinson, M. (2005). Maternal iron deficiency anaemia affects postpartum emotions and cognition. *Nutritional Epidemiology, 135*, 267–272.

Beck, A. T., Epstein, N., Brown, G., & Steer, R. A. (1988). An inventory for measuring clinical anxiety: Psychometric properties. *Journal of Consulting and Clinical Psychology, 56*, 893.

Beck, A. T., & Steer R. A. (1993). *Beck anxiety inventory manual*. San Antonio, TX: Harcourt Brace and Company.

Beck, A. T., Steer, R. A., & Brown, G. K. (1996). *Manual for the Beck depression inventory*-II. San Antonio, TX: Psychological Corporation.

Beck, A. T., Ward, C. H., Mendelson, M., Mock, J., & Erbaugh, J. (1961). An inventory for measuring depression. *Archives of General Psychiatry, 4*, 561–571.

Benton, D., & Cook, R. (1991). The impact of selenium supplementation on mood. *Biological Psychiatry, 29*, 109–1098.

Bjelland, I., Dahl, A. A., Tangen Haug, T., & Neckelmann, D. (2002). The validity of the Hospital Anxiety and Depression Scale: An updated literature review. *Journal of Psychosomatic Research, 52*, 69–77.

Blanchflower, D. G., Oswald, A. J., & Stewart-Brown, S. (2013). Is psychological well-being linked to the consumption of fruit and vegetables? *Social Indicators Research, 114*, 785–801.

Bond, A., & Lader, M. (1974). The use of analogue scales in rating subjective feelings. *The British Journal of Medical Psychology, 47*, 211–218.

Cagnacci, A., Arangino, S., Renzi, A., Zanni, A. L., Malmusi, S., & Volpe, A. (2003). Kava–Kava administration reduces anxiety in perimenopausal women. *Maturitas, 44*(2), 103–109.

Cantril, H. (1965). *The pattern of human concerns*. New Brunswick, NJ: Rutgers University Press.

Carr, A. C., Bozonet, S. M., Pullar, J. M., & Vissers, M. C. M. (2013). Mood improvement in young adult males following supplementation with gold kiwifruit, a high-vitamin C food. *Journal of Nutrition Science, 2*, 1–8.

Carroll, D., Ring, C., Suter, M., & Willemsen, G. (2000). The effects of an oral multivitamin combination with calcium, magnesium, and zinc on psychological well-being in healthy young male volunteers: A double-blind placebo-controlled trial. *Psychopharmacology, 150*(2), 220–225.

Carter, M. C., Burley, V. J., & Cade, J. E. (2013). Development of 'My Meal Mate' – A smartphone intervention for weight loss. *Nutrition Bulletin, 38*, 80–84.

Colangelo, L. A., He, K., Whooley, M. A., Daivglus, M. L., Morris, S., & Liu, K. (2014). Selenium exposure and depressive symptoms: The Coronary Artery Risk Development in Young Adults Trace Element Study. *NeuroToxicology, 41*, 167–174.

Conner, T., & Barrett, L. F. (2012). Trends in ambulatory self-report: Understanding the utility of momentary experiences, memories, and beliefs. *Psychosomatic Medicine, 74*, 327–337.

Conner, T. S., Brookie, K. L., Richardson, A. C., & Polak, M. A. (2014). On carrots and curiosity: Eating fruit and vegetables is associated with greater flourishing in daily life. *British Journal of Health Psychology.* Advance online publication. doi:10.1111/bjhp.12113

Conner, T. S., & Lehman, B. J. (2012). Getting started: Launching a study in daily life. In: M. R. Mehl & T. S. Conner. (Eds.), *Handbook of research methods for studying daily life.* New York: Guilford Press.

Cox, J. L., Holden, J. M., & Sagovsky, R. (1987). Detection of postnatal depression, Development of the 10-item Edinburgh Postnatal Depression Scale. *The British Journal of Psychiatry, 150,* 782–786.

Csikszentmihalyi, M., & Larson, R. (1987). Validity and reliability of the experience-sampling method. *The Journal of Nervous and Mental Disease, 175,* 526–536.

Deci, E. L., & Ryan, R. M. (2008). Hedonia, eudaimonia, and well-being: An introduction. *Journal of Happiness Studies, 9,* 1–11

Diener, E., Wirtz, D., Tov, W., Kim-Prieto, C., Choi, D. W., Oishi, S., & Biswas-Diener, R. (2010). New wellbeing measures: Short scales to assess flourishing and positive and negative feelings. *Social Indicators Research, 97,* 143–156.

Dye, L., Mansfield, M., Lasikiewicz, N., Mahawish, L., Schnell, R., Talbot, D., … Lawton, C. (2010). Correspondence of continuous interstitial glucose measurement against arterialised and capillary glucose following an oral glucose tolerance test in healthy volunteers. *British Journal of Nutrition, 103,* 134–140.

Fahrenberg, J., & Myrtek, M. (Eds.) (1996). *Ambulatory assessment. Computer-assisted psychological and psychophysiological methods in monitoring and field studies.* Seattle, WA: Hogrefe & Huber.

First, M. B., Spitzer, R. L., Gibbon, M., & Williams, J. B. W. (2002). *Structured clinical interview for DSM-IV-TR axis I disorders, research version, non-patient edition (SCID-I/ NP).* New York: Biometrics Research, New York State Psychiatric Institute.

Flint, A., Raben, A., Blundell, J. E., & Astrop, A. (2000). Reproducibility, power and validity of visual analogue scales in assessment of appetite sensations in single test meal studies. *International Journal of Obesity, 24,* 38–48.

Ford, P. A., Jaceldo-Siegl, K., Lee, J. W., Youngberg, W., & Tonstad, S. (2013). Intake of Mediterranean foods associated with positive affect and low negative affect. *Journal of Psychosomatic Research, 74,* 142–148.

Fordyce, M. W. (1988). A review of research on the happiness measure: A sixty second index of happiness and mental health. *Social Indicators Research, 20,* 355–381.

Gao, S., Jin, Y., Unverzagt, F. W., Liang, C., Hall, K. S., Cao, J., & Hendrie, H. C. (2012). Selenium level and depressive symptoms in a rural elderly Chinese cohort. *BMC Psychiatry, 12,* 1–8.

Gibson, J., McKenzie-McHarg, K., Shakespeare, J., Price, J., & Gray, R. (2009). A systematic review of studies validating the Edinburgh Postnatal Depression Scale in antepartum and postpartum women. *Acta Psychiatrica Scandinavica, 119,* 350–364.

Goldberg, D., & Williams, P. (1991). *General Health Questionnaire.* Hämtad från.

Gosney, M. A., Hammond, M. F., Shenkin, A., & Allsup, S. (2008). Effect of micronutrient supplementation on mood in nursing home residents. *Gerontology, 54,* 292–299.

Hamer, (2014). *European Journal of Nutrition* (in press).

Hamilton, M. (1959). The assessment of anxiety states by rating. *British Journal of Medical Psychology, 32,* 50–55.

Heuchert, J. P., & McNair, D. M. (2004). *Profile of mood states* (2nd ed.) (POMS 2). Toronto, Ontario, Canada: Multi-Health Systems Inc.

Jacka, F. N., Mykletun, A., Berk, M., Belland, I., & Tell, G. S. (2011). The association between habitual diet quality and the common mental disorders in community-dwelling adults: The Hordaland Health Study. *Psychosomatic Medicine, 73,* 483–490.

Jacka, F. N., Overland, S., Stewart, R., Tell, G. S., Bjelland, I., & Mykletun, A. (2009). Association between magnesium intake and depression and anxiety in community-dwelling adults: The Hordaland Health Study. *Australian and New Zealand Journal of Psychiatry, 43*, 45–52.

Jacka, F. N., Pasco, J. A., Mykletun, A., Williams, L. J., Hodge, A. M., O'Reilly, S. L., … Berk, M. (2010). Association of Western and traditional diets with depression and anxiety in women. *American Journal of Psychiatry, 167*(3), 305–311.

Jacka, F. N., Pasco, J. A., Williams, L. J., Mann, N., Hodge, A., Brazionis, L., & Berk, M. (2012a). Red meat consumption and mood and anxiety disorders. *Psychotherapy and Psychosomatics, 81*(3), 196–198.

Jacka, F. N., Pasco, J. A., Williams, L. J., Meyer, B. J., Digger, R., & Berk, M. (2012b). Dietary intake of fish and PUFA, and clinical depressive and anxiety disorders in women. *British Journal of Nutrition, 10*, 1–8.

Jackson, C. (2007). The general health questionnaire. *Occupational Medicine, 57*(1), 79–79.

Jezova, D, Makatsori, A., Smriga, M., Morinaga, Y., & Duncko, R. (2005). Subchronic treatment with amino acid mixture of L-lysine and L-arginine modifies neuroendocrine activation during psychosocial stress in subjects with high trait anxiety. *Nutrition Neuroscience, 8*, 155–160.

Johnson, L. A., Phillips, J. A., Mauer, C., Edwards, M., Hobson Balldin, V., Hall, J. R., & O'Bryant, S. E. (2013). *BMC Psychiatry, 13*, 1–8.

Kalliath, T. J., O'Driscoll, M. P., & Brough, P. (2004). A confirmatory factor analysis of the General Health Questionnaire-12. *Stress and Health, 20*, 11–20.

Lai, J. S., Hiles, S., Bisquera, A., Hure, A. J., McEvoy, M., & Attia, J. (2014). A systematic review and meta-analysis of dietary patterns and depression in community-dwelling adults. *American Journal of Clinical Nutrition, 99*, 181–197.

Lakhan, S. E., & Vieira, K. F. (2010). Nutritional and herbal supplements for anxiety and anxiety-related disorders: Systematic review. *Nutritional Journal, 9*, 42.

Lathia, N., Pejovic, V., Rachuri, K. K., Mascolo, C., Musolesi, M., & Rentfrow, P. J. (2013). Smartphones for large-scale behaviour change interventions. *IEEE Pervasive Computing* (May 2013).

Lenderking, W. R., Hu, M., Tennen, H., Cappelleri, J. C., Petrie, C. D., & Rush, A. J. (2008). Daily process methodology for measuring earlier antidepressant response. *Contemporary Clinical Trials, 29*, 867–877.

LiKamWa, R., Liu, Y., Lane, N. D., & Zhong, L. (2011, November). Can your smartphone infer your mood? In: *Proceedings of the PhoneSense Workshop*. Seattle, WA.

Lowe, M. R., & Fisher, E. B. (1983). Emotional reactivity, emotional eating, and obesity: A naturalistic study. *Journal of Behavioral Medicine, 6*, 135–49.

Lu, H., Frauendorfer, D., Rabbi, M., Mast, M. S., Chittaranjan, G. T., Campbell, A. T., & Choudhury, T. (2012, September). StressSense: Detecting stress in unconstrained acoustic environments using smartphones. In: *Proceedings of the 2012 ACM Conference on Ubiquitous Computing* (pp. 351–360). ACM. Pittsburgh, PA.

Lyubomirsky, S., & Lepper, H. S. (1999). A measure of subjective happiness: Preliminary reliability and construct validation. *Social Indicators Research, 46*, 137–155

Macht, M., Haupt, C., & Ellgring, H. (2005). The perceived function of eating is changed during examination stress: A field study. *Eating Behaviors, 6*, 109–112.

Mackinnon, A., Jorm, A. F., Christensen, H., Korten, A. E., Jacomb, P. A., & Rodgers, B. (1999). A short form of the Positive and Negative Affect Schedule: Evaluation of factorial validity and invariance across demographic variables in a community sample. *Personality and Individual Differences, 27*, 405–416

Maier, W., Buller, R., Philipp, M., & Heuser, I. (1988). The Hamilton Anxiety Scale: Reliability, validity and sensitivity to change in anxiety and depressive disorders. *Journal of Affective Disorders, 14*, 61–68.

Martin, C. K., Han, H., Coulon, S. M., Allen, H. R., Champagne, C. M., & Anton, S. D. (2009). A novel method to remotely measure food intake of free-living individuals in real time: The remote food photography method. *British Journal of Nutrition, 101*, 446–456.

Matthey, S., Henshaw, C., Elliott, S., & Barnett, B. (2006). Variability in use of cut-off scores and formats on the Edinburgh Postnatal Depression Scale – implications for clinical and research practice. *Archives of Women's Mental Health, 9*, 309–315.

McClung, J. P., Karl, J. P., Cable, S. J., Williams, K. W., Nindl, B. C., Young, A. J., & Lieberman, H. R. (2009). Randomized, double-blind, placebo-controlled trial of iron supplementation in female soldiers during military training: Effects on iron status, physical performance, and mood. *The American Journal of Clinical Nutrition, 90*, 124–131.

McConville, C., Simpson, E. E. A., Rae, G., Polito, A., Andriollo-Sanchez, M., Meunier, N., & Coudray, C. (2005). Positive and negative mood in the elderly: The ZENITH study. *European Journal of Clinical Nutrition, 59*, S22–S25.

McKnight, P. E., & Kashdan, T. B. (2009). Purpose in life as a system that creates and sustains health and well-being: An integrative, testable theory. *Review of General Psychology, 13*, 242–251.

McNair, D. M., Lorr, M., & Droppelman, L. F. (1971). *Manual for the profile of mood states*. San Diego, CA: Educational and Industrial Testing Service.

Mehl, M. R., Pennebaker, J. W., Crow, D. M., Dabbs, J., & Price, J. H. (2001). The Electronically Activated Recorder (EAR): A device for sampling naturalistic daily activities and conversations. *Behavior Research Methods, Instruments, & Computers, 33*, 517–523.

Miller, M. D., & Ferris, D. G. (1993). Measurement of subjective phenomena in primary care research. *The Visual Analogue Scale. Family Practice Research Journal, 13*, 15–24.

Mokhber, N., Namjoo, M., Tara, F., Boskabadi, H., Rayman, M. P., Ghayour-Mobarhan, M., & Ferns, G. (2011). Effect of supplementation with selenium on postpartum depression: A randomized double-blind placebo-controlled trial. *The Journal of Maternal-Fetal and Neonatal Medicine, 24*, 104–108.

Murakami, K., & Sasaki, S. (2010). Dietary intake and depressive symptoms: A systematic review of observational studies. *Molecular Nutrition & Food Research, 54*, 471–488.

Murray, D., & Cox, J. L. (1990). Screening for depression during pregnancy with the Edinburgh Depression Scale (EDDS). *Journal of Reproductive and Infant Psychology, 8*, 99–107.

Newman, E., O'Connor, D. B., & Conner, M. (2007). Daily hassles and eating behaviour: The role of cortisol reactivity status. *Psychoneuroendocrinology, 32*, 125–32.

Nezlek, J. B. (2012). Multi-level modeling analysis of diary-style data. In: M. R. Mehl & T. S. Conner. (Eds.), *Handbook of research methods for studying daily life*. New York: Guilford Press.

Nguyen, P. H., Grajeda, R., Melgar, P., Marcinkevage, J., DiGirolamo, A. M., Flores, R., & Martorel, R. (2009). Micronutrient supplementation may reduce symptoms of depression in Guatemalan women. *Archivos Latinoamericanos de Nutricion, 59*, 278–286.

OECD. (2013). *OECD Guidelines on measuring subjective well-being*. Paris, France: OECD Publishing.

Park, J. G., Patel, A., Curtis, D., Teller, S., & Ledlie, J. (2012, September). *Online pose classification and walking speed estimation using handheld devices*. In: *Proceedings of the 2012 ACM Conference on Ubiquitous Computing* (pp. 113–122). ACM. Pittsburgh, PA.

Parker, B. A., Sturm, K, MacIntosh, C. G., Feinle, C., Horowitz, M., & Chapman, I. M. (2004). Relation between food intake and visual analogue scale ratings of appetite and other sensations in healthy older and young subjects. *European Journal of Clinical Nutrition, 58*, 212–218.

Parkinson, B., Briner, R. B., Reynolds, S., & Totterdell, P. (1995). Time frames for mood: Relations between momentary and generalized ratings of affect. *Personality and Social Psychology Bulletin, 21*, 331–339.

Pastore, D. R., Fisher, M., & Friedman, S. B. (1996). Abnormalities in weight status, eating attitudes, and eating behaviors among urban high school students: Correlations with self-esteem and anxiety. *Journal of Adolescent Health, 18*, 312–319.

Pavot, W., & Diener, E. (1993). Review of the satisfaction with life scale. *Psychological Assessment, 5*, 164–172.

Pipingas, A., Camfield, D. A., Stough, C., Cox, K. H. M., Fogg, E., Tiplady, B., ... Scholey, A. B. (2013). The effects of multivitamin supplementation on mood and general well-being in healthy young adults. A laboratory and at-home mobile phone assessment. *Appetite, 6*, 123–136.

Polak, M. A., Conner, T.S., Haszard, J.J., Harper, M. J., & Houghton, L. A. (in preparation). Suitability of vitamin D3 supplementation over winter in healthy premenopausal women to ward off the 'winter blues'.

Polak, M. A., Houghton, L. A., Reeder, A. I., Harper, M. J., & Conner, T. S. (2014). Serum 25-hydroxyvitamin D concentrations and depressive symptoms among young adult men and women. *Nutrients, 6*, 4720–4730.

Poslusna, K., Ruprich, J., de Vries, J. H., Jakubikova, M., & van't Veer, P. (2009). Misreporting of energy and micronutrient intake estimated by food records and 24 hour recalls, control and adjustment methods in practice. *British Journal of Nutrition, 101*, S73-S85.

Rachuri, K. K. (2012). Smartphones based Social Sensing: Adaptive Sampling, Sensing and Computation Offloading. University of Cambridge. Cambridge, U.K. Retrieved from https://www.cl.cam.ac.uk/~cm542/phds/kiranrachuri.pdf. Accessed online May 8, 2014.

Rachuri, K. K., Mascolo, C., Musolesi, M., & Rentfrow, P. J. (2011, September). Sociable Sense: Exploring the trade-offs of adaptive sampling and computation offloading for social sensing. In: *Proceedings of the 17th Annual International Conference on Mobile Computing and Networking* (pp. 73–84). ACM. Las Vegas, NV.

Radloff, L. S. (1977). The CES-D Scale: A self-report depression scale for research in the general population. *Applied Psychological Measurement, 1*, 385–401

Rahe, C., Unrath, M., & Berger, K. (2014). Dietary patterns and the risk of depression in adults: A systematic review of observational studies. *European Journal of Nutrition, 53*, 997–1013.

Richter, P., Werner, J., Heerlein, A., Kraus, A., & Sauer, H. (1998). On the validity of the Beck Depression Inventory. *Psychopathology, 31*, 160–168

Rooney, C., McKinley, M. C., & Woodside, J. V. (2013). The potential role of fruit and vegetables in aspects of psychological well-being: A review of the literature and future directions. *The Proceedings of the Nutrition Society, 72*, 420–432.

Rucklidge, J. J., & Kaplan, B. J. (2013). Broad-spectrum micronutrient formulas for the treatment of psychiatric symptoms: A systematic review. *Expert Review of Neurotherapeutics, 13*, 49–73.

Russell, J. A. (2003). Core affect and the psychological construction of emotion. *Psychological Review, 110*, 145–172.

Ryan, R. M., Huta, V., & Deci, E. L. (2008). Living well: A self-determination theory perspective on eudaimonia. *Journal of Happiness Studies, 9*, 139–170.

Ryff, C. D., & Keyes, C. L. M. (1995). The structure of psychological well-being revisited. *Journal of Personality and Social Psychology, 69*, 719–727.

Sarris, J., McIntyre, E., & Camfield, D. A. (2013). Plant-based medicines for anxiety disorders, part 2: A review of clinical studies with supporting preclinical evidence. *CNS Drugs, 27*(4), 301–319.

Sayegh, R., Schiff, I., Wurtman, J., Spiers, P., McDermott, J., & Wurtman, R. (1995). The effect of a carbohydrate-rich beverage on mood, appetite, and cognitive function in women with premenstrual syndrome. *Obstetrics & Gynecology, 86*, 520–528.

Schlotz, W. (2011). Ambulatory psychoneuroendocrinology: Assessing salivary cortisol and other hormones in daily life. In: M. R. Mehl & T. S. Conner. (Eds.), *Handbook of research methods for studying daily life*. New York: Guilford Press.

Shiffman, S., Stone, A., & Hufford, M. R. (2008). Ecological momentary assessment. *Annual Review of Clinical Psychology, 4*, 1–32

Shrout, P. E., & Lane, S. P. (2012). Psychometrics. In: M. R. Mehl & T. S. Conner. (Eds.), *Handbook of research methods for studying daily life*. New York: Guilford Press.

Smriga, M., Ando, T., Akutsu, M., Furukawa, Y., Miwa, K., & Morinaga, Y. (2007). Oral treatment with L-lysine and L-arginine reduces anxiety and basal cortisol levels in healthy humans. *Biomedical Research (Tokyo, Japan), 28*, 85–90.

Spielberger, C. D. (1983). *Manual for the state-trait anxiety inventory: STAI (Form Y)*. Palo Alto, CA: Consulting Psychologists Press.

Spielberger, C. D., Gorsuch, R. L., Lushene, R., Vagg, P. R., & Jacobs, G. A. (1983). *Manual for the state-trait anxiety inventory*. Palo Alto, CA: Consulting Psychologists Press.

Stein, R. I., Kenardy, J., Wiseman, C. V., Dounchis, J. Z., Arnow, B. A., & Wilfley, D. E. (2007). What's driving the binge in binge eating disorder? A prospective examination of precursors and consequences. *International Journal of Eating Disorders, 40*, 195–203.

Stone, A. A., Kessler, R. C., & Haythomthwatte, J. A. (1991). Measuring daily events and experiences: Decisions for the researcher. *Journal of Personality, 59*, 575–607.

Tanskanen, A., Hibbeln, J. R., Tuomilehto, J., Uutela, A., Haukkala, A., Vilnamäki, H., & Vartianinen, E. (2001). Fish consumption and depressive symptoms in the general population in Finland. *Psychiatric Services, 52,* 529–531.

Tennant, R., Hiller, L., Fishwick, R., Platt, S., Joseph, S., Weich, S., ... Stewart-Brown, S. (2007). The Warwick-Edinburgh Mental Wellbeing Scale (WEMWBS): Development and UK validation. *Health and Quality of Life Outcomes, 5*, doi:10.1186/1477-7525-5-63

Tomiyama, A. J., Mann, T., & Comer, L. (2009). Triggers of eating in everyday life. *Appetite, 52*, 72–82.

Tugade, M. M., Conner, T., & Feldman Barrett, L. (2007). Assessment of mood. In: S. Ayers, C. McManus, S. Newman, K. Wallston, J. Weinman, & R. West (Eds.), *The Cambridge handbook of psychology, health, and medicine*. Cambridge, U.K.: Cambridge University Press.

Vahdat Shariatpanaahi, M., Vahdat Shariatpanaahi, Z., Moshtaaghi, M., Shahbaazi, S. H., & Abadi, A. (2007). The relationship between depression and serum ferritin level. *European Journal of Clinical Nutrition, 61*, 532–535.

Veenhoven, R. (2003). Hedonism and happiness. *Journal of Happiness Studies, 4*, 437–457.

Watkins, L. L., Connor, K. M., & Davidson, J. R. (2001). Effect of kava extract on vagal cardiac control in generalized anxiety disorder: Preliminary findings. Journal of *Psychopharmacology, 15*, 283–286.

Watson, D., & Clark, L. A. (1994). *The PANAS-X: Manual for the positive and negative affect schedule-expanded form*. Ames, IA: The University of Iowa.

Watson, D., Clark, L. A., & Tellegen, A. (1988). Development and validation of brief measures of positive and negative affect: The PANAS scales. *Journal of Personality and Social Psychology, 54,* 1063–1070.

White, B. A., Horwath, C. C., & Conner, T. S. (2013). Many apples a day keep the blues away – Daily experiences of negative and positive affect and food consumption in young adults. *British Journal of Health Psychology, 18*, 782–98.

Williams, E., Stewart-Knox, B., McConville, C., Bradbury, I., Armstrong, N. C., & McNulty, H. (2008). Folate status and mood: Is there a relationship? *Public Health Nutrition, 11*, 118–123.

Woo, J., Lynn, H., Lau, W. Y., Leung, J., Lau, E., Wong, S. Y. S., & Kwok, T. (2006). Nutrient intake and psychological health in an elderly Chinese population. International *Journal of Geriatric Psychiatry, 21*, 1036–1043.

Yannakoulia, M., Panagiotakos, D. B., Pitsavos, C., Tsetsekou, E., Fappa, E., Papageorgiou, C., & Stefanadis, C. (2008). Eating habits in relations to anxiety symptoms among apparently healthy adults. A pattern analysis from the ATTICA Study. *Appetite, 51*, 519–525.

Yesavage, J. A., Brink, T. L., Rose, T. L., Lum, O., Huang, V., Adey, M., & Otto Leirer, V. (1983). Development and validation of a Geriatric Depression Scale: A preliminary report. *Journal of Psychiatric Research, 17*, 37–49.

Yi, S., Nanri, A., Poudel-Tandukar, K., Nonaka, D., Matsushita, Y., Hori, A., & Mizoue, T. (2011). Association between serum ferritin concentrations and depressive symptoms in Japanese municipal employees. *Psychiatry Research, 189*, 368–372.

Zigmond, A. S., & Snaith, R. P. (1983). The hospital anxiety and depression scale. *Acta Psychiatrica Scandinavica, 67*, 361–370.

# Section III

*The Story So Far: Foods and Nutrition for Performance across the Lifespan*

# 6 Glycaemic Control and Cognition

## Evidence across the Lifespan

*Sandra I. Sünram-Lea, Lauren Owen*
*and Bernadette Robertson*

## CONTENTS

## SUMMARY

There has been increasing interest in the effects of nutrition on cognitive performance and more specifically how cognitive performance can be optimised using nutritional interventions. The macronutrient glucose has particularly received attention and is perhaps most thoroughly researched in terms of its effects on cognition. The notion that oral glucose administration might facilitate mental performance was first proposed in the 1950s. Hafermann (1955) investigated the effects of glucose administration on school children and observed a distinct increase in cognitive performance, including performance in mathematics, and generally improved concentration. However, it was not until the mid-1980s that glucose effects on cognitive performance became more widely investigated (Gold, 1986).

In this chapter the impact of glucose administration and glucose regulation on cognitive processes across the lifespan will be reviewed. We describe the ways by which glucose might facilitate cognitive performance and evaluate potential nutritional and lifestyle interventions that may be beneficial to optimising cognitive performance and/or prevent cognitive decline. We begin, however, by discussing some of the features of glucose metabolism that are important for the understanding of its role in cognitive performance.

## 6.1   GLUCOSE: FUNCTION AND METABOLISM

Glucose is one of the most important monosaccharides (basic carbohydrate unit) in terms of mammalian metabolism and one of the most abundant sugars in our diet representing 80% of the final products of carbohydrate digestion. In humans and most animals, adenosine triphosphate (ATP) works as the main carrier of chemical energy. The human body uses three types of molecules to yield the necessary energy to drive ATP synthesis: fats, proteins and carbohydrates (see Figure 6.1). Lipids are broken down into fatty acids, proteins into amino acids and carbohydrates into glucose. Via a series of oxidation–reduction reactions, mitochondria degrade fatty acids, amino acids and pyruvate (the end product of glucose degradation in the cytoplasm) into several intermediate compounds. The intermediates enter the Krebs or citric acid cycle (also known as the tricarboxylic acid cycle). These reduced electron carriers are themselves oxidised via the electron transport chain, with concomitant consumption of oxygen and ATP synthesis. This process is called oxidative phosphorylation.

Over a hundred ATP molecules are synthesised from the complete oxidation of one molecule of fatty acid, and almost 40 ATP molecules result from amino acid and pyruvate oxidation. Two ATP molecules are synthesised in the cytoplasm via the conversion of glucose molecules to pyruvate. Both the enzymes and the physical environment necessary for the oxidation of these molecules are contained in the mitochondria.

In addition to being the major source of biological energy, aerobic carbohydrate metabolism is the main source of energy available for brain tissue, and glucose and oxygen are the sole metabolic energy source that can cross the blood–brain barrier (BBB) and hence be utilised by brain cells to form ATP (Thompson, 1967). All processes of cells (including nerve cells) require energy. This energy is available in the form of the cellular energy-carrying molecule ATP, most of which is generated in the Krebs/citric acid cycle, the aerobic pathway of carbohydrate and glucose metabolism and the major source of biological free energy in higher organisms.

In most meals (as opposed to pure glucose loads studied in experimental situations), digestible carbohydrates pass through the intestines where they are converted to glucose, which is immediately absorbed into the bloodstream. At this post-absorptive state, blood glucose levels are at their highest. The resulting rise in blood glucose levels stimulates the pancreatic islets of Langerhans beta cells to release insulin. Insulin lowers circulating glucose in two ways: it prevents the liver from releasing additional glucose and it causes muscle and fat cell uptake for glycogenesis (production of glycogen). As blood glucose levels decrease, the negative feedback of glucose causes beta cells to stop secreting insulin and the body's metabolism returns to basal state. When ambient glucose levels are high, that is, when glucose is not immediately required for energy, upon leaving the intestine excess glucose is actively transported to the absorptive cells of the intestinal mucosa and absorbed from the intestine into the portal vein, which carries glucose to the liver. Glucose is then

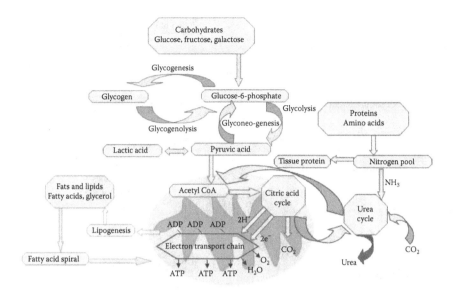

**FIGURE 6.1** The generation of energy from organic compounds. *Carbohydrate* catabolism is the breakdown of carbohydrates into smaller units. Carbohydrates are usually taken into cells once they have been digested into monosaccharides. The major route of breakdown is glycolysis, where sugars such as glucose and fructose are converted into pyruvate and some ATP is generated. Pyruvate is an intermediate in several metabolic pathways, but the majority is converted to acetyl-CoA and fed into the citric acid cycle. Although some more ATP is generated in the citric acid cycle, most of it is generated in the electron transport chain in the mitochondrion, which is the site of oxidative phosphorylation in eukaryotes. Here NADH and succinate generated in the citric acid cycle are oxidised, providing energy to power ATP synthase. In anaerobic conditions, glycolysis produces lactate, through the enzyme lactate dehydrogenase for re-use in glycolysis. *Fats* are catabolised by hydrolysis to free fatty acids and glycerol. The glycerol enters glycolysis and the fatty acids are broken down by beta-oxidation to release acetyl-CoA, which then is fed into the citric acid cycle. Fatty acids release more energy upon oxidation than carbohydrates. Lipogenesis is the process by which acetyl-CoA is converted to fatty acids for storage in the form of fats. *Proteins and amino acids* are either used to synthesise proteins and other biomolecules or oxidised to urea and carbon dioxide as a source of energy. Dietary proteins are first broken down to individual amino acids by various enzymes and hydrochloric acid present in the gastrointestinal tract. These amino acids are further broken down to $\alpha$-keto acids which can be recycled in the body for generation of energy and production of glucose or fat or other amino acids. This breakdown of amino acids to $\alpha$-keto acids occurs in the liver by a process known as transamination.

stored for later use as polymerised glucose or glycogen in the liver and muscle cells, or converted to fat by the liver and adipose cells and then stored in the adipocytes (Guyton, 1991). Conversely, when blood glucose is low, the secretion of the opposing pancreatic hormone glucagon is induced. Glucagon induces the breakdown of liver glycogen to glucose and increases gluconeogenesis in the liver. Gluconeogenesis is the biosynthesis of a carbohydrate from simpler, non-carbohydrate precursors such as pyruvate (Purves et al., 2001).

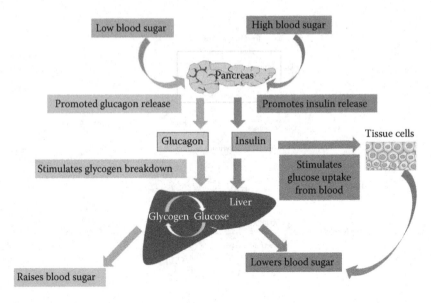

**FIGURE 6.2** The homeostatic control of blood glucose. Following a meal, glucose levels increase and high blood sugar levels stimulate the pancreatic islets of Langerhans beta cells to release insulin. Insulin lowers circulating glucose in two ways: it prevents the liver from releasing additional glucose and it promotes storage of glucose as glycogen or by conversion to fat by the liver and adipose cells and then stored in the adipocytes. As blood glucose levels decrease, the negative feedback of glucose causes beta cells to stop secreting insulin and the body's metabolism returns to basal state. Conversely, when blood glucose is low, the secretion of the opposing pancreatic hormone glucagon is induced. Glucagon induces the breakdown of liver glycogen to glucose and increases gluconeogenesis in the liver. Gluconeogenesis is the biosynthesis of a carbohydrate from simpler, non-carbohydrate precursors such as pyruvate.

These complex hormonal feedback systems (see Figure 6.2) ensure that the concentration of glucose in the blood plasma is tightly regulated to stay within the normal range of 4–6 mmol/L (72–108 mg/dL). When blood glucose drops below 4 mmol/L (72 mg/dL; hypoglycaemic condition), it can cause discomfort, confusion, coma, convulsions or even death in extreme conditions (Nelson and Cox, 2005). Persistent blood glucose concentrations above the normal range (hyperglycaemic condition) can also have damaging physiological effects. Because glucose exerts osmotic pressure in the extracellular fluid (ECF), extremely high blood glucose concentrations can cause cellular dehydration. An excessively high level of blood glucose concentration also causes loss of glucose in the urine, which can affect kidney function and deplete the body's supply of fluids and electrolytes (Guyton, 1991).

## 6.2  GLUCOSE AS FUEL FOR THE BRAIN

The central significance of glucose as the major nutrient of the brain, its metabolism and control, have been well documented. Brain tissue is absolutely dependent upon the oxidative metabolism of glucose for energy. Associated measurements of oxygen and glucose levels in blood sampled upon entering and leaving the brain in humans show that almost all the oxygen utilised by the brain can be accounted for by the oxidative metabolism of glucose (McIlwain, 1959).

Since relatively little glucose can be stored, the brain is reliant on a continuous supply of glucose as its primary fuel, delivered via the bloodstream. Although small molecules, such as oxygen, can pass readily through the BBB, most of the larger molecules required by brain cells must be actively taken up by special transport mechanisms (Iversen, 1979). The entry of glucose into the brain is mediated by the family of glucose (GLUT) transporters which are adapted to the metabolic needs of the tissue in which it is found. The primary GLUT isoforms in the brain are GLUT1 and GLUT3, but others have been detected in different brain regions, at a low level of expression. As mentioned earlier, compared with other organs, the brain possesses paradoxically limited stores of glycogen, which without replenishment are exhausted in up to 10 min. In nervous tissue, glycogen is stored in astrocytes. Astrocytes participate significantly in brain glucose uptake and metabolism, and due to their location and metabolic versatility, they may be the 'fuel-processing plants' within the central nervous system (CNS) (Lehninger et al., 2005). Glucose deprivation in astroglial cultures results in reduction in the ATP/ADP ratio and membrane depolarization (Wiesinger et al., 1997) or rapid depletion of glycogen stores (Kauppinen et al., 1988).

The immense expenditure of energy by the brain relative to its weight and volume is thought to be due to the need to maintain ionic gradients across the neuronal membrane, on which the conduction of impulses in billions of brain neurons depends. In addition, there is no break from the brain's energy demand as the rate of brain metabolism is relatively steady day and night and may even increase slightly during the dreaming phases of sleep. Thus, the energy requirements of brain tissue are exceptionally constant (Iversen, 1979), and glucose deprivation can severely disrupt neuronal activity, producing EEG patterns characteristic of lowered cognitive functioning (Holmes et al., 1983).

## 6.3   GLUCOSE METABOLISM: CHANGES ACROSS THE LIFESPAN

Age-related changes can be observed in glucose brain metabolism across the lifespan. Initially, there is a rise in the rate of glucose utilisation from birth until about age four years, at which time the child's cerebral cortex uses more than double the amount of glucose compared to adults. Childhood is a time of intense learning, and this high rate of glucose utilisation is maintained from age 4 to 10 years coinciding with a period of one of the most metabolically expensive cognitive processes (Haymond, 1989). The increased energy demand of children's brains requires the use of the majority of hepatically generated plasma glucose (Haymond & Sunehag, 1999). Glucose supply needs to be particularly stable as impairments occur at a much higher plasma glucose level (4.2 mmol/L) (Jones et al., 1995). After this period, there is a gradual decline in glucose metabolic rates, which reach adult values by age 16–18 years (see, e.g. Harry & Chugani, 1998). This is followed by a plateau phase until middle age after which a significant age-related decline in cerebral glucose metabolism can be observed (see, e.g. Moeller et al., 1996). This age-specific metabolic pattern of glucose consumption has not been observed in other species, and it has been argued that this could be a driver or a consequence of human cognition (Caravas & Wildman, 2014).

Most children and young adults maintain circulating glucose within the normal range throughout cycles of feeding and fasting and balanced alterations in secretions of regulatory hormones. In contrast, older adults have a broader range over which circulating glucose is maintained and in addition have attenuated counterregulatory responses. Circulating insulin levels tend to be elevated with age (approx. 8% higher than in young adults) and are indicative of reduced insulin sensitivity (Melanson et al., 1998). Reduced insulin sensitivity or insulin resistance is a condition where individuals develop resistance to the cellular actions of insulin, characterised by an impaired ability of insulin to inhibit glucose output from the liver and to promote glucose uptake in fat and muscle. Both effects of insulin insensitivity on liver and muscle tissue cause elevations in peripheral blood glucose levels. Changes in insulin action have been observed at different stages of the development. Basal insulin secretion increases during puberty, falling back to prepubertal levels in adulthood (Caprio et al., 1989). Yet fasting glucose levels remain constant, implying an increase in tissue resistance to insulin coinciding with puberty (Savage et al., 1992). It is commonly in middle age when insulin resistance and poor glucose tolerance become a greater issue. Given that the brain uses glucose as a primary substrate for cognitive activity, it is perhaps not surprising that conditions that affect peripheral and central glucose regulation and utilisation may also affect cognitive functioning. Moreover, based on the aforementioned evidence, there might be 'critical periods' in which alterations in cerebral glucose supply might have more pronounced effects on cognitive performance.

In summary, the brain has a high metabolic rate and its metabolism is almost entirely restricted to oxidative utilisation of glucose. These factors emphasise the extreme dependence of neural tissue on a stable and adequate supply of glucose and account for the fact that brain function is far more rapidly and profoundly impaired by conditions such as hypoglycaemia than other organ systems. The consequences of fluctuations in central glucose availability have begun to be better understood. Whereas initially it was thought that only glucose deprivation (i.e. under hypoglycaemic conditions) can affect brain function, it has become apparent that low-level fluctuations in central availability can affect neural and, consequently, cognitive performance. In the next section, we will review work into the phenomenon of cognitive enhancement following a glucose load.

## 6.4   GLUCOSE AND COGNITIVE FUNCTION

The effect of glucose on cognition has been extensively studied in an acute, short-term context in which a glucose load is administered and cognitive performance assessed shortly afterwards. Beneficial effects of glucose administration have been observed across different populations using this experimental paradigm. For example, glucose administration can enhance learning and memory in healthy young and aged animals and humans and may improve several cognitive functions in subjects with severe cognitive pathologies, including individuals with Alzheimer's disease and Down's syndrome (see Messier, 2004; Smith et al., 2011 for reviews).

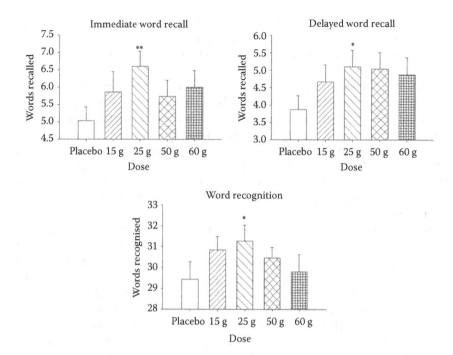

**FIGURE 6.3** Dose–response relationship for declarative memory tasks, with significant glucose facilitation observed following administration of 25 g of glucose. These results confirm that this appears to be the optimal dose for most memory tasks for younger populations. (From Sünram-Lea, S.I. et al., *J. Psychopharmacol.*, 25(8), 1076, 2011.)

Facilitation of cognitive performance induced by elevations in plasma glucose levels has also been reported in patients with schizophrenia (Fucetola, 1999; Newcomer et al., 1999). As with many substances affecting cognitive performance, glucose displays an inverted U-shaped dose–response curve, and its effect is time dependent (Gold, 1986; Sünram-Lea et al., 2011). For young adults, 25 g seems to most reliably facilitate cognitive performance (see Figure 6.3). However, there is some evidence suggesting that the optimal dose may be dependent upon age, inter-individual difference in glucose metabolism and the cognitive domain being assessed (Sünram-Lea et al., 2011).

The clearest enhancement effects of increased glucose supply have been observed for verbal declarative memory over a variety of conditions and paradigms (for review, see Hoyland et al., 2008). These findings suggest that glucose facilitation may be particularly pronounced in tasks that pertain to the hippocampal formation, which is strongly involved in declarative memory (Sünram-Lea et al., 2001). The level of task demand is a further moderating factor for cognitive enhancement by increased glucose availability. Tasks that are more cognitively demanding appear to be more sensitive to the effect of glucose loading (Kennedy & Scholey, 2000; Scholey, 2001; Sünram-Lea et al., 2002). In addition, 'depletion' of episodic memory capacity and/ or glucose resources in the brain due to performing a concomitant cognitive task might be crucial to the demonstration of a glucose facilitation effect. Although the exact underlying mechanisms for this are still unclear, animal research has demonstrated selective reduction in extracellular hippocampal glucose concentrations as a function of the cognitive demand associated with different memory tasks (McNay et al., 2000).

Although there is considerable evidence suggesting possible hippocampal mediation for the glucose facilitation effect in both cognitive and physiological terms, the facilitation effect of glucose appears to be multifarious rather than restricted solely to one brain area, that is, the hippocampus. For example, glucose administration has resulted in enhancement of central processing speed and reaction times (Benton et al., 1994), working memory performance (Kennedy & Scholey, 2000; Martin & Benton, 1999; Sünram-Lea et al., 2001, 2002b) and attention (Messier et al., 1997). When looking at the beneficial effect on non-mnemonic tasks, the factor that appears to be of particular relevance is whether these tasks are cognitively demanding. The energy cost for effortful, controlled or executive processes appears to be significantly higher than that for automatic or reflexive processes (Gailliot & Baumeister, 2007). Effortful, controlled or executive processes are processes that are reliant on the central executive, in which thoughts, behaviours and actions are coordinated to allow goal-directed and purposeful behaviour (Miller & Wallis, 2009), while automatic and reflexive behaviours are evolutionarily predisposed or learned behaviours elicited by environmental stimuli. Indeed, lowered peripheral glucose levels following performance of a cognitively demanding task have been reported (Fairclough & Houston, 2004; Scholey et al., 2001). These results indicate that cognitively demanding tasks and in particular those relying on executive functions are also sensitive to changes in glucose. One crucial function of executive control is to enable self-control, the ability to inhibit ones automatic or habitual responses. Controlling ones desires, emotions, thoughts and behaviours is vital for successful societal functioning. A series of experiments has explored that relationship, and there is evidence that acts of self-control use relatively large amounts of glucose and that glucose administration can improve self-control (see Gailliot and Baumeister, 2007, for review).

In summary, glucose administration is one of the few interventions with demonstrated benefits on certain aspects of cognitive performance across the lifespan. Investigating the effects of glucose on cognitive performance through acute administration of a glucose load has served as a prototypical experimental model by which to research the nutrition–behaviour axis. These investigations have increased our knowledge of those aspects of cognition that are particularly susceptible to plasma glucose fluctuations as well as our understanding the potential underlying mechanisms involved, which will be reviewed in the next section.

## 6.5 MECHANISMS

The precise mechanisms by which increased peripheral and/or central glucose availability affects cognitive processes are still unclear. There are two broad theoretical approaches: energetic demand models and domain-specific models. However, as will become clear these different approaches are by no means mutually exclusive, their relative explanatory value depending on the cognitive task and brain structure.

Glucose metabolism does not only vary across the lifespan but also varies throughout tissue/cell types of the brain, with a clearly established correlation between increased energy metabolism and increased neuronal activity and energy metabolism (Sokoloff, 1999). Both the rate of blood to brain glucose transport (Lund-Anderson, 1979) and glucose metabolism (Reivich & Alavi, 1983) are stimulated in different areas in the brain during cognitive tasks relevant to that area. It is usually thought that an increase in glucose consumption in certain parts of the brain is counterbalanced by reductions elsewhere (Seitz & Roland, 1992). However, there is evidence that performing cognitively demanding tasks increases total brain consumption by as much as 12% (Madsen et al., 1995). It takes about 4–6 s following neural activation for blood flow to increase, which suggests that a temporary energy shortage in neurons may occur (Raichle & Mintun, 2006). This (temporary) insufficiency has been suggested to underlie the improvement effect of glucose ingestion upon cognition, particularly memory (McNay et al., 2000).

Glucose exerts robust effects on long-term memory tasks, in particular declarative memory. The hippocampus is the brain region most strongly implicated in long-term memory performance (Aggleton & Brown, 1999). Microdialysis measurements of brain glucose have shown a large decrease in hippocampal ECF (32% ± 2%) in rats tested for spontaneous alternation on a four-arm maze (a difficult memory task), while a smaller decrease (11% ± 2%) was seen in rats tested on a simpler three-arm maze, suggesting that the changes observed in ECF glucose are related to task difficulty. The fall in ECF can be prevented by administration of glucose, which in turn leads to enhanced memory performance (McNay et al., 2000). There is some evidence that the concentration of extracellular glucose in the brain after its transfer across the BBB from plasma glucose varies with the brain region from 1.3 mmol/L in the hippocampus to 0.3–0.5 mmol/L in the striatum (for review, see McNay et al., 2001). These findings suggest that the hippocampal area is particularly sensitive to energy fluctuations. However, the hippocampus has comparatively high stores of glycogen suggesting that it has evolved some protection against temporary deficits (13 mmol/L compared to 5–6 mmol/L in the cerebral cortex; Dalsgaard et al., 2007). However, arguably this protection only works if cerebral glucose metabolism is not compromised.

Based on the 'last-in, first-out rule', cognitive abilities that developed last ontogenetically are likely the first to become impaired when cognitive and/or physiological resources are compromised. Evolutionary pressures forced the development of ever more integrative neural structures able to process increasingly complex information. This, in turn, led to increased behavioural flexibility and adaptability. The cerebral cortex, and in particular the prefrontal cortex, is at the top of that hierarchy, representing the neural basis of higher cognitive functions (e.g. Frith & Dolan, 1996; Fuster, 2002). Aspects of higher-level cognition include executive function and inhibition (self-control), which were probably one of the last cognitive abilities to develop and may be one of the first to show impairments when cognitive and/or fuel resources are limited.

To summarise, there is evidence that certain brain structures and certain cognitive tasks require more energetic fuel than others. The question is, how can the brain adjust its energy supply to its varying energy needs and under which conditions is optimal fuel supply of particular importance? From an evolutionary perspective, energy mobilisation is of particular importance in times of stress in order to prepare the body for the 'fight or flight' response. Exposure to threats or stressors results in activation of two major endocrine systems, the hypothalamic–anterior pituitary–adrenocortical axis (HPA) and the sympatho-adrenomedullary axis (SAM axis). A major physiological role of activation of both endocrine systems is considered to be a temporary increase in energy production and more specifically provision of additional metabolic fuel through increase in glucose availability (Evans et al., 1986). Consequently, additional metabolic resources allow the organism to adapt rapidly to environmental challenges.

It has been suggested that the brain controls allocation of energy resources via both physiology and behaviour, to support its own dominant energy needs (Peters et al., 2004). This energy allocation is proposed to be governed by a balance between excitatory and inhibitory neurones in corticolimbic networks, which are differentially sensitive to brain ATP levels. With moderately low energy, or ATP levels, excitatory glutamatergic neuronal activity dominates and signals a need for more energy, but with high levels of ATP, as might follow a high glucose load, inhibitory neuronal activity predominates. According to that concept, the brain regulates cerebral energy homeostasis by actively demanding energy from the body. Activation of the aforementioned stress system (SAM and HPA axis) and the concomitant increase in glucose availability therefore function to procure fuel for the brain when needed. These changes appear to modulate brain processes to ensure optimal adaptation, which includes effective storage of these significant events (memory).

Moreover, there is evidence indicating that glucose affects cognitive processes, in particular memory through an enhancement of brain acetylcholine synthesis and/or its release (see Messier, 2004, for review). Endogenous processes (including hormonal responses and differences in neurotransmitter availability and/or binding) could modulate memory strength in terms of recall probability to training and contribute to memory formation by selectively promoting the storage of significant events and not trivial ones (Gold, 1991; Gold & McGaugh, 1975). Consequently, such endogenous processes can act as relevance moderators of the 'print-now' signal by regulating encoding and synaptic plasticity (Sandberg et al., 2001). Sandberg et al. (2001) described a model of an autoassociative network with plasticity modulation that produced an inverted U-shaped curve to overall plasticity similar to the one commonly observed in arousal–performance or glucose dose–response plots. Applied to glucose facilitation of memory, the observed dose–response curve could be explained in terms of lower plasticity at low glucose availability (the network learns slowly), while at high levels, high plasticity (or hyperexcitability) leads to the network learning quickly, but there will be a memory decline due to fast forgetting.

In addition, elevated insulin in response to hyperglycaemia rather than glucose levels *per se* may moderate memory performance (see Watson & Craft, 2004, for review). Originally, insulin was considered only as a peripheral hormone, unable to cross the BBB and to affect the CNS. However, there is now increasing evidence that neuronal glucose metabolism is antagonistically controlled by insulin and cortisol (see Duarte et al., 2012, for review). Insulin present in adult CNS is primarily derived from pancreatic β-cells and is transported by cerebrospinal fluid (CSF) into the brain. It is also partially formed in pyramidal neurons, such as those in the hippocampus, prefrontal cortex, entorhinal cortex and the olfactory bulb, but not in glial cells (Hoyer, 2003). The suggestion that glucose administration and/or impairments in glucoregulatory mechanisms exert the most profound effects on medial temporal regions is supported by functional characteristics associated with these areas such as high density of insulin receptors in the hippocampus (see, e.g. Messier, 2004) which are known to promote cellular glucose uptake (see, e.g. Watson and Craft, 2004). Insulin-sensitive glucose transporters such as GLUT4 (which mediate passive diffusion of glucose through the BBB) are also enriched in the hippocampus (though the highest concentration is in the cerebellum; see McEwen and Reagan, 2004).

Given the established role of the hippocampus in memory, elevated insulin in response to hyperglycaemia may boost glucose utilisation in the hippocampus and result in improved performance (Craft et al., 1993). Indeed, at the molecular level, insulin and/or insulin receptors seem to contribute to the regulation of learning and memory via the activation of specific signalling pathways, one of which is shown to be associated with the formation of long-term memory (for a more detailed account, see Zhao and Alkon, 2001).

Finally, glucose might also act via peripheral physiological mechanisms, which in turn facilitate central mechanisms involved in cognition. It has been suggested that important players in this peripheral route are the liver and the vagus nerve. Messier and White (1987) and White (1991) suggested that changes in cell membrane transport in the liver following administration of high doses of glucose and fructose (>1000 mg/kg) are detected by the coeliac ganglion, then transformed into neural signals and finally carried via the vagus nerve to the brain. In accordance with this suggestion, coeliac ganglion lesions (which block most of the efferents of the liver) have been shown to abolish the mnemonic effect of glucose (White, 1991). Although to date there is no concrete information available concerning how this proposed neural signal from the liver might influence memory performance when it reaches the brain, White (1991) suggests that the hippocampus might be potentially involved in both central and peripheral memory facilitating actions of glucose. The nucleus of the solitary tract in the brainstem is the main relay station for afferent vagal nerve fibres. This nucleus has widespread projections to numerous areas in the forebrain as well as the brainstem, including areas involved in learning and memory formation (amygdala, hippocampus). Stimulation of the vagus nerve induces changes in the electrophysiological and metabolic profile of these brain structures (Clark et al., 1999).

In summary, the research is not yet conclusive but suggests that the underlying mechanism is multifarious rather than particular. The most likely scenario is that glucose provides additional metabolic fuel under high-demand conditions and that certain areas of the brain are more susceptible to limitations in fuel supply or are evolutionarily programmed to react to an endogenous rise in plasma glucose levels. It is important to understand these mechanisms as they provide insight into factors mediating optimal cognitive performance across the lifespan.

## 6.6   GLYCAEMIC CONTROL AND COGNITION: SHORT TERM

The investigations into the effects of administration of a glucose load have been important in elucidating the potential underlying mechanisms. However, it is important to note that ingestion of a glucose load is not a valid nutritional intervention to optimise cognitive performance in the long term or indeed to alleviate cognitive deficits. Administration of a glucose load leads to a sharp rise in blood glucose levels followed by a decline, which can decrease to a value lower than fasting levels due to insulin secretion. As outlined earlier, the relationship between plasma glucose and cognitive performance follows an inverted U-shaped dose–response curve, with low levels and high levels impairing cognition. Consequently, nutritional interventions that avoid peaks and troughs in glucose availability should be optimal for food-induced cognitive enhancement.

When considering the nature of glucose availability, the rate at which food increases and maintains blood glucose, that is, 'the glycaemic index' (GI) appears to be an important modulating factor. Shortly after intake of a high-GI food, there is a relatively rapid rise in blood glucose levels followed by a corresponding rapid decrease, whereas after the intake of a low-GI food, there is a relatively smaller rise in blood glucose followed by more stable blood glucose concentration. Although the effect of glucose administration has been extensively studied in an acute, short-term context, much remains to be done in order to establish the cognitive effects associated with foods of low or high GI.

In general, it appears that although a rise in blood glucose levels leads to immediate short-term benefits, over longer periods of time (i.e. over the morning), low-GI foodstuff appear to be more beneficial to cognitive performance (e.g. Benton et al., 2003; Mahoney, 2005; Ingwersen et al., 2007). Most studies examining the effects of GI on cognition have focused on the effect of breakfast on children's cognitive performance. It has been shown that children at risk for malnourishment have improved cognition and learning at school if provided with breakfast (see Hoyland et al., 2009, for a review of the literature). Moreover, in developed countries, it has been found that skipping breakfast can result in impaired cognitive performance (Benton & Parker, 1998; Hoyland et al., 2009). This suggests that increased plasma glucose availability due to breakfast consumption leads to better cognitive performance. Investigating the optimal rate of glucose supply following breakfast consumption, Mahoney et al. (2005) compared a low-GI breakfast with a high-GI breakfast and found that when children consumed the low-GI food, they remembered significantly more than when they ate the high-GI breakfast. Ingwersen et al. (2007) compared the cognitive effects of a low-GI breakfast and a high-GI breakfast across the morning and found that performance on attention tasks was poorer 130 min after the high-GI breakfast compared to the low-GI breakfast. Furthermore, the low-GI breakfast prevented a decline in memory performance. Overall, the results of studies assessing GI in children suggest that lower-GI breakfasts may be protective against a decline in memory and attention throughout the morning (over 2 h).

Few studies have looked at the effects of GI in adolescent populations and the results are somewhat contradictive. Wesnes et al. (2003) found that a low-GI breakfast resulted in better memory performance and attention, but the age range used in this study was quite large (6–16 years). Other studies found performance benefits following a high-GI intervention when assessing memory performance (Micha et al., 2010; Smith & Foster, 2008), whereas a low-GI intervention proved to be beneficial for measures of attention/information processing (Micha et al., 2010). Cooper et al.

(2012) found no difference between high GI and low GI on reaction times, but better performance on an executive function task following low GI (Cooper et al., 2012). In adult populations, the outcome of investigating the effects of GI has also been somewhat inconsistent. Some show beneficial effects on cognitive performance of low-GI foods (Benton et al., 2003; Nilsson et al., 2009, 2012), whereas others show no such effects (Dye et al., 2010; Kaplan et al., 2000).

Glycaemic load (GL) (as opposed to GI) has also been shown to affect cognitive performance (Benton & Jarvis, 2007). GL takes into account the amount of carbohydrates consumed and is calculated by multiplying the amount of available carbohydrate in a food item by the GI of the food and dividing this by 100. Benton et al. (2007) compared three breakfasts varying in GL from 2·5 to 17·86 and found that the higher GL foods led to poorer memory performance. To date, only a few studies have been carried out into the effect of low-GI and low-GL foods on glycaemic control and cognition in type 2 diabetes. One study showed that consuming a low-GI carbohydrate meal, relative to a high-GI carbohydrate meal, resulted in better cognitive performance in the postprandial period in adults with type 2 diabetes (Papanikolaou et al., 2006), whereas two recent studies by Lamport et al. (2013, 2014) did not find any benefits following consumption of a low-GL breakfast. All three of these studies investigated the acute effects of postprandial glycaemic manipulation, and it may be the case that cognitive effects will only be evident with chronic improvements in glycaemic control. Indeed dietary interventions (combined with exercise interventions) have been shown to result in improved cognitive performance in adults with impaired glucose control and type 2 diabetes when they were implemented for 12 months and 2 years, respectively (Watson et al., 2006; Yamamoto et al., 2009).

In conclusion, it appears that a quick rise in blood glucose levels has some short-term benefits, most notably on memory performance, whereas over longer periods of time (i.e. throughout the morning), a more stable blood glucose profile seems to be more beneficial. In normoglycaemic samples, effects of low-GI and/or low-GL foods were usually observed in the late postprandial period (75–222 min) where they seem to prevent a decline in attention and memory (e.g. Benton et al., 2003; Ingwersen et al., 2007; Mahoney, 2005). In populations with abnormalities in glucose regulation, benefits of low-GI foods have been reported, in particular following longer term intervention.

## 6.7 GLYCAEMIC CONTROL AND COGNITION: LONG TERM

The aforementioned findings show that cognition can be affected by changes in glucose levels within a fairly small plasma glucose range. As a result, the ability to regulate levels of plasma glucose and ensure optimal peripheral and central availability might be important for optimal cognition. Due to the complex relationship between glucose administration, glucose metabolism and cognition, inducement of repeated hyperglycaemic conditions would eventually result in performance decrements as it affects glycaemic control. For the purpose of this chapter, glycaemic control is defined as the ability of the body to effectively regulate blood glucose levels and to remove glucose from the blood. Blood glucose levels of healthy

**TABLE 6.1**

**WHO (2006) Recommendations for the Diagnostic Criteria for Diabetes and Intermediate Hyperglycaemia**

| | Diabetes | Impaired Glucose Tolerance | Impaired Fasting Glucose | Normal Glucose Tolerance |
|---|---|---|---|---|
| Fasting plasma glucose | ≥7.0 mmol/L (126 mg/dL) | <7.0 mmol/L (126 mg/dL) and | 6.1–6.9 mmol/L (110–125 mg/dL) | <6.1 mmol/L (110 mg/dL) |
| 2 h plasma glucose[a] | or ≥11.1 mmol/L (200 mg/dL) | ≥7.8 and <11.1 mmol/L (140 and 200 mg/dL) | and (if measured) <7.8 mmol/L (140 mg/dL) | and <7.8 mmol/L (140 mg/dL) |

[a] Venous plasma glucose 2 h after ingestion of 75 g oral glucose load. If 2 h plasma glucose is not measured, status is uncertain as diabetes or IGT cannot be excluded.

individuals respond to glucose ingestion by rising for roughly half an hour and then returning to near baseline measures within 2 h, whereas in individuals with poor glucose control, blood glucose levels commonly peak quickly and then fall more slowly. Conditions in which glycaemic control is severely compromised are diabetes, impaired glucose tolerance (IGT), and impaired fasting glucose (IFG). The clinical criteria as defined by the World Health Organization (WHO) for these conditions are shown in Table 6.1.

Impairments in glucose and insulin regulation lead to increases in plasma glucose levels (see Table 6.1) but decreased glucose utilisation due to insulin resistance. Given the dependence of the brain on glucose for optimal functioning and the evidence showing that acute glucose administration can influence cognitive function, it is not surprising that impaired glycaemic control may contribute to cognitive impairments (see Lamport et al., 2009, for a review of the literature).

Cognitive impairments were indeed one of the earliest recognised neurological complications associated with diabetes (Miles and Root, 1922). To date, numerous studies have compared cognitive functioning in diabetic patients with nondiabetic controls (Brands et al., 2005). Although these studies differed widely with respect to patient characteristics (age and duration of type of diabetes) and cognitive tests used, the majority of these studies demonstrated cognitive impairments in this population which included decreased performance on various attention and memory tasks (Awad et al., 2004; Brands et al., 2004; Tun et al., 1990; Lamport et al., 2013; van den Berg et al., 2009). Tun et al. (1990) argued that performance of complex cognitive tasks appear to be more impaired, whereas performance of less demanding tasks seems to be comparable to controls. This pattern parallels the cognitive changes of normal ageing, where age differences are insignificant on less demanding immediate memory tasks but more pronounced on secondary or long-term memory tasks (Perlmutter et al., 1984). Risk factors associated with cognitive complications in diabetes appear to be (1) degree of metabolic control (Meuter et al., 1980) and (2) repeated episodes of hypoglycaemia (Auer 1986). It is therefore not surprising that in children diagnosed with type 1 diabetes before age 10 years, cognitive complications are generally only observed if they have a history of hypoglycaemic seizures (Kaufman et al., 1999).

Poor metabolic control is not only a risk factor for cognitive performance in diabetic patients, as recent investigations have shown that subclinical changes in glucose tolerance can impact upon cognition (see Awad et al., 2004 and Lamport et al., 2009, for reviews). As mentioned earlier, impairments in glucose tolerance become a larger issue in middle age, and consequently, it is likely that the negative cognitive impact of abnormalities in glucose tolerance increases with age. Cognitive decline over the ageing process has been well documented, and it has been suggested that normal ageing may represent a condition in which there is greater vulnerability to disrupted glucose regulation (see, e.g. Gold & Stone, 1988). Indeed, evidence to support this hypothesis is provided by the finding that memory performance in elderly participants with poor glucose regulation is impaired relative to elderly participants with good glucose regulation (Craft et al., 1992, 1994; Hall et al., 1989; Messier et al., 2003). Moreover, age-related changes in glucose metabolism have been identified as a risk factor for Alzheimer's disease (Hoyer, 2000; Messier, 2004; Watson & Craft, 2004). Consistent with this notion is the finding that hyperglycaemia (induced through oral and intravenous glucose administration) can facilitate memory performance in Alzheimer's patients, at least in the early stages of the disease (Craft et al., 1998). Interestingly, alterations in blood glucose regulation seem to depend on the severity of the disease process. More specifically, high insulin levels are observable at the very early (very mild) stages and decline as dementia progresses. Moreover, memory facilitation can be achieved through glucose administration in the early stages and the degree of facilitation decreases at more advanced stages of the disease (Craft et al., 1993).

However, and perhaps more worryingly, performance decrements due to poor glucose regulation have also been reported in younger individuals (see Awad et al., 2004; Lamport et al., 2009, for reviews). For example, recent studies have shown that even in a healthy young student population, those with better glucose regulation (those who had the smallest blood glucose rise following glucose ingestion) perform better on tests of memory (Awad et al., 2002; Benton & Owens, 1998; Donohoe & Benton, 1999; Messier et al., 1999; Owen et al., 2013; Sünram-Lea et al., 2011), vigilance (Benton & Owens, 1998; Donohoe & Benton, 1999), planning (Donohoe and Benton, 1999) and dichotic listening (Parker & Benton, 1995) compared to those with poorer glucose regulation. In addition, glucose administration preferentially improved performance in those with poorer glucose regulation, and the effects are less likely to be observed in good glucose regulators in both old and young populations (Messier, 2004). This would suggest that glucose control or tolerance is associated with cognition throughout the lifespan. Overall there appears to be some evidence that glucoregulation may exert direct effects on cognitive function in that those with poor glucoregulation may demonstrate mild cognitive deficit compared with good glucoregulation. Furthermore, glucoregulation may modulate the glucose facilitation effect by attenuating deficits in those with poor glucoregulation. However, research in young adults is limited; furthermore, the methodologies for determining glucoregulatory control have been varied. Only a few studies have used a standardised oral glucose tolerance test (OGTT) for the evaluation of glucose tolerance in healthy young adults (e.g. Donohoe and Benton; 2000; Owen et al., 2013). The OGTT involves administration of a 75 g glucose load after a minimum 8 h fast and is the gold standard test for the diagnosis of diabetes mellitus (WHO, 1999). Moreover, the majority of studies have only assessed one specific measurement of glucose tolerance. There is currently no consensus as to which glucoregulatory index is the best predictor of cognitive performance in normoglycaemic samples, that is, populations with normal glucose tolerance as defined by the WHO. Several glucoregulatory indices have been previously evaluated for their relationship with cognitive performance in younger and older participants. These include fasting levels, peak glucose levels, recovery and evoked glucose to baseline levels and incremental area under the curve (AUC) (see Owen et al., 2013). At a younger age, the deficits associated with poor glucoregulation may be minimal and hard to detect; therefore, it is important to identify the most sensitive marker. A recent study in our laboratory found AUC, which takes baseline blood glucose levels into account (AUC with respect to ground; see Pruessner et al., 2003, for calculations), to be the best predictor of cognitive performance, whereas the most commonly used incremental AUC did not show a strong association (Owen et al., 2013). This suggests that overall circulating glucose levels may be an important factor in the assessment of glucoregulation in populations with normal glucose tolerance as defined by the WHO.

To summarise, there is a relatively large body of evidence demonstrating that cognitive decline accompanies certain metabolic health conditions such as type 2 diabetes. However there is less evidence for the potential modification of cognitive function by glucose control in relatively 'normal' health young samples. The very fact that glucose is capable of moderating cognitive performance and that these effects are moderated by individual differences demonstrates how susceptible brain function is to even small metabolic fluctuations. In health terms and for diagnostic purposes, diseases such as diabetes are categorised by whether an individual's glucoregulation falls between various ranges and cut-off points. However, these disease states are progressive and thus it seems important to think of our metabolic profile in terms of a continuum rather than whether an individual fits within diagnostic ranges, particularly since these disease states are preventable. Finding that subclinical impairments can result in impairments suggests that WHO criteria appear to be less suitable to predict cognition. These diagnostic glucose concentration thresholds were derived from estimates of the level at which they are associated with an increased risk of disease, including cardiovascular and retinal complications, but appear to lack sensitivity in terms of the cognitive effects of impairments in glycaemic control. This highlights the need to re-evaluate what is considered healthy blood glucose levels and consider the role of higher than normal blood glucose levels as a risk factor for neural health and cognition.

## 6.8  CONCLUSION AND NUTRITIONAL RECOMMENDATIONS

In terms of nutritional recommendations, based on the evidence in the preceding text, it is clear that avoiding peaks and troughs in glucose availability is key to optimal cognitive performance. Administration of a glucose load does not represent a viable strategy over any prolonged time frame since consistently elevated blood glucose leads to insulin resistance. Diets that are rich in refined/simple carbohydrates also lead to high blood glucose. As we saw earlier, following ingestion of low-GI and/or low-GL food, there is a relatively smaller rise in blood glucose followed by more stable blood glucose concentration. Nutritional compounds that alter the rate of carbohydrate degradation during digestion and consequently affect regulation of postprandial blood glucose and insulin levels are, for example, fibres and proteins. A lowering of glycaemic response has been found when purified extracts of fibre are added to a test food in sufficient quantity (Doi et al., 1979; Jenkins et al., 1976; Tappy et al., 1996; Wolever et al., 1991). Moreover, high-fibre diets have been shown to decrease postprandial blood glucose levels (Post et al., 2012), improve glycaemic control in diabetic populations and decrease the risk of type 2 diabetes (Eshak et al., 2010; Lattimer & Haub, 2010; Papathanasopoulos & Camilleri, 2010; Sierra et al., 2002). Similarly, dietary proteins have been found to have positive effects on insulin production in populations with normal glucose metabolisms as well as type 2 diabetes (Frid et al., 2005; Nilsson et al., 2004; Östman et al., 2001). Another factor that appears to be important is the amount and the type of fat consumed. Evidence suggests that the risk of type 2 diabetes is associated with a high *trans* fatty acid intake and a low poly-unsaturated to saturated fat intake ratio (Manco et al., 2004). There are reports stating that saturated and trans fatty acids increase insulin resistance, whereas poly-unsaturated fats decrease resistance and offer protection against disease (see Martins et al., 2006). Consequently, diets high in saturated fats or trans fats should be avoided as they are likely to interfere with glucose tolerance and insulin sensitivity.

In conclusion, a habitual diet that secures optimal glucose delivery to the brain in the fed and fasting states should be most advantageous for the maintenance of cognitive function. This can be achieved by adhering to a low saturated fat and low-GL diet, especially when combined with sufficient physical exercise, which has also been shown to significantly reduce the risk of developing impairments in glucose metabolism (see, e.g. Goodyear & Kahn, 1998). This combination of diet and exercise has been demonstrated to have cognitive and metabolic benefits (improved glucose and insulin metabolism) in adults with type 2 diabetes and IGT (Watson et al., 2006; Yamamoto et al., 2009). Dietary lifestyle changes can have a positive impact throughout the lifespan and appear to not only reduce the risk of acquiring cognitive impairments but can also attenuate existing impairments. For example, a recent study showed that a 4-week low saturated fat/low-GI diet resulted in improved memory performance and insulin metabolism in adults with amnestic mild cognitive impairment (Bayer-Carter et al., 2011).

## 6.9 LIMITATIONS AND FUTURE RESEARCH

There is some evidence suggesting that simple carbohydrates including glucose have an immediate effect on cognition: diets high in complex carbohydrates are associated with better cognitive function and a lower risk of cognitive impairments in the longer term. Acute administration of a glucose load has been shown to benefit cognitive performance. This can be advantageous in conditions where there is a need for fast 'fuel refill', for example, in situations of stress combined with physical performance (see, e.g. Sünram-Lea et al., 2012). However, the relationship between plasma glucose and cognitive performance follows an inverted U-shaped dose–response curve, with low levels and high levels impairing cognition. Moreover, inducement of repeated hyperglycaemic conditions is likely to result in progressive glucoregulatory impairments with ensuing cognitive performance decrements. Therefore, administration of simple carbohydrates is not a viable nutritional recommendation for improving cognitive function in the long term. Although the evidence to date is promising, there is an urgent need for hypothesis-driven, randomised controlled trials that evaluate the role of different glycaemic manipulations on cognition. A recent review into the effects of carbohydrates on cognition in older individuals identified only one study that fulfilled these criteria (Ooi et al., 2011). The study that was included investigated the acute effects of a glucose drink (Gagnon et al., 2010), whereas studies investigating more complex carbohydrates were not included. Future research comparing the effects of different types of carbohydrates, with differing glycaemic profiles, is clearly needed. What limits our ability to draw strong conclusions from the findings of previous studies is the fact that they often differ widely with respect to subject characteristics and cognitive tests used. Future research needs to carefully consider conceptual and methodological factors including potential inter-individual differences, adequate selection of tests and control of extraneous (confounding) variables.

The rise in obesity, diabetes and metabolic syndrome in recent years highlights the need for targeted dietary and lifestyle strategies to promote healthy lifestyle and brain function across the lifespan and for future generations. The data indicate that modifiable lifestyle factors and most notably dietary changes may contribute significantly to optimal cognition across the lifespan. Consequently, the therapeutic effects of longer term dietary intervention may be a promising avenue of exploration. Lifestyle changes are difficult to execute and to maintain but present an exciting potential for optimising cognitive performance across the lifespan.

### TOP 4 SUMMARY POINTS FROM THE CHAPTER

- The brain is largely dependent on a steady supply of glucose for optimal performance.
- Acute administration of a glucose load has some short-term benefits on memory and demanding cognitive tasks, but in the long term, a more stable blood glucose profile seems to be more beneficial.
- The mechanisms enabling increased peripheral and/or central glucose availability to influence cognitive processes are unclear. They are likely to include provision of additional metabolic fuel (ATP), neurotransmitter synthesis and insulin signalling, as well as the possible involvement of peripheral mechanisms.
- Cognitive decline accompanies certain metabolic health conditions such as type 2 diabetes, but non-clinical impairments in glucose regulation have also been shown to affect cognition.

## RECOMMENDATIONS

- Acute administration of a glucose load has been shown to benefit cognitive performance. This can be advantageous in conditions where there is a need for fast 'fuel refill'; however, it does not represent a viable long-term strategy to improve cognition as this can lead to impairments in glucose control (hyperglycaemia and insulin resistance).
- A habitual diet that secures optimal glucose delivery to the brain should be most advantageous for optimal cognitive performance and maintenance of cognitive function across the lifespan.
- This can be achieved by consumption of foods rich in fibres and with a low GI and reduction in intake of saturated fats or trans fats as they are likely to interfere with glucose tolerance and insulin sensitivity.
- Data suggest that it is never too late for dietary changes to confer cognitive benefits.

## WHERE TO FROM HERE?

- The rise in obesity, diabetes and metabolic syndrome highlights the need for targeted dietary and lifestyle strategies to promote healthy lifestyle and brain function across the lifespan
- The data indicate that modifiable lifestyle factors, and most notably dietary changes, may contribute significantly to optimal cognition across the lifespan.
- Although the evidence to date is promising, it is insufficient to allow firm and evidence-based nutritional recommendations.
- There is an urgent need for hypothesis-driven, randomised controlled trials that evaluate the role of different glycaemic manipulations on cognition.

## REFERENCES

Aggleton, J. P., & Brown, W. B. (1999). Episodic memory, amnesia and the hippocampal-anterior thalamic axis. *Behavioral and Brain Sciences, 22*, 425–486.

Auer, R. N. (1986). Progress review: Hypoglycemic brain damage. *Stroke, 17*(4), 699–708.

Awad, N., Gagnon, M., Desrochers, A., Tsiakas, M., & Messier, C. (2002). Impact of peripheral glucoregulation on memory. *Behavioral Neuroscience, 116*(4), 691–702.

Awad, N., Gagnon, M., & Messier, C. (2004). The relationship between impaired glucose tolerance, type 2 diabetes, and cognitive function. *Journal of Clinical and Experimental Neuropsychology, 26*(8), 1044–1080.

Bayer-Carter, J. L., Green, P. S., Montine, T. J., VanFossen, B., Baker, L. D., Watson, G. S., ... Craft, S. (2011). Diet intervention and cerebrospinal fluid biomarkers in amnestic mild cognitive impairment. *Archives of Neurology, 68*(6), 743–752.

Benton, D., & Jarvis, M. (2007). The role of breakfast and a mid-morning snack on the ability of children to concentrate at school. *Physiology and Behavior, 90,* 382–385.

Benton, D., Maconie, A., & Williams, C. (2007). The influence of the glycaemic load of breakfast on the behaviour of children in school. *Physiology & Behavior, 92,* 717–724.

Benton, D., Owens, D. S., & Parker, P. Y. (1994). Blood glucose influences memory and attention in young adults. *Neuropsychologia, 32*(5), 595–607.

Benton, D., & Parker, P. Y. (1998). Breakfast, blood glucose and cognition. *The American Journal of Clinical Nutrition, 67*(suppl), 772S–778S.

Benton, D., Ruffin, M. P., Lassel, T., Nabb, S., Messaoudi, M., Vinoy, S., ... Lang, V. (2003). The delivery rate of dietary carbohydrates affects cognitive performance in both rats and humans. *Psychopharmacology, 166,* 86–90.

Brands, A. M., Biessels, G. J., de Haan, E. H., Kappelle, L. J., Kessels, R. P. (2005). The effects of type 1 diabetes on cognitive performance: A meta-analysis. *Diabetes Care, 28*(3) 726–735.

Brands, A. M. A., Kessels, R. P. C., de Haan, G. H. F., Kappelle, L. J., & Jan Biessels, G. (2004). Cerebral dysfunction in type 1 diabetics: effects of insulin, vascular risk factors and blood-glucose levels. *European Journal of Pharmacology, 490*(1–3), 159–168.

Caprio, S., Plewe, G., Diamond, M. P., Simonson, D. C., Boulware, S. D., Sherwin, R. S., & Tamborlane, W. V. (1989). Increased insulin secretion in puberty: A compensatory response to reductions in insulin sensitivity. *The Journal of Pediatrics, 114*(6), 963–967.

Caravas, J., & Wildman, D. E. (2014). A genetic perspective on glucose consumption in the cerebral cortex during human development. *Diabetes, Obesity and Metabolism, 16*(S1), 21–25.

Clark, K. B., Naritolu, D. K., Smith, D. C., Browning, R. A., & Jensen, R. A. (1999). Enhanced recognition memory following vagus nerve stimulation in human subjects. *Nature Neuroscience, 2,* 94–98.

Cooper, S. B., Bandelow, S., Nute, M. L., Morris, J. G., Nevill, M. E. (2012). Breakfast glycaemic index and cognitive function in adolescent school children. *British Journal of Nutrition, 107*(12), 1823–1832.

Craft, S., Dagogo-Jack, S. E., Wiethop, B. V., Murphy, C., Nevins, R. T., Fleischman, S., Rice, V., ... Cryer, P. E. (1993). Effects of hyperglycemia on memory and hormone levels in dementia of the Alzheimer type: A longitudinal study. *Behavioral Neuroscience, 207,* 926–940.

Craft, S., Murphy, C., & Wemstrom, J. (1994). Glucose effects on complex memory and non memory tasks: The influence of age, sex and glucoregulatory response, *22*(2), 95–105.

Craft, S., Peskind, E., Schwartz, M. W., Schellenberg, G. D., Raskind, M., & Porte, Jr. D. (1998). Cerebrospinal fluid and plasma insulin levels in Alzheimer's disease: relationship to severity of dementia and apolipo-protein ε genotype. *Neurology, 50,* 164–168.

Craft, S. Zallen, G., & Baker, L. D. (1992). Glucose and memory in mild senile dementia of the Alzheimer type. *Journal of Clinical and Experimental Neuropsychology, 14*(2), 253–267.

Dalsgaard, M. K., Madsen, F. F., Secher, N. H., Laursen, H., & Quistorff, B. (2007). High glycogen levels in the hippocampus of patients with epilepsy. *Journal of Cerebral Blood Flow and Metabolism, 27,* 1137–1141.

Doi, K., Matsuura, M., Kawara, A., & Baba, S. (1979). Treatment of diabetes with glucomannan (konjacmannan). *Lancet, 1,* 987–988.

Donohoe, R. T., & Benton, D. (1999). Declining blood glucose levels after a cognitively demanding task predict subsequent memory. *Nutritional Neuroscience, 2,* 413–424.

Donohoe R. T., & Benton, D. (2000). Glucose tolerance predicts performance on tests of memory and cognition. *Physiology and Behavior, 71*(3–4), 395–401.

Duarte, A. I., Moreira, P. I., & Oliveira, C. R. (2012). Insulin in central nervous system: More than just a peripheral hormone. *Journal of Aging Research, 2012.*

Dye, L., Gilsenan, M. B., Quadt, F., Martens, V. E. G., Bot, A., Lasikiewicz, N., Cambridge, D., Croden, F., & Lawton, C. (2010). Manipulation of glycemic responses with iso-maltulose in a milk-based drink does not affect cognitive performance in healthy adults. *Molecular Nutrition and Food Research, 54*(4), 506–515.

Evans, W. J., Meredith, C. N., Cannon, J. G., Dinarello, C. A., Frontera, W. R., Hughes, V. A., … Knuttgen, H. G. (1986). Metabolic changes following eccentric exercise in trained and untrained men. *Journal of Applied Physiology, 61,* 1864–1868.

Fairclough, S. H., & Houston, K. (2004). A metabolic measure of mental effort. *Biological Psychology, 66,* 177–190.

Fird, A. H., Nilsson, M., Holst, J. J., & Björck, I. M. E. (2005). Effect of whey on blood glu-cose and insulin responses to composite breakfast and lunch meals in type 2 diabetic subjects. *The American Journal if Clinical Nutrition, 82,* 1246–1253.

Frith, C. D., & Dolan, R. (1996). The role of the prefrontal cortex in higher cognitive func-tions. *Cognitive Brain Research, 5,* 175–181.

Fucetola, R., Newcomer, J. W., Craft, S., & Melson, A. K. (1999). Age-and dose-dependent glucose-induced increases in memory and attention in schizophrenia. *Psychiatry Research, 88*(1), 1–13.

Fuster, J. M. (2002). Frontal lobe and cognitive development. *Journal of Neurocytology, 31,* 373–385.

Gagnon, C., Greenwood, C. E., & Bherer, L. (2010). The acute effects of glucose ingestion on attentional control in fasting healthy older adults. *Psychopharmacology, 211,* 337–46.

Galliot, M. T., & Baumeister, R. F. (2007). The physiology of willpower: Linking blood glu-cose to self-control. *Personality and Social Psychology Review, 11*(4), 303–327.

Goodyear, L. J., & Kahn, B. B. (1998). Exercise, glucose transport, and insulin sensitivity. *Annual Review of Medicine, 49*(1), 235–261.

Gold, P. E. (1986). Glucose modulation of memory storage processing. *Behavioural and Neural Biology, 45,* 342–349.

Gold, P. E. (1991). An integrated memory regulation system: From blood to brain. In: R. C. A. Frederickson, J. L. McGaugh, & D. L. Felten (Eds.), *Peripheral signaling of the brain: role in neural-immune interactions and learning and memory* (pp. 391–419). Toronto, Ontario, Canada: Hogrefe & Huber.

Gold, P. E., & McGaugh, J. L. (1975). A single-trace, two-process view of memory storage processes. In: D. Deutsch & A. J. Deutsch, (Eds.), *Short term memory* (pp. 355–390). New York: Academic Press.

Gold, P. E. & Stone, W. S. (1988). Neuroendocrine factors in age-related memory dysfunc-tions: Studies in animals and humans. *Neurobiology of Aging, 9,* 709–717.

Guyton, A. C. (1991). *Textbook of medical physiology* (8th ed.). Philadelphia, PA: W. B. Saunders Company.

Hafermann, G. (1955). Schulmüdigkeit und Blutzuckerverhalten. *Öffentlicher Gesundheitsdienst, 17,* 1.

Hall, J. L., Gonder-Frederick, L. A., Chewning, W. W., Silveira, J., & Gold, P. E. (1989). Glucose enhancement of performance on memory tests in young and aged humans. *Neuropsychologia, 27*(9), 1129–1138.

Harry, T., & Chugani, M. D. (1998). A critical period of brain development: Studies of cerebral glucose utilization with PET. *Preventive Medicine, 27*(2) 184–188.

Haymond, M. W. (1989). Hypoglycemia in infants and children. *Endocrinology and Metabolism Clinics of North America, 18*(1), 211–252.

Haymond, M. W., & Sunehag, A. (1999). Controlling the sugar bowl. Regulation of glucose homeostasis in children. *Endocrinology and Metabolism Clinics of North America, 28,* 663–694.

Holmes, C.S., Hayford, J.T., Gonzalez, J.L., & Weydert, J.A. (1983). A survey of cognitive functioning at different glucose levels in diabetic persons. *Diabetes Care, 6:* 180–185.

Hoyer, S. (2000). Brain glucose and energy metabolism abnormalities in sporadic Alzheimer disease. Causes and consequences: an update. *Experimental Gerontology, 3*(9–10), 1363–1372.

Hoyer, S. (2003). Memory function and brain glucose metabolism. *Pharmacopsychiatry, 36*(1), S62–S67.

Hoyland, A., Dye, L., & Lawton, C. L. (2009). A systematic review of the effect of breakfast on the cognitive performance of children and adolescents. *Nutrition Research Reviews, 22*(2), 220–243.

Hoyland, A., Lawton, C., & Dye, L. (2008). Acute effects of macronutrient manipulations on cognitive test performance in healthy young adults: A systematic research review. *Neuroscience & Biobehavioral Reviews, 32*, 72–85.

Ingwersen, J., Defeyter, M. A., Kennedy, D. O., Wesnes, K. A., & Scholey, A. B. (2007). A low glycaemic index breakfast cereal preferentially prevents children's cognitive performance from declining throughout the morning. *Appetite, 49*(1), 240–244.

Iversen, L. I. (1979). The chemistry of the brain. In: D. Flanagan, F. Bello, & P. Morrison (Eds.), *The brain. A scientific American book* (pp. 70–83). San Francisco, CA: W. H. Freeman and Company.

Jenkins, D. J., Leeds, A. R., Wolever, T. S., Goff, D., George, K., Alberti, M. M., … Hockaday, R. (1976). Unabsorbable carbohydrates and diabetes: Decreased post-prandial hyperglycaemia. *Lancet, 308*(7978), 172–174.

Jones, K. L., Horowitz, M., & Wishart, J. M. (1995). Relationships between gastric-emptying, intragastric meal distribution and blood-glucose concentrations in diabetes-mellitus. *Journal of Nuclear Medicine, 36*(12), 2220–2228.

Kaplan, R. J., Greenwood, C. E., Winocur, G., & Wolever, T. M. S. (2000). Cognitive performance is associated with glucose regulation in healthy elderly persons and can be enhanced with glucose and dietary carbohydrates. *The American Journal of Clinical Nutrition, 72*(3), 825–836.

Kaufman, F. R., Epport, K., Engilman, R., & Halvorson, M. (1999). Neurocognitive functioning in children diagnosed with diabetes before age 10 yrs. *Journal of Diabetes and its Complications, 13*(1), 21–38.

Kauppinen, R., McMahon, H., & Nicholls, D. (1988). $Ca^{2+}$-dependent and $Ca^{2+}$-independent glutamate release, energy status and cytosolic free $Ca^{2+}$ concentration in isolated nerve terminals following metabolic inhibition: Possible relevance to hypoglycaemia and anoxia. *Neuroscience, 27*, 175–182.

Kennedy, D., & Scholey, A. (2000). Glucose administration, heart rate and cognitive performance: Effects of increasing mental effort. *Psychopharmacology, 149*, 63–71.

Lamport, D. J., Dye, L., Mansfield, M. W., & Lawton, C. L. (2013). Acute glycaemic load breakfast manipulations do not attenuate cognitive impairments in adults with type 2 diabetes. *Clinical Nutrition, 32*(2), 265–272.

Lamport, D. J., Lawton, C. L., Mansfield, M. W., & Dye, L. (2009). Impairments in glucose tolerance can have a negative impact on cognitive function: A systematic research review. *Neuroscience & Biobehavioral Reviews, 33*(3), 394–413.

Lamport, D. J., Lawton, C. L., Mansfield, M. W., Moulin, C. A., & Dye, L. (2014). Type 2 diabetes and impaired glucose tolerance are associated with word memory source monitoring recollection deficits but not simple recognition familiarity deficits following water, low glycaemic load, and high glycaemic load breakfasts. *Physiology & Behavior, 124*, 54–60.

Lattimer, L., & Haub, M. (2010). Effects of dietary fiber and its components on metabolic health. *Nutrients, 2*(12), 1266–1289.

Lehninger, A. L., Nelson, D. L., & Cox, M. M. (2005). *Lehninger principles of biochemistry*. New York: W. H. Freeman and Company.

Lund-Andersen, H. (1979). Transport of glucose from blood to brain. *Physiological Reviews, 59*(2), 305–352.

Madsen, P. L., Hasselbalch, S. G., Hagemann, L. P., Olsen, K. S., Bulow, J., Holm S., ... Lassen, N. A. (1995). Persistent resetting of the cerebral oxygen/glucose uptake ratio by brain activation: Evidence obtained with the Kety-Schmidt technique. *Journal of Cerebral Blood Flow & Metabolism, 15*, 485–491.

Mahoney, C. R., Taylor, H. A., Kanarck, R. B., & Samuel, P. (2005). Effect of breakfast composition on cognitive processes in elementary school children. *Physiology and Behavior, 85*(5), 635–645.

Manco, M., Menotti, C., & Mingrone, G. (2004). Effects of dietary fatty acids on insulin sensitivity and secretion. *Diabetes, Obesity and Metabolism, 6*(6), 402–413.

Martin, P. Y., & Benton, D. (1999). The influence of a glucose drink on a demanding working memory task. *Physiology and Behavior, 67*(1), 69–74.

Martins, I. J., Hone, E., Foster, J. K., Sünram-Lea, S. I., Gnjec, A., Nolan, D., ... Martins, R. N. (2006). Apolipoprotein E, cholesterol metabolism, diabetes, and the convergence of risk factors for Alzheimer's disease and cardiovascular. *Molecular Psychiatry, 11*(8), 721–736.

McEwen, B. S., & Reagan, L. P. (2004). Glucose transporter expression in the central nervous system: relationship to synaptic function. *European Journal of Pharmacology, 490*(1–3), 13–24.

McIlwain, H. (1959). *Biochemistry and the Central Nervous System* (2nd ed.). London, U.K.: J & A Churchill.

McNay, E. C., Fries, T. M., & Gold, P. E. (2000). Decreases in rat extracellular hippocampal glucose concentration associated with cognitive demand during a spatial task. *Proceedings of the National Academy of Sciences, 97*(6), 2881–2885.

McNay, E. C., McCarty, R. C., & Gold, P. E. (2001). Fluctuations in brain glucose concentration during behavioral testing: Dissociations between brain areas and between brain and blood. *Neurobiology of Learning and Memory, 75*(3), 325–337.

Melanson, K. J., Greenberg, A. S., Ludwig, D. S., Saltzman, E., Dallal, G. E., & Roberts, S. B. (1998). Blood glucose and hormonal responses to small and large meals in healthy young and older women. *The Journals of Gerontology Biological Sciences & Medical Sciences Series A, 53*, B299–B305.

Messier, C. (2004). Glucose improvement of memory: A review. *European Journal of Pharmacology, 490*(1), 33–57.

Messier, C., Desrochers, A., Gagnon, M (1999). Effects of glucose, glucose regulation and word imagery value on human memory. *Behavioral Neuroscience, 113*(3), 431–438.

Messier, C., Gagnon, M., & Knott, V. (1997). Effect of glucose and peripheral glucose regulation on memory in the elderly. *Neurobiology of Aging, 18*(3), 297–304.

Messier, C., Tsiakas, M., Gagnon, M., Desrochers, A., & Awad, N. (2003). Effect of age and glucoregulation on cognitive performance. *Neurobiology of Aging, 24*(7), 985–1003.

Messier, C., & White, N. M. (1987). Memory improvement by glucose, fructose and two glucose analogy: A possible effect on peripheral glucose transport. *Behavioral and Neural Biology, 48*(1), 104–127.

Meuter, F., Thomas, W., Gruneklee, D., Gries, F. A., & Lohman, R. (1980). Psychometric evaluation of performance in diabetes. *Hormone and Metabolic Research, 9*, 9–17.

Micha, R., Rogers, P. J., & Nelson, M. (2010). The glycaemic potency of breakfast and cognitive function in school children. *European Journal of Clinical Nutrition, 64*, 948–957.

Miles, W. R., & Root, H. F. (1922). Psychologic tests applied to diabetic patients. *Archives of Internal Medicine, 30*(6), 767–777.

Miller, E. K., & Wallis, J. D. (2009). Executive function and higher-order cognition: Definition and neural substrates. *Encyclopedia of Neuroscience, 4*, 99–104.

Moeller, J. R., Ishikawa, T., Dhawan, V., Spetsieris, P., Mandel, F., Al-Expander, G. E., ... Eidelberg, D. (1996). The metabolic topography of normal aging. *Journal of Cerebral Blood Flow & Metabolism, 16*, 385–398.

Nelson, D. L., & Cox, M. M. (2005). *Lehninger principles of biochemistry* (4th ed.). New York: W. H. Freeman and Company.

Newcomer, J. W., Craft, S., Fucetola, R., Moldin, S. O., Selke, G., Paras, L., & Miller, R. (1999). Glucose induced increase in memory performance in patients with schizophrenia. *Shizophrenia Bulletin, 25*(2), 321–335.

Nilsson, A., Radeborg, K., & Björck, I. (2009). Effects of differences in postprandial glycaemia on cognitive functions in healthy middle-aged subjects. *European Journal of Clinical Nutrition, 63,* 113–120.

Nilsson, A., Radeborg, K., & Björck, I. (2012). Effects on cognitive performance of modulating the postprandial blood glucose profile at breakfast. *European Journal of Clinical Nutrition, 66,* 1039–1043.

Nilsson, M., Stenberg, M., Frid, A. H., Holst, J. J., & Björck, I. M. E. (2004). Glycemia and insulinemia in healthy subjects after lactose equivalent meals of milk and other food proteins: the role of plasma amino acids and incretins. *The American Journal of Clinical Nutrition, 80,* 1246–1253.

Ooi, C. P., Loke, S. C., Yassin, Z., & Hamid, T. A. (2011). Carbohydrates for improving the cognitive performance of independent-living older adults with normal cognition or mild cognitive impairment. *Cochrane Database of Systematic Reviews, 13*(4), 1–31. doi: 10.1002/14651858.CD007220.pub2.

Östman, E. M., Elmståhl, H. G. M. L., & Björck, M. E. (2001). Inconsistency between glycemic and insulinemic responses to regular and fermented milk products. *The American Journal of Clinical Nutrition, 74*(1), 96–100.

Owen, L., Scholey, A., Finnegan, Y., & Sünram-Lea, S. I. (2013). Response variability to glucose facilitation of cognitive enhancement. *British Journal of Nutrition, 110*(10), 1873–1884.

Owen, L., & Sünram-Lea, S. I. (2011). Metabolic agents that enhance ATP can improve cognitive functioning: A review of the evidence for glucose, oxygen, pyruvate, creatine, and L-carnitine. *Nutrients, 3*(8), 735–755.

Papanikolaou, Y., Palmer, H., Binns, M. A., Jenkins, D. J. A. & Greenwood, C. E. (2006). Better cognitive performance following a low-glycaemic-index compared with a high-glycaemic-index carbohydrate meal in adults with type 2 diabetes. *Diabetologia, 49*(5), 855–862.

Papathanasopoulos, A., & Camilleri, M. (2010). Dietary fiber supplements: Effects in obesity and metabolic syndrome and relationship to gastrointestinal functions. *Gastroenterology, 138*(1), 65–72.

Parker, P. Y., & Benton, D. (1995). Blood glucose levels selectively influence memory for word lists dichotically presented to the right ear. *Neuropsychologia, 33*(7), 843–854.

Perlmutter, L. C., Hakami, M. K., Hodgson-Harrington, C., Ginsberg, J., Katz, J., Singer, D. E., & Nathan, D. M. (1984). Decreased cognitive function in aging non-insulin dependent diabetic patients. *American Journal of Medicine, 77*(6), 1043–1048.

Peters, A., Schweiger, U., Pellerin, L., Hubold, C., Oltmanns, K. M., Conrad, M., Schultes, B., Born, J., & Fehm, H. L. (2004). The selfish brain: competition for energy resources. *Neuroscience and Biobehavioral Reviews, 28,* 143–180.

Post, R. E., Mainous, A. G., King, D. E., & Simpson, K. N. (2012). Dietary fiber for the treatment of type 2 diabetes mellitus: A meta-analysis. *The Journal of the American Board of Family Medicine, 25*(1), 16–23.

Pruessner, J. C., Kirschbaum, C., Meinlschmid, G., & Hellhammer, D. H. (2003). Two formulas for computation of the area under the curve represent measures of total hormone concentration versus time-dependent change. *Psychoneuroendocrinology, 28*(7), 916–931.

Purves, W. K., Sadava, D., Orians, G. H., & Heller, H. C. (2001). *Life: The science of biology* (6th ed.). Sunderland, MA: Sinauer Associates, Inc.

Raichle, M. E., & Mintun, M. A. (2006). Brain work and brain imaging. *Annual Review of Neuroscience, 29,* 449–476.

Reivich, M., Gur, R., & Alavi, A. (1983). Positron emission tomographic studies of sensory stimuli, cognitive processes and anxiety. *Human Neurobiology, 2*, 25–33.

Sandberg, A., Lansner, A., & Petersson, K.M. (2001). Selective enhancement of recall through plasticity modulation in an autoassociative memory. *Neurocomputing, 38–40*, 867–873.

Savage, M. O., Smith, C. P., Dunger, D. B., Gale, E. A., Holly, J. M., & Preece, M. A. (1992). Insulin and growth factors adaptation to normal puberty. *Hormonal Research, 37*(3), 70–73.

Scholey, A. B., Harper, S., & Kennedy, D. O. (2001). Cognitive demand and blood glucose. *Physiology & Behavior, 73*, 585–592.

Seitz, R. J., & Roland, P. E. (1992). Vibratory stimulation increases and decreases the regional cerebral blood flow and oxidative metabolism: A positron emission tomography (PET) study. *Acta Neurologica Scandinavica, 86*(1), 60–67.

Sierra, M., Garcia, J. J., Fernandez, N., Diez, M. J., & Calle, A. P. (2002). Therapeutic effects of psyllium in type 2 diabetic patients. *European Journal of Clinical Nutrition, 56*(9), 830–842.

Smith, M. A., & Foster, J. K. (2008). The impact of a high versus a low glycaemic index breakfast cereal meal on verbal episodic memory in healthy adolescents. *Nutritional Neuroscience, 11*(5), 219–227.

Smith, M. A., Riby, L. M., Eekelen, J. A., & Foster, J. K. (2011). Glucose enhancement of human memory: A comprehensive research review of the glucose memory facilitation effect. *Neuroscience & Biobehavioral Reviews, 35*(3), 770–783.

Sokoloff, L. (1999). Energetics of functional activation in neural tissues. *Neurochemical Research, 24*(2), 321–329.

Sünram-Lea, S. I., Foster, J. K., Durlach, P., & Perez, C. (2001). Glucose facilitation of cognitive performance in healthy young adults: Examination of the influence of fast-duration, time of day and pre-consumption plasma glucose levels. *Psychopharmacology, 157*(1), 46–54.

Sünram-Lea, S. I., Foster, J. K., Durlach, P. & Perez, C. (2002a). Investigation into the significance of task difficulty and divided allocation of resources on the glucose memory facilitation effect. *Psychopharmacology, 160*(4), 387–397.

Sünram-Lea, S. I., Foster, J. K., Durlach, P., & Perez, C. (2002b). The effect of retrograde and anterograde glucose administration on memory performance in healthy young adults. *Behavioural Brain Research, 134*(1–2), 505–516.

Sünram-Lea, S. I., Owen, L., Finnegan, Y., & Hu, H. (2011). Dose–response investigation into glucose facilitation of memory performance and mood in healthy young adults. *Journal of Psychopharmacology, 25*(8), 1076–1087.

Sünram-Lea, S. I., Owen-Lynch, J., Robinson, S. J., Jones, E., & Hu, H. (2012). The effect of energy drinks on cortisol levels. *Psychopharmacology, 219*(1), 83-97.

Tappy, L., Gugolz, E., & Wursch, P. (1996). Effects of breakfast cereals containing various amounts of beta-glucan fibers on plasma glucose and insulin responses in NIDDM subjects. *Diabetes Care, 19*, 831–834.

Thompson, R. T. (1967). *Foundations of physiological psychology*. New York: Harper International.

Tun, P. A., Nathan, D. M., & Perlmuter, L. C. (1990). Cognitive and affective disorders in elderly diabetics. *Clinical Geriatric Medicine, 6*(4), 731–746

van den Berg, E., Kloppenborg, R. P., Kessels, R. P., Kappelle, L. J., & Biessels, G. J. (2009). Type 2 diabetes mellitus, hypertension, dyslipidemia and obesity: A systematic comparison of their impact on cognition. *Biochimica et Biophysica Acta (BBA)-Molecular Basis of Disease, 1792*(5), 470–481.

Watson, G., & Craft, S. (2004). Modulation of memory by insulin and glucose: Neuropsychological observations in Alzheimer's disease. *European Journal of Pharmacology, 490*(1), 97–113.

Watson, G. S., Reger, M. A., Baker, L. D., McNeely, M. J., Fujimoto, W. Y., Kahn, S. E., ...
    & Craft, S. (2006). Effects of exercise and nutrition on memory in Japanese Americans
    with impaired glucose tolerance. *Diabetes care, 29*(1), 135–136.
Wesnes, K. A., Pincock, C., Richardson, D., Helm, G., & Hails, S. (2003). Breakfast reduces
    declines in attention and memory over the morning in schoolchildren. *Appetite, 41*(3),
    329–331.
White, N. M. (1991). Peripheral and central memory enhancing actions of glucose. In:
    Frederickson, R. C. A., McGaugh, J. L., & Felton, D. L. (Eds.), *Peripheral signalling of
    the brain: role on neural-immune interactions and learning and memory* (pp. 421–441).
    Hognefe and Humber, Toronto.
WHO, (1999). Definition, diagnosis and classification of diabetes mellitus and its complica-
    tions. Report of a WHO Consultation, Part 1: Diagnosis and Classification of Diabetes
    Mellitus, Geneva 1999, World Health Organization.
Wiesinger, H., Hamprecht, B., & Dringen, R. (1997). Metabolic pathways for glucose in astro-
    cytes. *Glia, 21*, 22–34.
Wolever, T. M., Vuksan, V., Eshuis, H., Spadafora, P., Peterson, R. D., Chao, E. S., ... Jenkins,
    D. J. (1991). Effect of method of administration of psyllium on glycaemic response
    and carbohydrate digestibility. *Journal of the American College of Nutrition, 10*(4),
    364–371.
Yamamoto, N., Yamanaka, G., Takasugi, E., Ishikawa, M., Yamanaka, T., Murakarmi, S.,
    Hanafusa, T., Matsubayashi, K., & Otsuka, K. (2009). Lifestyle intervention reversed
    cognitive function in aged people with diabetes mellitus: Two-year follow up. *Diabetes
    Research and Clinical Practice, 85*(3), 343–346.
Zhao, W-Q., & Alkon, D. L. (2001). Role of insulin and insulin receptor in learning and mem-
    ory. *Molecular and Cellular Endocrinology, 177*(1–2), 125–134.

# 7 Role of Long-Chain Omega-3 Fatty Acids in Cognitive and Emotional Development

*Robert K. McNamara and Christina J. Valentine*

## CONTENTS

## SUMMARY

Long-chain omega-3 ($n - 3$) fatty acids including docosahexaenoic acid (DHA) have anti-inflammatory, neurotrophic and neuroprotective properties. DHA accumulates in the brain during critical periods of perinatal cortical expansion and maturation. Reductions in perinatal rat brain DHA accrual are associated with delays in neuronal migration and arborization, synaptic pathology as well as neurocognitive deficits and elevated behavioural indices of aggression and depression. Primates raised on an $n - 3$ fatty acid–deficient diet exhibit hyperactivity, impairments in visual attention and functional connectivity deficits within frontal cortical networks. Preterm delivery is associated with robust deficits in fetal cortical DHA accrual and reduced connectivity within cortical networks. Children and adolescents born preterm are at increased risk for developing psychiatric disorders associated with functional connectivity deficits within frontal cortical networks. Moreover, youth with cognitive and mood disorders exhibit reversible DHA deficits associated with symptom severity. Maternal and infant formula DHA supplementation may be associated with better neurocognitive outcomes in healthy developing children though this remains controversial. While these associations provide general support for a role of DHA in the maturation of cortical networks mediating cognitive and emotional processes, additional prospective longitudinal studies are needed to inform optimal intake levels during critical periods of neurodevelopment.

## 7.1  INTRODUCTION

Long-chain omega-3 (LC$n$ − 3) fatty acids, including eicosapentaenoic acid (EPA; 20:5$n$ − 3) and DHA (22:6$n$ − 3), are 'essential' nutrients because mammals are completely dependent on dietary sources to procure and maintain adequate concentrations in peripheral and central tissues. The principle LC$n$ − 3 fatty acid found in mammalian brain grey matter is DHA, which represents approximately 15% of total fatty acid composition which varies by age and brain region (Carver et al., 2001; Diau et al., 2005; McNamara et al., 2008a; Xiao et al., 2005). The precursors of DHA including α-linolenic acid (ALA; 18:3$n$ − 3) and EPA (20:5$n$ − 3) comprise <1% of total brain fatty acid composition due in part to rapid oxidization (Chen et al., 2013). The rate-limiting enzymes regulating biosynthesis of DHA and EPA from ALA include delta-6 desaturase (delta6-desaturase, *FADS2*) and delta-5 desaturase (delta5-desaturase, *FADS1*) (Reardon & Brenna, 2013), and the final synthesis of DHA additionally requires β-oxidation within peroxisomes (Wanders, 2013). However, the limited capacity of humans to biosynthesise DHA from ALA and EPA (Brenna et al., 2009) suggests that the accrual and maintenance of optimal DHA levels in cortical membranes require intake of preformed DHA from fish, fish oil (FO) supplements or algal sources.

Human childhood and adolescence are critical developmental periods associated with the establishment of structural and functional connectivity between frontal lobe regions that mediate attention and executive function with limbic structures that mediate emotion and mood (Giedd et al., 1999, 2009; Paus et al., 1999; Sowell et al., 1999). During this period, DHA concentrations in the frontal cortex may play an important role in cortical circuit maturational processes. This is supported in part by findings that psychiatric disorders characterized by frontal circuit maturation deficits and cognitive and emotional dysregulation are associated with robust DHA deficits. Moreover, emerging neuroimaging evidence suggests that DHA status is positively correlated with frontal cortex structural and functional integrity in healthy subjects across the lifespan (McNamara, 2013b). Developing a more comprehensive understanding of the requirement for LC$n$ − 3 fatty acids including DHA during child and adolescent brain development could therefore have significant implications for informing recommendations for optimal intake during critical periods of neurodevelopment.

Over the past 30 years, evidence has emerged from both animal and clinical research that suggests that normal brain development requires optimal DHA levels. This chapter provides an overview of evidence from rodent, non-human primate and human studies investigating the role of LC$n$ − 3 fatty acids in normal brain development. We additionally review evidence implicating DHA deficits in the pathophysiology of psychiatric disorders that initially emerge in childhood and adolescence including attention deficit/hyperactivity disorder (ADHD) and bipolar disorder.

## 7.2  RODENT NEURODEVELOPMENT

Animal studies have provided important insight into the role of dietary LC$n$ − 3 fatty acids in normal brain development. The advantage of animal feeding studies is the ability to systematically control a myriad of extraneous variables that frequently confound interpretation of clinical studies and permit invasive investigation of brain neurochemistry, neuroanatomy and gene expression. Rodents, unlike humans, are very efficient at biosynthesizing DHA from ALA, which is the sole source of $n$ − 3 fatty acids in rodent chow. Studies have typically utilized a 'perinatal' feeding paradigm in which female rats receive either ALA-fortified diet or ALA-free diet for some period (e.g. 2 months) prior to mating and during pregnancy and lactation, and offspring are maintained on the maternal diet post weaning into adulthood. This feeding paradigm leads to large (~70%) DHA deficits in frontal cortex membranes in adult offspring (McNamara et al., 2009a). Alternatively, the 'post-weaning' or 'peri-adolescent' deficiency model involves placing the offspring of mothers receiving an ALA-fortified diet on an ALA-free diet immediately following weaning into adulthood. This paradigm leads to moderate DHA deficits (~25%) in central membranes (Figure 7.1). Both the perinatal and post-weaning models lead to increases in the ratio of DHA to the LC$n$ − 6 fatty acid arachidonic acid (AA) (i.e. AA/DHA) as well as increases in the LC$n$ − 6 fatty acid docosapentaenoic acid (DPA; 22:5$n$ − 6). Other studies have investigated maternal and neonatal dietary FO supplementation during perinatal development, which increases (~10%) central greater membrane DHA levels compared with rats maintained on ALA-fortified diet (Chalon et al., 1998). Peri-adolescent dietary FO supplementation increases (~5%) central DHA levels compared with rats maintained on ALA-fortified diet (Figure 7.1).

In studies of female rats maintained on standard ALA-fortified chow, a positive association exists between ovarian hormones and blood and brain DHA composition (Childs et al., 2008; McNamara et al., 2009b). Moreover, low maternal dietary $n$ − 3 fatty acid composition and pregnancy interact to reduce maternal peripheral and central DHA composition (Levant et al., 2006a,b). During early perinatal rodent brain development, fetal cortical DHA concentrations increase during active periods of neurogenesis, neuroblast migration, neuronal differentiation and synaptogenesis (Green & Yavin, 1996). Moreover, the increase in frontal cortex DHA during the peri-adolescent period (Figure 7.1a) coincides with substantial (~50%) pruning of glutamatergic connections between the frontal cortex and amygdala (Cressman et al., 2010). In general, feeding studies have demonstrated that DHA positively regulates cortical neurogenesis (Beltz et al., 2003; Coti Bertrand et al., 2006; Kawakita et al., 2006), neuroblast migration (Yavin et al., 2009), neuronal differentiation and

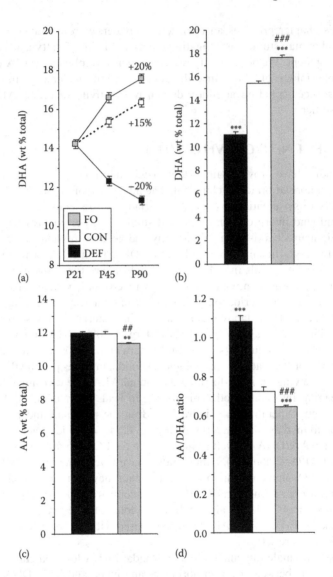

**FIGURE 7.1**   Effects of peri-adolescent dietary $n-3$ fatty acid intake on young adult rat frontal cortex DHA and AA compositions and the AA/DHA ratio. Rats were fed one of three diets during peri-adolescent development (P21–P90): (1) ALA ($18:3n-3$)-fortified diet (control [CON]), (2) ALA-free diet (deficient [DEF]) or (3) diet containing FO in place of ALA. During peri-adolescent development, frontal cortex DHA levels increase sharply in rats maintained on the CON (+15%) and FO (+20%) diets, and feeding the DEF diet leads to a sharp decline in DHA (−20%) (a). Young adult rats maintained on the DEF diet during peri-adolescent development exhibit 30% lower cortical DHA composition (b), and a 33% greater AA/DHA ratio (d), compared with controls. Rats maintained on the FO-fortified diet exhibit 15% greater frontal cortex DHA composition, 5% lower AA composition (c) and 15% lower AA/DHA ratio (d) compared with controls. These data demonstrate that dietary $n-3$ fatty acid intake during peri-adolescent development is an important determinant of frontal cortex DHA status in young adulthood.

arborization (Calderon & Kim, 2004), neurotrophic factor (NGF, BDNF) expression (Ikemoto et al., 2000; Rao et al., 2007) and nerve growth factor-induced neurite outgrowth and synaptogenesis (Cao et al., 2009; Ikemoto et al., 1997; Innis et al., 2001a; Martin & Bazan, 1992). However, maternal FO supplementation, as well as maternal $n - 3$ fatty acid deficiency, during pregnancy and lactation, has also been found to impair auditory brainstem responses in neonates which suggest slowed neural transmission (Church et al., 2008, 2009). These and other data suggest that there are optimal cortical DHA levels required for normal cortical synaptic maturation and functional connectivity.

In addition to neurotrophic effects, DHA and its bioactive metabolites are neuroprotective against a variety of insults associated with oxidative stress and lipid peroxidation in the fetal rat brain (Green et al., 2001; Yavin et al., 2002). In adult rodents DHA has been found to be neuroprotective against focal and global ischemia (Belayev et al., 2009; Blondeau et al., 2002), glutamate excitotoxicity (Blondeau et al., 2002; Hogyes et al., 2003; Ozyurt et al., 2007), traumatic brain injury (Wu et al., 2004) and chronic neuroinflammation (Orr et al., 2013). Increasing dietary LC$n - 3$ fatty acid status is also protective against inflammation- (Tuzun et al., 2012) and trauma-induced (Bailes & Mills, 2010) axonal white matter injury in adult rats and is protective against histopathological features in the experimental autoimmune encephalomyelinitis model of multiple sclerosis (Kong et al., 2011). Additionally, dietary-induced elevations in rodent brain DHA can prevent or attenuate neurodegenerative features associated with age-related cognitive decline (Calon & Cole, 2007). This body of evidence suggests that DHA has protective effects in the fetal and adult rat brain which may be mediated by anti-inflammatory and anti-oxidative mechanisms.

Perinatal $n - 3$ fatty acid deficiency is not associated with gross neuronal lamination abnormalities or neuronal loss in the adult rat cortex (Ahmad et al., 2002; Salem et al., 2001). However, perinatal $n - 3$ fatty acid deficiency is associated with reductions in hippocampal neuronal size (Ahmad et al., 2002) and reductions in hippocampal volume as well as lateral ventricle enlargement (Figure 7.2). Additionally, perinatal $n - 3$ fatty acid deficiency is associated with microstructural alterations in synaptic morphology (Yoshida et al., 1997; Zimmer et al., 2000a) and dysregulation in multiple neurotransmitter systems (Chalon, 2006). Within the brain DHA preferentially accumulates in synaptic membranes within phosphatidylethanolamine and phosphatidylserine phospholipids (Suzuki et al., 1997). Perinatal deficits in DHA accrual are associated with selective reductions in neuronal membrane phosphatidylserine concentrations (Hamilton et al., 2000), whereas perinatal FO supplementation increases phosphatidylserine concentrations (Chalon et al., 1998). Phosphatidylserine mediates the binding of several structural and signal transduction proteins that regulate synaptic transmission and structural plasticity, and reductions in synaptic membrane phosphatidylserine concentrations would be anticipated to lead to a general dysregulation in synaptic connectivity and function (McNamara et al., 2006). Because synaptic neurotransmission is critical for the establishment of cortical networks that regulate cognitive and emotional processes, the role of DHA in the maturation and resilience of different neurotransmitter systems is reviewed in greater detail in the following text.

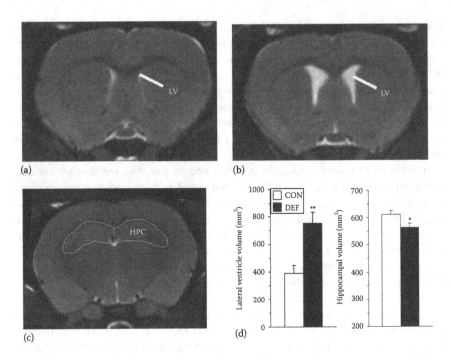

**FIGURE 7.2** Chronic $n-3$ fatty acid deficiency during perinatal development reduces bilateral dorsal hippocampal volumes and increases lateral ventricle (LV) volumes in young adult rats. Representative coronal MRI images from adult CON (a) and perinatal $n-3$ DEF (b) rats obtained with a 7T Bruker Biospec Imaging System and a coronal image illustrating the boundaries of the dorsal hippocampus (c). Quantitative analysis of bilateral hippocampus and LV volumes are presented in (d). Values are expressed as group mean ± S.E.M.

## 7.2.1 GLUTAMATE

A persistent enhancement of glutamatergic synaptic efficacy exemplified by long-term potentiation (LTP) is thought to mediate the formation of new synaptic connections and requires activation of $N$-methyl-D-aspartate (NMDA) receptors. An early ex vivo study found that DHA enhances the function of glutamate receptor channels (Nishikawa et al., 1994), though the effects of exogenous application of DHA on LTP induction are pathway specific (Fujiti et al., 2001; Itokazu et al., 2000; Mirnikjoo et al., 2001). Nevertheless, $n-3$ fatty acid deprivation during perinatal development is associated with decreases of NMDA receptor NR2A subunit expression, reductions in glutamatergic synapses and impaired LTP in the rat hippocampus (Cao et al., 2009). It is also relevant that dietary-induced restoration of DHA deficits in the aged rat brain is associated with the normalization of lower NR2B subunit expression and hippocampal LTP deficits (Dyall et al., 2007; Martin et al., 2002; McGahon et al., 1999). FO fortification attenuates impairment of pre-pulse inhibition following treatment with the NMDA receptor antagonist ketamine (Gama et al., 2012; Zugno et al., 2014) but not histopathological features induced by chronic NMDA treatment (Keleshian et al., 2014). Together, these findings suggest that the accrual and maintenance of cortical DHA are required for optimal glutamatergic synaptic neurotransmission, plasticity and resilience. NMDA receptor-dependent LTP is also thought to mediate the consolidation and storage of new memories (Morris, 2013). Consistent with impaired glutamatergic synaptic plasticity, deficits in brain DHA accrual are associated with impairments in hippocampus-dependent spatial learning which are attenuated with dietary $n-3$ fatty acid fortification (Fedorova et al., 2009; Moriguchi et al., 2000; Moriguchi & Salem, 2003). Perinatal deficits in brain DHA accrual are also associated with learning impairments on olfactory discrimination tasks (Greiner et al., 1999, 2001; Hichami et al., 2007) and the persistence of long-term memories in an inhibitory avoidance task (Bach et al., 2014). In the latter study, memory impairments in $n-3$ fatty acid–deficient rats were associated with reductions in NMDA NR2B subunit expression. An ultrastructural study found that $n-3$ fatty acid deprivation led to abnormal decreases in vesicle densities in hippocampal glutamatergic synapses following learning (Yoshida et al., 1997). Naturally occurring reductions in aged rat brain DHA levels are associated with impaired learning performance (Ulmann et al., 2001), and dietary-induced restoration of aged brain DHA content is associated with improvements in hippocampus-dependent learning performance (Carrie et al., 2002). These and other data suggest that cortical DHA accrual and maintenance are required for optimal associative learning performance in rodents over the lifespan.

## 7.2.2 ACETYLCHOLINE

Acetylcholine plays a critical role in neurocognitive processes in rodents and humans (Everitt & Robbins, 1997; Sarter & Bruno, 2000). Rodent studies have demonstrated that perinatal deficits in cortical DHA accrual significantly blunt potassium chloride–evoked release of acetylcholine in the hippocampus and increase spontaneous acetylcholine release (Aid et al., 2003). In the latter study, DHA deficiency was also associated with a reduction in cholinergic muscarinic receptor binding, whereas acetylcholinesterase activity and the vesicular acetylcholine transporter were not altered. In contrast, rodent maternal dietary FO supplementation throughout gestation and lactation significantly decreased spontaneous acetylcholine release and enhanced stimulated acetylcholine release (Aid et al., 2005). Dietary-induced restoration of aged rat brain DHA content is associated with increased spontaneous and evoked acetylcholine release in the hippocampus (Favreliere et al., 2003). Maternal FO supplementation protected developing cholinergic neurons in the infant rat brain against NMDA-induced excitotoxicity (Hogyes et al., 2003). Moreover, hippocampal cell loss in response to acute treatment with an epileptic dose of pilocarpine, a cholinergic muscarinic receptor agonist, was attenuated in FO-supplemented rats (Ferrari et al., 2008). Lastly, deficits in spatial learning resulting from treatment with scopolamine, a cholinergic muscarinic receptor antagonist, are attenuated in rats supplemented with phosphatidylserine-bound DHA (Vaisman & Pelled, 2009). Collectively, these data suggest that cortical DHA levels play an important role in acetylcholine synaptic function as well as resilience of cholinergic neurons to excitotoxic degeneration.

### 7.2.3 DOPAMINE

Deficits in mesocorticolimbic dopamine neurotransmission are thought to contribute to impairments in attention and executive function (Ernst et al., 1998; Rosa Neto et al., 2002; Volkow et al., 2007) and reward (Nestler & Carlezon, 2006; Stein, 2008). Rat studies have demonstrated that deficits in brain DHA accrual during perinatal development are associated with a significant loss of dopamine neurons in the ventral tegmental area, the source of mesolimbic and mesocortical dopamine projections (Ahmad et al., 2008). Perinatal deficits in brain DHA accrual are also associated with increased expression of tyrosine hydroxylase, the rate-limiting enzyme in dopamine biosynthesis, in the dorsal striatum of adolescent but not adult rats (Bondi et al., 2014). Perinatal deficits in brain DHA accrual are associated with significant deficits in basal and tyramine-stimulated extracellular dopamine concentrations in the frontal cortex of young adult rats (Kodas et al., 2002a; Zimmer et al., 1998). Importantly, deficits in tyramine-stimulated dopamine release are reversible with early (P0–P14), but not later (P21), postnatal $n-3$ fatty acid supplementation (Kodas et al., 2002a). Rats subjected to perinatal deficits in brain DHA accrual also exhibit deficits in mesolimbic dopamine neurotransmission (Zimmer et al., 2000b, 2002). Perinatal deficits in brain DHA accrual also leads to alterations in dopamine $D_1$ and $D_2$ receptor expression and binding (Delion et al., 1996; Kuperstein et al., 2008; Zimmer et al., 2000b) but does not significantly alter the density or function of dopamine transporters (Kodas et al., 2002b). Maternal dietary FO supplementation throughout gestation and lactation significantly increases dopamine concentrations in the frontal cortex of adult offspring (Chalon et al., 1998). These findings suggest that early perinatal brain DHA accrual is critical for the functional maturation of mesocortical and mesolimbic dopamine pathways.

Pharmacological studies have additionally found that deficits in perinatal brain DHA accrual are associated with altered responses to drugs that target dopamine neurotransmission and commonly used to treat ADHD (amphetamine) and psychosis (haloperidol). For example, amphetamine-induced locomotor activity was significantly enhanced in $n-3$ fatty acid–deficient rats (Levant et al., 2004), and amphetamine-induced behavioural sensitization is significantly augmented in $n-3$ fatty acid–deficient adult C57BL/6J mice (McNamara et al., 2008b). Moreover, amphetamine-induced behavioural sensitization was significantly augmented by $n-3$ fatty acid deficiency in a 'sensitization-resistant' inbred mouse strain (DBA/2J) (McNamara et al., 2008c). In the latter study, augmented sensitization was associated with greater amphetamine-induced mesolimbic dopamine activity. Perinatal deficits in cortical DHA accrual are associated with significant decrements in catalepsy induced by the dopamine $D_2$ receptor antagonist haloperidol (Levant et al., 2004). Sensorimotor gating as measured by pre-pulse inhibition of the acoustic startle response is impaired by amphetamine (Mansbach et al., 1988) and perinatal deficits in brain DHA accrual (Fedorova et al., 2009). Therefore, pharmacological studies further suggest that $n-3$ fatty acid deficiency leads to abnormal dopamine neurotransmission.

Constitutive or strain-dependent variations in rat brain DHA status may also influence dopamine-mediated processes including spontaneous locomotor activity, performance on attention tasks and sensorimotor gating. For example, rats displaying greater spontaneous nocturnal activity and activity in response to a novel environment exhibited lower frontal cortex DHA levels compared with rats with lower activity levels despite being fed identical diets (Vancassel et al., 2007). Similarly, inbred C57BL/6J mice exhibit significantly lower regional constitutive DHA levels, and a greater AA/DHA ratio, and exhibit greater spontaneous and amphetamine-induced activity relative to inbred DBA/2J mice despite being fed identical diets (McNamara et al., 2009c). Spontaneously hypertensive rats, an animal model of ADHD, exhibit a greater AA/DHA ratio and deficits on an attentional set-shifting task (Cao et al., 2013). These preliminary findings suggest that constitutive differences in brain DHA status are an important determinant of dopamine-mediated neurocognitive and motor processes in rodents independent of diet.

### 7.2.4 SEROTONIN

Maternal dietary FO fortification significantly increases serotonin (5-hydroxytryptamine [5-HT]) concentrations in the frontal cortex (Chalon et al., 1998) and attenuates reductions in frontal cortex serotonin content in response to chronic stress (Vancassel et al., 2008) in yough adult offspring. Conversely, perinatal deficits in cortical DHA accrual are associated with impaired fenfluramine-induced elevations in extracellular serotonin concentrations (Kodas et al., 2004); reductions in midbrain expression of tryptophan hydroxylase-2, the rate-limiting enzyme in serotonin biosynthesis (McNamara et al., 2009a); and elevations in $5-HT_{2A}$ receptor binding density in the rat frontal cortex (Delion et al., 1996). The 5-hydroxyindoleacetic acid (5-HIAA)/5-HT ratio, an index of serotonin turnover, was significantly increased in the frontal cortex, hypothalamus and ventral striatum of adult perinatal $n - 3$–deficient rats and was prevented by early normalization of $n - 3$ fatty acid status (McNamara et al., 2010a). Importantly, the increase in the 5-HIAA/5-HT ratio observed in the perinatal DHA-deficient rat brain is opposite to that produced by the selective serotonin reuptake inhibitor (SSRI) antidepressant medication fluoxetine (McNamara et al., 2013a). Together this evidence suggests that $LCn - 3$ fatty acid status during development is an important determinant of central serotonin neurotransmission in adult rats.

Consistent with clinical evidence implicating a dysregulation in serotonin neurotransmission in the pathophysiology and treatment of depression and aggression (Arango et al., 2002; Coccaro et al., 1997; Vaswani et al., 2003), post-weaning deficits in cortical DHA accrual are associated with elevated behavioural indices of aggression and depression in rats (DeMar et al., 2006). Interestingly, dietary FO fortification significantly decreases depression-like behaviour similar to SSRI medications in the forced swim test (Carlezon et al., 2005; Huang et al., 2008). Moreover, the combination of dietary FO supplementation and fluoxetine is significantly more effective than fluoxetine treatment alone for reducing depression-like behaviour in the forced swim test (Laino et al., 2010; Lakhwani et al., 2007). Although post-weaning deficits in cortical DHA accrual are not associated with diminished SSRI efficacy in female rats in the forced swim test (McNamara et al., 2013a), it is associated with abnormal behavioural activation in the forced swim test in male rats (Able et al., 2014). It is also relevant that the Flinders sensitive line rats, an inbred rat model of depression, exhibit constitutive increases in regional brain AA/DHA ratio (Green et al., 2005). These findings suggest that cortical DHA status is an important determinant of behaviours regulated by serotonin including depression and aggression.

## 7.3   NON-HUMAN PRIMATE NEURODEVELOPMENT

Similar to humans, dietary DHA intake is more effective than is dietary ALA for increasing cortical DHA levels in developing non-human primates (Anderson et al., 2005; Connor et al., 1990; Hsieh et al., 2007; Su et al., 1999). In the developing monkey brain, frontal cortex DHA concentrations represent ~15% of total fatty acids at birth and, between birth and 22 months of age, increase to comprise ~22% of total fatty acids (Anderson et al., 2005; Neuringer et al., 1986). Feeding studies have found that a maternal diet low in ALA beginning 2 months prior to conception is associated with reduced neonatal monkey prefrontal cortex DHA concentrations at birth compared with neonates whose mothers were maintained on a standard diet containing higher levels of ALA (Anderson et al., 2005; Neuringer et al., 1986). Postnatal dietary FO fortification leads to a progressive increase in prefrontal cortex DHA concentrations in DHA-deficient neonatal monkeys, reaching control levels after approximately 10–15 weeks (Connor et al., 1990). Baboons born preterm exhibit cortical DHA deficits compared with term births, and 4-week feeding with DHA-fortified human infant formula is more efficient for normalizing cortical DHA levels compared with human infant formula not fortified with DHA (Sarkadi-Nagy et al., 2003, 2004). These studies suggest that gestational length and maternal DHA status, as well as postnatal neonate dietary DHA intake, are important determinants of cortical DHA status of young adult non-human primates.

Primate perinatal $n - 3$ fatty acid deficiency is associated with deficits in visual attention (Reisbick et al., 1997), polydipsia (excessive thirst) (Reisbick et al., 1990) and deficits in visual acuity and electroretinogram abnormalities (Anderson et al., 2005; Neuringer et al., 1986). Electroretinogram abnormalities have also been observed in neonatal baboons born preterm (Diau et al., 2003). Consistent with elevated mesolimbic dopamine activity, perinatal $n - 3$ fatty acid deficiency is associated with increased home cage stereotypy and locomotion bouts (Reisbick et al., 1994). A positron emission tomography study demonstrated that dietary supplementation with DHA improves the age-related impairment in cerebral blood flow in the somatosensory cortex in response to tactile stimulation (Tsukada et al., 2000). Furthermore, a recent neuroimaging study found that resting-state functional connectivity among prefrontal cortical networks was deficient in monkeys raised on an $n - 3$ fatty acid–deficient diet compared with monkeys raised on an FO-fortified diet (Grayson et al., 2014). These findings provide functional evidence that lower cortical DHA status is associated with a range of neurodevelopmental abnormalities in young adult non-human primates.

## 7.4   HUMAN NEURODEVELOPMENT

During pregnancy the developing human fetus acquires DHA from maternal stores, and DHA is preferentially transported across the human placenta by fatty acid transport proteins (Dutta-Roy, 2000; Koletzko et al., 2007). Emerging clinical evidence suggests that ovarian hormones positively regulate ALA → DHA conversion (Bakewell et al., 2006; Burdge & Wooton, 2002; Giltay et al., 2004;

Sumino et al., 2003) and that ALA → DHA biosynthesis is more efficient in pregnant women and infants compared with healthy adult human subjects (Brenna et al., 2009; Otto et al., 2001). Supplementation studies have demonstrated that preformed DHA is significantly more effective than ALA for increasing erythrocyte (Barceló-Coblijn et al., 2008) and breast milk (Francois et al., 2003; Valentine et al., 2013) DHA composition. Higher maternal DHA and fetal status during pregnancy is an important determinant of gestational length and intrauterine growth (Carlson et al., 2013; Cetin et al., 2002; Olsen et al., 1992, 2007; Salvig & Lamont, 2011). Uncorrected reductions in maternal DHA stores may be associated with increased risk for perinatal depression (Hibbeln, 2002; Markhus et al., 2013; Otto et al., 2003). Some but not all trials have found that maternal LC$n-3$ fatty acid supplementation is protective against perinatal depression (Freeman et al., 2008; Makrides et al., 2010; Miller et al., 2013; Su et al., 2008).

During human neonatal development, DHA accumulates in brain tissue at an increased rate during the third trimester in association with active periods of neurogenesis, neuroblast migration, differentiation and synaptogenesis (Clandinin et al., 1980a; Martinez, 1992). Some observational studies suggest that higher maternal DHA status or higher seafood intake during pregnancy has a beneficial effect on term infant neurodevelopmental outcomes, including more mature sleep patterns, higher visual acuity, faster processing speed, lower distractibility and higher stereoacuity and cognitive function (Cheruku et al., 2002; Colombo et al., 2004; Helland et al., 2003; Innis et al., 2001b; Jacobson et al., 2008; Williams et al., 2001). However, recent controlled trials have found that maternal DHA supplementation during pregnancy did not have a significant impact on visual acuity (Smithers et al., 2011) or neurocognitive outcomes (Makrides et al., 2010) in term infants at 18 months of age.

As observed in non-human primates, human infants born preterm exhibit lower erythrocyte and postmortem cortical DHA concentrations compared with term infants fed with the same ALA-fortified formula postpartum (Clandinin et al., 1980a; Farquharson et al., 1992, 1995; Martinez, 1992; Martinez & Mougan, 1998). Preterm infants fed formulas without DHA also had lower erythrocyte and postmortem cerebral cortex DHA levels compared with preterm infants fed human milk (Carlson et al., 1986; Farquharson et al., 1992, 1995; Martinez, 1992). Structural imaging studies have also found that children and adolescents born preterm exhibit significant reductions in regional cortical grey matter volumes, reduced amygdala and hippocampal volumes, reduced corpus callosum and white matter volumes and larger cerebral ventricles relative to age- and sex-matched term born controls (Kesler et al., 2008; Ment et al., 2009; Nagy et al., 2003; Nosarti et al., 2002; Peterson et al., 2000; Stewart et al., 1999). More recent imaging studies have also found that children, adolescents and adults born preterm exhibit decreased white matter tract integrity and reduced connectivity within cortical networks (Constable et al., 2008; Gozzo et al., 2009; Lubsen et al., 2011; Mullen et al., 2011; Schafer et al., 2009; Smyser et al., 2013; White et al., 2014). Children and adolescents born preterm also exhibit a significantly higher incidence of attention deficits, impulsivity, learning disability, language impairments, hyperactivity, anxiety, motor impairments and poor social functioning relative to age- and sex-matched term children/adolescents (Bhutta et al., 2002; Botting et al., 1997; Cherkes-Julkowski, 1998; Cooke & Foulder-Hughes, 2003; Foulder-Hughes & Cooke, 2003; Lawson & Ruff, 2004; Olsen et al., 1998; Salt & Redshaw, 2006; Schothorst & van Engeland, 1996).

Randomized studies have observed beneficial effects of DHA supplementation on visual acuity and visual attention processes in preterm infants (Carlson & Neuringer, 1999; Carlson & Werkman, 1996; Clandinin et al., 2005; Gibson et al., 2001; Werkman & Carlson, 1996) as well as psychomotor development scores at 2.5 years of age (SanGiovanni et al., 2000). A placebo-controlled structural MRI study found that postnatal DHA supplementation did not significantly alter age-related increases in white matter volume in premature infants (van Wezel-Meijler et al., 2002). A meta-analysis observed no clear long-term benefits on weight, length or head circumference in preterm infants receiving LC$n$ − 3−supplemented formula (Schulzke et al., 2011). Moreover, feeding preterm infants LC$n$ − 3−supplemented milk containing higher DHA levels did not influence language development or behaviour in early childhood (Smithers et al., 2010). Therefore, the role of deficits in early fetal DHA accrual on neurodevelopmental outcomes in children and adolescents born preterm remains to be established. However, it is important to note that non-human primate feeding studies suggest that normalization of cortical DHA deficits in human preterm infants would require long-term high-dose dietary DHA supplementation.

The role of DHA in human fetal brain development is further suggested for infants with generalized peroxisomal biogenesis disorders. The final synthesis of DHA additionally requires beta-oxidation within peroxisomes (Wanders, 2013), and neonates with peroxisomal biogenesis disorders exhibit robust erythrocyte and postmortem cortex DHA deficits (Martinez, 1995). Neonates with peroxisomal disorders exhibit abnormalities in neuronal migration, deficits in central myelinogenesis and pervasive neurological impairment (Powers et al., 1998). Preliminary DHA intervention studies have observed improvements in visual function (Martinez, 1996; Martinez et al., 2000; Noguer & Martinez, 2010) and brain white matter volumes (Martinez & Vazquez, 1998) in patients with peroxisomal disorders. However, peroxisomal disorders are also associated with other lipid abnormalities, including elevated very-long-chain fatty acid levels, which may contribute to abnormalities in neurodevelopmental outcomes.

Postpartum, the human fetal brain continues to grow from ~350 g at birth to ~925 g at 1 year of age (Dobbing & Sands, 1973), during which DHA represents approximately 9% of the total cortical fatty acid composition (Carver et al., 2001; Clandinin et al., 1980b). Postpartum neonates are reliant on maternal breast milk (or formula) as the sole source of DHA. Human breast milk DHA concentrations are highly correlated with maternal dietary DHA but not ALA intake (Francois et al., 2003; Innis, 2004; Jensen et al., 2000; Lauritzen et al., 2002), vary widely across different countries in accordance with habitual dietary fish consumption (Brenna et al., 2007) and are influenced by FADS genotype (Molto-Puigmarti et al., 2010). Consistent with primate studies (Sarkadi-Nagy et al., 2003, 2004), the human infant frontal cortex accumulates DHA faster over the course of postnatal development when breastfed compared with feeding DHA-free formula (Gibson et al., 1996). Term infants fed formulas without DHA consistently exhibit significantly lower erythrocyte or postmortem brain cortex DHA concentrations relative to breastfed infants or infants fed formula containing DHA (Auestad et al., 1997; Byard et al., 1995; Farquharson et al., 1995; Gibson et al., 1996; Jamieson et al., 1999; Makrides et al., 1994; Putnam et al., 1982; Sanders & Naismith, 1979). The effect of postnatal DHA supplementation on neurocognitive development in term infants has been reviewed in detail previously (Carlson, 2009; Carlson & Neuringer, 1999; Lauritzen & Carlson, 2011; Scholtz et al., 2013; Uauy et al., 2001). Although controversial, studies have found that infants fed formulas without DHA exhibit several neurological and neurocognitive 'soft signs' in infancy and childhood relative to infants fed formulas with DHA or maternal breast milk, including lower visual acuity, slower processing speed on tests of visual recognition memory and more mature motor movement, problem-solving and psychomotor function. Based on this body of evidence, in 2002, infant formula fortified with DHA became widely available in the United States.

During early childhood development, DHA levels continue to increase in the frontal cortex (Carver et al., 2001) in association with linear increases in frontal cortex grey matter expansion (Giedd et al., 1999, 2009; Paus et al., 1999; Sowell et al., 1999) and the maturation of frontal-mediated neurocognitive processes involving attention and executive function (Conklin et al., 2007). A controlled fMRI study found that DHA supplementation significantly increased prefrontal cortex activation during performance of a sustained attention task in healthy children 8–10 years of age and that erythrocyte DHA composition was positively correlated with prefrontal activation at baseline and study end point (McNamara et al., 2010b). A recent observational study found that greater LC$n$ − 3 fatty acid intake measured by questionnaire was associated with better hippocampus-dependent relational memory performance in 52 children aged 7–9 years of age (Baym et al., 2014). However, the results of acute LC$n$ − 3 fatty acid supplementation trials have in general not observed significant neurocognitive benefits in healthy developing children (Ryan et al., 2010). For example, a controlled trial of 450 healthy children 8–10 years of age found that 16-week treatment with 400 mg FO did not significantly impact performance across several cognitive tasks (Kirby et al., 2010). A more recent placebo-controlled trial of 362 healthy children 7–9 years of age found that 16-week treatment with 600 mg DHA did not influence teacher-rated behaviour or working memory performance but was associated with improved reading performance in a subgroup of 224 children with poor reading ability (Richardson et al., 2012). In the latter study, DHA supplementation was associated with reduced parent-rated ADHD-type symptoms including oppositional behaviour and hyperactivity. The results from these and other short-term LC$n$ − 3 fatty acid supplementation trials suggest no robust neurocognitive benefits in healthy developing children, though additional longer dose-ranging studies in children with initially low DHA status are warranted.

Prospective longitudinal studies have begun to investigate the relationship between maternal or fetal (cord blood) LC$n$ − 3 fatty acid status and neurodevelopmental outcomes in older children. One study found that supplementing pregnant and lactating women with FO resulted in higher IQ scores at 4 years of age compared with maternal supplementation with corn oil (Helland et al., 2003). However, a follow-up study found that maternal FO supplementation during pregnancy and lactation did not impact IQ at 7 years of age (Helland et al., 2008). Another study found that maternal FO supplementation during the first 4 months of lactation did not result in statistically significant effects at 7 years of age on neurocognitive outcomes including working memory and inhibitory control compared with olive oil supplementation (Cheatham et al., 2011). Moreover, a large trial found that maternal DHA supplementation during pregnancy did not significantly impact cognition, language and executive function at 4 years of age (Makrides et al., 2014). However, the Avon Longitudinal Study of Parents and Children found that higher fish consumption during pregnancy was associated with higher scores of fine motor skills, verbal IQ, social development and pro-social behaviour in children 7–8 years of age (Hibbeln et al., 2007). Prospective longitudinal studies have found that higher cord blood DHA levels are associated with higher movement scores but not neurocognitive scores at 7 years of age (Bakker et al., 2003, 2009), better visual function at 5 years of age (Jacques et al., 2011) and better recognition memory and associated event-related potentials at ~11 years of age (Boucher et al., 2011). While these data suggest that higher fetal DHA status may have long-term beneficial effects on neurocognitive outcomes in childhood, variability in dietary DHA intake during the intervening period may contribute to variability between studies.

Adolescence is a period of increasing dietary autonomy and surveys have found that a large percentage of adolescents residing in western countries consume low quantities of LC$n$ − 3 fatty acids in their habitual diet (Clayton et al., 2009a; Harel et al., 2001; Lauritzenet et al., 2012; Sichert-Hellertet et al., 2009). For example, a survey of 1,117 ninth-grade adolescents (average age 15 years) in the United States found that only 36% consumed fish at least once a week, 29% consumed fish once a month, and 35% consumed fish <3 times per year (Harel et al., 2001). In adolescents, low LC$n$ − 3 fatty acid status is associated with higher cardiovascular disease risk factors (Dangardt et al., 2010; O'Sullivan et al., et al., 2011). During adolescent development cortical DHA levels continue to increase to ~15% total cortical fatty acids in young adulthood (Carver et al., 2001), and this increase coincides with frontal cortex synaptic pruning (Glantz et al., 2007; Huttenlocher, 1979; Petanjek et al., 2011), white matter expansion and frontal lobe functional connectivity (Ducharme et al., 2012; Giedd et al., 1999, 2009; Paus et al., 1999; Sowell et al., 1999; Tisserand et al., 2002) (Figure 7.3). Although there is currently little known about the importance of LC$n$ − 3 fatty acid intake during childhood on cognitive outcomes in adolescence, a longitudinal cohort study found that greater fish intake (>1 time per week) at 15 years of age was associated with higher scores in composite IQ and verbal performance and visuospatial performance at 18 years of age compared with adolescents consuming fish >1 time per week (Aberg et al., 2009). As discussed in the following section, emerging evidence suggests that low LC$n$ − 3 fatty acid status in adolescents is also associated with emotional dysregulation and mood symptoms.

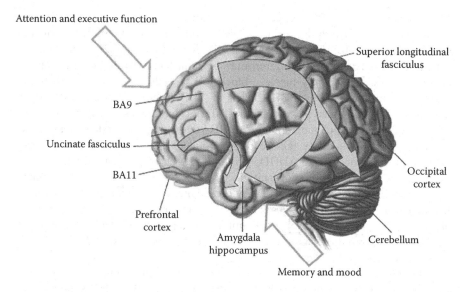

Attention and executive function

Superior longitudinal
fasciculus

BA9

Uncinate fasciculus

BA11

Occipital
cortex

Prefrontal
cortex

Amygdala
hippocampus

Cerebellum

Memory and mood

**FIGURE 7.3**   Diagram illustrating connectivity between frontal lobe regions, including the dorsolateral prefrontal cortex (Brodmann area 9 [BA9]) and orbitofrontal cortex (BA11), which regulates attention and executive function and temporal lobe structures including the amygdala and hippocampus which regulate mood and memory. Frontal lobe connectivity with limbic structures is mediated in part by the uncinate fasciculus and superior longitudinal fasciculus which becomes established during childhood and adolescence. Reduced frontal circuit connectivity is exhibited by DHA-deficient non-human primates, children and adolescents born preterm, and patients with psychiatric disorders associated with DHA deficiency including ADHD and bipolar disorder.

## 7.5   COGNITIVE AND EMOTIONAL PATHOLOGY

Human childhood and adolescence are developmental periods associated with the maturation of frontal cortical regions that mediate attention and executive functions and the establishment of structural and functional connectivity between frontal regionals and limbic structures that mediate emotion and mood (Giedd et al., 1999, 2009; Paus et al., 1999; Sowell et al., 1999). Major psychiatric disorders that initially emerge in childhood and adolescence, including ADHD and bipolar disorder, are associated with blood DHA deficits as well as aberrant brain organization compared with healthy developing youth (Menon, 2011). Moreover, emerging neuroimaging evidence suggests that LCn − 3 fatty acid status is positively correlated with frontolimbic structural and functional integrity in healthy subjects across the lifespan (McNamara, 2013b). These associations suggest that deficits in human brain DHA accrual may represent a modifiable neurodevelopmental risk factor for suboptimal cortical circuit development and associated cognitive and emotional dysregulation (McNamara & Carlson, 2006).

Several cross-sectional studies have shown that children with ADHD exhibit significantly lower erythrocyte or plasma DHA levels compared with healthy typically developing children (Antalis et al., 2006; Chen et al., 2004; Mitchell et al.,

1987; Stevens et al., 1995). A recent meta-analysis of nine cross-sectional studies observed significantly lower blood DHA levels in ADHD children compared with healthy controls (Hawkey & Nigg, 2014). While the aetiology of blood DHA deficits observed in ADHD children may be multifactorial, dietary FO supplementation dose dependently increase blood DHA levels (Flock et al., 2013) and is sufficient to increase blood DHA levels in ADHD patients (Milte et al., 2012). Several small randomized placebo-controlled trials have investigated the effects of LC$n$ − 3 fatty acid supplementation in ADHD youth, and independent meta-analyses found that LC$n$ − 3 fatty acid treatment produces a modest but significant benefit over placebo for treating ADHD symptoms (Bloch & Qawasmi, 2011; Hawkey & Nigg, 2014). However, homogeneity in trial designs and concomitant treatment with psychostimulant medications likely contribute to discrepancies in outcomes. It remains to be determined whether earlier long-term LC$n$ − 3 fatty acid supplementation is protective against the initial development of ADHD and whether established abnormalities in cortical circuits can be normalized by LC$n$ − 3 fatty acid supplementation.

Although it is not currently known whether low DHA intake during fetal and neonatal development contributes to the emergence of ADHD symptoms in childhood, a retrospective study found that children with ADHD had a significantly shorter duration of breastfeeding compared with children without ADHD (Kadziela-Olech & Piotrowska-Jastrzebska, 2005). Moreover, preterm birth is associated with early deficits in cortical DHA accrual and increased risk for ADHD children (Bhutta et al., 2002; Foulder-Hughes & Cooke, 2003). Similar to children born preterm, ADHD children exhibit significantly smaller frontal and temporal cortex grey and white matter volumes, reduced corpus callosum volumes and enlarged cerebral ventricles (Castellanos et al., 2002; Hill et al., 2003; Lyoo et al., 1996; Sowell et al., 2003), though these volume reductions are smaller than those typically observed in children born preterm (Peterson et al., 2000). Also similar to children and adolescents born preterm, youth with ADHD exhibit decreased white matter tract integrity (Chuang et al., 2013; Lawrence et al., 2013) and reduced connectivity within frontal lobe cortical networks (Cao et al., 2009; Sun et al., 2012; Tian et al., 2006). To date there have been no longitudinal prospective intervention trials conducted to evaluate whether low prenatal or perinatal accrual of brain DHA accrual in children born preterm represents a modifiable risk factor for ADHD.

In addition to the core symptoms of attentional impairment and motor hyperactivity, ADHD is frequently associated with emotion dysregulation. ADHD is highly co-morbid with disorders including conduct disorder and oppositional defiant disorder, and ADHD youth frequently exhibit callous antisocial traits and abnormalities in emotion-elicited event-related potentials which are correlated with blood LC$n$ − 3 fatty acid levels (Gow et al., 2013a,b). Moreover, paediatric bipolar disorder, which is typically characterized by recurrent mood (depression and mania) episodes, has a very high rate of ADHD co-morbidity, and the initial onset of mania is frequently preceded by symptoms of inattention and hyperactivity (Singh et al., 2006). Importantly, longitudinal prospective evidence also suggests that children with ADHD are more likely to develop mood disorders in young adulthood (Biederman et al., 2010, 2012). These data suggest that the presence of ADHD and/or attentional symptoms during childhood may be an important antecedent of emotional dysregulation emerging in adolescence and young adulthood.

Accumulating evidence suggests that dietary LC$n-3$ fatty acid insufficiency may contribute to the pathoaetiology of emotional dysregulation. In adolescents, lower LC$n-3$ fatty acid intake is associated with depressive symptoms (Allen et al., 2013; Murakami et al., 2010; Oddy et al., 2011; Swenne et al., 2011). Moreover, cross-sectional studies have found that adult (Lin et al., 2010), as well as paediatric and adolescent (Clayton et al., 2008; McNamara et al., 2014; Pottala et al., 2012), patients with mood disorders exhibit erythrocyte DHA deficits compared with healthy controls. Additionally, first-episode adolescent manic patients exhibit lower erythrocyte DHA levels compared with healthy adolescents (McNamara et al., 2011), suggesting this deficit precedes or coincides with the initial onset of mood dysregulation. Erythrocyte DHA levels are positively correlated with frontal cortex DHA levels (Connor et al., 2009), and some (Conklin et al., 2010; McNamara et al., 2007, 2008d, 2013c) but not all (Igarashi et al., 2010; Lalovic et al., 2007) postmortem studies have observed DHA deficits in the prefrontal cortex or anterior cingulate of adult patients with mood disorders. The age-related increase in DHA and decrease in the AA/DHA observed in the prefrontal cortex of healthy developing adolescents was not observed in adolescent suicide victims (McNamara et al., 2009c). Moreover, the sharp increase in prefrontal cortex DHA composition between adolescence and young adulthood in healthy subjects was significantly blunted in suicide victims (McNamara, 2013d). Together these data suggest that mood disorders are associated with deficits in the normal age-related increase in peripheral and central LC$n-3$ fatty acid status.

While the aetiology of blood and postmortem brain DHA deficits in patients with mood disorders is poorly understood, erythrocyte DHA composition is positively correlated with fish consumption (Sands et al., 2005) and dietary FO supplementation is sufficient to increase blood DHA levels in youth with mood disorders (Clayton et al., 2009b; McNamara et al., 2014; Wozniak et al., 2007). Preliminary trials have found that LC$n-3$ fatty acid supplementation significantly reduces depression and manic symptom severity in paediatric and adolescent patients (Clayton et al., 2009b; McNamara et al., 2014; Nemets et al., 2006; Wozniak et al., 2007) as well as in depressive symptoms in adult patients (Grosso et al., 2014). Although there have been no longitudinal prospective studies conducted to determine whether low DHA intake during fetal and neonatal development contributes to the emergence of mood symptoms in adolescence, preterm birth is associated with increased risk for mood and psychotic disorders in adolescence and young adulthood (Nosarti et al., 2012). Similar to children and adolescents born preterm and ADHD patients, youth with bipolar disorder exhibit decreased white matter tract integrity and reduced connectivity within frontal lobe cortical networks (Dickstein et al., 2010; Strakowski et al., 2012; Wang et al., 2012).

Cross-national epidemiological surveys have found a significant inverse correlation between per capita fish or seafood consumption and lifetime prevalence rates of bipolar disorder and depression (Hibbeln, 1998; Noaghiul & Hibbeln, 2003). It is relevant therefore that adolescent and young adult females with mood disorders exhibit significant blood DHA deficits (McNamara et al., 2010c, 2014) and are at increased risk for preterm delivery (Lee & Lin, 2010). LC$n$ – 3 fatty acid deficiency in mothers with mood disorders may therefore increase risk for preterm birth, lower breast milk DHA levels, increase neonatal deficits in cortical DHA accrual and increase risk for mood disorders in offspring. Longitudinal prospective studies will be required to determine whether maternal and offspring LC$n$ – 3 fatty acid supplementation can reduce the risk of developing mood disorders in youth with a family history of psychopathology.

## 7.6  SUMMARY AND CONCLUSIONS

Over the past 30 years, a body of evidence has emerged from animal and clinical studies which supports the general assertion that normal brain development requires optimal DHA levels. Rodent studies suggest that cortical DHA has neurotrophic and neuroprotective properties and that reductions in perinatal rat brain DHA accrual are associated with delays in neuronal migration and arborization, synaptic pathology and deficits in multiple neurotransmitter systems. Deficits in perinatal rat brain DHA accrual also lead to neurocognitive impairments and elevated behavioural indices of depression and aggression. It is important to note, however, that the dietary manipulations used in many rodent studies lead to peripheral and central DHA deficits that are substantially greater than those observed in human patients with psychiatric disorders. Nevertheless, other studies have found that smaller decreases in brain DHA levels, resulting from constitutive strain differences or dietary manipulations, are also associated with relevant behavioural abnormalities. Non-human primate studies further suggest a link between $n$ – 3 fatty acid deficiency and perinatal development that are associated with long-standing deficits in functional connectivity within prefrontal cortical networks, hyperactivity and impairments in visual attention. In general, results from animal studies provide strong evidence for a critical role of perinatal DHA accrual for the normal maturation of neural circuits mediating cognitive and emotional processes.

Human studies suggest that preterm birth, which results in deficits in third trimester fetal cortical DHA accrual, is associated with enduring abnormalities in brain structure and function, a spectrum of enduring neurocognitive deficits and enduring connectivity abnormalities within cortical networks. Preterm birth is also associated with increased risk for psychiatric disorders which is also associated with deficits in functional connectivity within prefrontal cortical networks including ADHD and mood disorders. While these associations suggest that third trimester cortical DHA accrual may play a critical role in cognitive and emotional development of offspring in later life, the impact of other variables associated with preterm birth may also contribute. However, early postnatal DHA supplementation has been found in some studies to improve visual acuity and visual attention processes in infants and children born preterm. Nevertheless, prospective longitudinal studies are needed to evaluate whether early LC*n* − 3 fatty acid supplementation can reduce the risk of developing cognitive and emotional dysregulation of children and adolescence born preterm.

Although observational studies suggest that higher maternal and fetal DHA status may be associated with better neurodevelopmental outcomes in infants and children, results from recent controlled maternal LC*n* − 3 fatty acid supplementation trials have not consistently observed robust benefits in neurocognitive outcomes in healthy children. Similarly, acute controlled LC*n* − 3 fatty acid supplementation trials have not observed robust improvements in neurocognitive outcomes in healthy developing children. Discrepancies between observational studies and controlled LC*n* − 3 fatty acid supplementation trials may indicate that longer exposure periods are required before modifications in cortical structure and function become evident. Moreover, these findings suggest that the LC*n* − 3 fatty acid status of healthy developing youth is sufficient to prevent robust perturbations in neurodevelopment. Indeed, LC*n* − 3 fatty acid supplementation has been found to have benefits for cognitive and mood symptoms in children and adolescents with ADHD or mood disorders associated with significant blood DHA deficits. Therefore, more robust effects of LC*n* − 3 fatty acid supplementation on cognitive and emotional processes may become apparent in children and adolescents with low blood DHA levels.

The effects of LC*n* − 3 fatty acid supplementation on cognitive and emotional outcomes likely first require changes in established cortical circuitry. While it is not currently known whether LC*n* − 3 fatty acid supplementation alone is sufficient to modify functional connectivity within established cortical networks, it appears to play a critical role in their initial development. This is supported by a recent non-human primate study finding that *n* − 3 fatty acid deficiency during perinatal development is associated with long-standing hypoactivity in functional connectivity within prefrontal cortical (Grayson et al., 2014). Moreover, emerging neuroimaging evidence indicates that psychiatric disorders that initially emerge in childhood and adolescence are also associated with frontal structural and functional connectivity deficits and low blood DHA levels compared with healthy developing youth. While these translational findings suggest a potential link between low LC*n* − 3 fatty acid status and deficits in the development of functional connectivity within prefrontal cortical networks, deficits in frontolimbic circuit maturation may represent a permanent neurodevelopmental 'scar' that is potentially irreversible once established, suggesting that early intervention may have the greatest impact. Additional neuroimaging studies will be required to determine whether long-term LC*n* − 3 fatty acid supplementation can restore normal prefrontal cortical networks and associated cognitive and emotional dysregulation in youth with psychiatric disorders.

In conclusion, the role of perinatal brain DHA accrual on cognitive and emotional development is only beginning to be fully understood. While extant evidence from translational studies suggest that optimal brain development and function requires an optimal level of LC*n* − 3 fatty acids during perinatal development, LC*n* − 3 fatty acid supplementation may have limited additional benefit for neurocognitive outcomes in healthy mothers and their offspring. However, under conditions of maternal and offspring LC$n$ – 3 fatty acid deficiency, as observed in psychiatric disorders, early and long-term LC$n$ – 3 fatty acid supplementation may be required to reduce the risk of preterm birth, deficits in fetal frontolimbic functional connectivity and ensuing cognitive impairment and emotional dysregulation. Developing a more comprehensive understanding of the requirement for LC$n$ – 3 fatty acids during normal human perinatal brain development could have significant implications for informing optimal intake levels during critical periods of neurodevelopment as well as potential preventative strategies for at-risk youth.

## ACKNOWLEDGEMENTS

This work was supported in part by National Institute of Health grants MH083924, AG034617 and DK097599 to RKM and AT006880 to CJV. RKM has received research support from NARSAD, Martek Biosciences Inc., the Inflammation Research Foundation (IRF), Ortho-McNeil Janssen, AstraZeneca and Eli Lilly and was a member of the IRF scientific advisory board. CJV has received research support from Nestle Nutrition and the Perinatal Institute at Cincinnati Children's Hospital.

### TOP 5 SUMMARY POINTS FROM THE CHAPTER

- Long-chain omega-3 (LC$n$ – 3) fatty acids including DHA are primarily acquired via dietary intake and accumulate in the rodent, primate and human brain during development.
- Rodent studies provide critical evidence and insight into the role of LC$n$ – 3 fatty acids in neurodevelopment. These studies have shown that LC$n$ – 3 fatty acids have anti-inflammatory, neurotrophic and neuroprotective properties and play a role in cortical synaptic maturation and regional connectivity.
- Evidence for a role of DHA in the maturation of different neurotransmitter systems, including glutamate, acetylcholine, dopamine and serotonin, support a potential link with cognitive and emotional processes.
- Clinical studies show that DHA from both maternal and dietary sources plays an important role in the neurodevelopment of infants as well as children and adolescents. Emerging evidence suggests that deficits in human brain DHA accrual may represent a modifiable risk factor for suboptimal cortical circuit development and associated cognitive and emotional dysregulation.
- Future research integrating neuroimaging technology and prospective longitudinal designs are required to provide a comprehensive understanding of optimal maternal and offspring LC$n$ – 3 fatty acid intake and status to inform potential preventative strategies for psychopathology.

## REFERENCES

Aberg MA, Aberg N, Brisman J, Sundberg R, Winkvist A, Torén K. Fish intake of Swedish male adolescents is a predictor of cognitive performance. *Acta Paediatr.* 2009;98:555–560.

Able JA, Liu Y, Jandacek R, Rider T, Tso P, McNamara RK. Omega-3 fatty acid deficient male rats exhibit abnormal behavioral activation in the forced swim test following chronic fluoxetine treatment: Association with altered 5-HT1A and alpha2A adrenergic receptor expression. *J Psychiatr Res.* 2014;50:42–50.

Ahmad A, Murthy M, Greiner RS, Moriguchi T, Salem N Jr. A decrease in cell size accompanies a loss of docosahexaenoate in the rat hippocampus. *Nutr Neurosci.* 2002;5:103–113.

Ahmad SO, Park JH, Radel JD, Levant B. Reduced numbers of dopamine neurons in the substantia nigra pars compacta and ventral tegmental area of rats fed an n − 3 polyunsaturated fatty acid-deficient diet: A stereological study. *Neurosci Lett.* 2008;438:303–307.

Aïd S, Vancassel S, Linard A, Lavialle M, Guesnet P. Dietary docosahexaenoic acid [22:6(n − 3)] as a phospholipid or a triglyceride enhances the potassium chloride-evoked release of acetylcholine in rat hippocampus. *J Nutr.* 2005;135:1008–1013.

Aïd S, Vancassel S, Poumès-Ballihaut C, Chalon S, Guesnet P, Lavialle M. Effect of a diet-induced n − 3 PUFA depletion on cholinergic parameters in the rat hippocampus. *J Lipid Res.* 2003;44:1545–1551.

Allen KL, Mori TA, Beilin L, Byrne SM, Hickling S, Oddy WH. Dietary intake in population-based adolescents: Support for a relationship between eating disorder symptoms, low fatty acid intake and depressive symptoms. *J Hum Nutr Diet.* 2013;26:459–469.

Anderson GJ, Neuringer M, Lin DS, Connor WE. Can prenatal N − 3 fatty acid deficiency be completely reversed after birth? Effects on retinal and brain biochemistry and visual function in rhesus monkeys. *Pediatr Res.* 2005;58:865–872.

Antalis CJ, Stevens LJ, Campbell M, Pazdro R, Ericson K, Burgess JR. Omega-3 fatty acid status in attention-deficit/hyperactivity disorder. *Prostaglandins Leukot Essent Fatty Acids.* 2006;75:299–308.

Arango V, Underwood MD, Mann JJ. Serotonin brain circuits involved in major depression and suicide. *Prog Brain Res.* 2002;136:443–453.

Auestad N, Montalto MB, Hall RT, Fitzgerald KM, Wheeler RE, Connor WE, Neuringer M, Connor SL, Taylor JA, Hartmann EE. Visual acuity, erythrocyte fatty acid composition, and growth in term infants fed formulas with long chain polyunsaturated fatty acids for one year. Ross Pediatric Lipid Study. *Pediatr Res.* 1997;41:1–10.

Bach SA, de Siqueira LV, Müller AP, Oses JP, Quatrim A, Emanuelli T, Vinadé L, Souza DO, Moreira JD. Dietary omega-3 deficiency reduces BDNF content and activation NMDA receptor and Fyn in dorsal hippocampus: Implications on persistence of long-term memory in rats. *Nutr Neurosci.* 2014;17:186–192.

Bailes JE, Mills JD. Docosahexaenoic acid reduces traumatic axonal injury in a rodent head injury model. *J Neurotrauma.* 2010;27:1617–1624.

Bakewell L, Burdge GC, Calder PC. Polyunsaturated fatty acid concentrations in young men and women consuming their habitual diets. *Br J Nutr.* 2006; 96:93–99.

Bakker EC, Ghys AJ, Kester AD, Vles JS, Dubas JS, Blanco CE, Hornstra G. Long-chain polyunsaturated fatty acids at birth and cognitive function at 7 y of age. *Eur J Clin Nutr.* 2003;57:89–95.

Bakker EC, Hornstra G, Blanco CE, Vles JS. Relationship between long-chain polyunsaturated fatty acids at birth and motor function at 7 years of age. *Eur J Clin Nutr.* 2009;63:499–504.

Barceló-Coblijn G, Murphy EJ, Othman R, Moghadasian MH, Kashour T, Friel JK. Flaxseed oil and fish-oil capsule consumption alters human red blood cell n − 3 fatty acid composition: A multiple-dosing trial comparing 2 sources of n − 3 fatty acid. *Am J Clin Nutr.* 2008;88:801–809.

Baym CL, Khan NA, Monti JM, Raine LB, Drollette ES, Moore RD, Scudder MR, Kramer AF, Hillman CH, Cohen NJ. Dietary lipids are differentially associated with hippocampal-dependent relational memory in prepubescent children. *Am J Clin Nutr.* 2014;99:1026–1032.

Belayev L, Khoutorova L, Atkins KD, Bazan NG. Robust docosahexaenoic acid-mediated neuroprotection in a rat model of transient, focal cerebral ischemia. *Stroke.* 2009;40:3121–3126.

Beltz BS, Tlusty MF, Benton JL, Sandeman DC. Omega-3 fatty acids upregulate adult neurogenesis. *Neurosci Lett.* 2007;415:154–158.

Bhutta AT, Cleves MA, Casey PH, Cradock MM, Anand KJ. Cognitive and behavioral outcomes of school-aged children who were born preterm: A meta-analysis. *JAMA.* 2002;288:728–737.

Biederman J, Petty CR, Monuteaux MC, Fried R, Byrne D, Mirto T, Spencer T, Wilens TE, Faraone SV. Adult psychiatric outcomes of girls with attention deficit hyperactivity disorder: 11-year follow-up in a longitudinal case-control study. *Am J Psychiatry.* 2010;167:409–417.

Biederman J, Petty CR, Woodworth KY, Lomedico A, Hyder LL, Faraone SV. Adult outcome of attention-deficit/hyperactivity disorder: A controlled 16-year follow-up study. *J Clin Psychiatry.* 2012;73:941–950.

Bloch MH, Qawasmi A. Omega-3 fatty acid supplementation for the treatment of children with attention-deficit/hyperactivity disorder symptomatology: Systematic review and meta-analysis. *J Am Acad Child Adolesc Psychiatry.* 2011;50:991–1000.

Blondeau N, Widmann C, Lazdunski M, Heurteaux C. Polyunsaturated fatty acids induce ischemic and epileptic tolerance. *Neuroscience.* 2002;109:231–241.

Bondi CO, Taha AY, Tock JL, Totah NK, Cheon Y, Torres GE, Rapoport SI, Moghaddam B. Adolescent behavior and dopamine availability are uniquely sensitive to dietary omega-3 fatty acid deficiency. *Biol Psychiatry.* 2014;75:38–46.

Botting N, Powls A, Cooke RW, Marlow N. Attention deficit hyperactivity disorders and other psychiatric outcomes in very low birthweight children at 12 years. *J Child Psychol Psychiatry.* 1997;38:931–941.

Boucher O, Burden MJ, Muckle G, Saint-Amour D, Ayotte P, Dewailly E, Nelson CA, Jacobson SW, Jacobson JL. Neurophysiologic and neurobehavioral evidence of beneficial effects of prenatal omega-3 fatty acid intake on memory function at school age. *Am J Clin Nutr.* 2011;93:1025–1037.

Brenna JT, Salem N Jr, Sinclair AJ, Cunnane SC; International Society for the Study of Fatty Acids and Lipids, ISSFAL. alpha-Linolenic acid supplementation and conversion to n − 3 long-chain polyunsaturated fatty acids in humans. *Prostaglandins Leukot Essent Fatty Acids.* 2009;80(2–3):85–91.

Brenna JT, Varamini B, Jensen RG, Diersen-Schade DA, Boettcher JA, Arterburn LM. Docosahexaenoic and arachidonic acid concentrations in human breast milk worldwide. *Am J Clin Nutr.* 2007;85:1457–1464.

Burdge GC, Wootton SA. Conversion of alpha-linolenic acid to eicosapentaenoic, docosapentaenoic and docosahexaenoic acids in young women. *Br J Nutr.* 2002;88:411–420.

Byard RW, Makrides M, Need M, Neumann MA, Gibson RA. Sudden infant death syndrome: Effect of breast and formula feeding on frontal cortex and brainstem lipid composition. *J Paediatr Child Health.* 1995;31:14–16.

Calderon F, Kim HY. Docosahexaenoic acid promotes neurite growth in hippocampal neurons. *J Neurochem.* 2004;90:979–988.

Calon F, Cole G. Neuroprotective action of omega-3 polyunsaturated fatty acids against neurodegenerative diseases: Evidence from animal studies. *Prostaglandins Leukot Essent Fatty Acids.* 2007;77:287–293.

Cao AH, Yu L, Wang YW, Wang GJ, Lei GF. Composition of long chain polyunsaturated fatty acids (LC-PUFAs) in different encephalic regions and its association with behavior in spontaneous hypertensive rat (SHR). *Brain Res*. 2013;1528:49–57.

Cao D, Kevala K, Kim J, Moon HS, Jun SB, Lovinger D, Kim HY. Docosahexaenoic acid promotes hippocampal neuronal development and synaptic function. *J Neurochem*. 2009;111:510–521.

Cao X, Cao Q, Long X, Sun L, Sui M, Zhu C, Zuo X, Zang Y, Wang Y. Abnormal resting-state functional connectivity patterns of the putamen in medication-naïve children with attention deficit hyperactivity disorder. *Brain Res*. 2009;1303:195–206.

Carlezon WA Jr, Mague SD, Parow AM, Stoll AL, Cohen BM, Renshaw PF. Antidepressant-like effects of uridine and omega-3 fatty acids are potentiated by combined treatment in rats. *Biol Psychiatry*. 2005;57:343–350.

Carlson SE. Docosahexaenoic acid supplementation in pregnancy and lactation. *Am J Clin Nutr*. 2009;89:678S–684S.

Carlson SE, Colombo J, Gajewski BJ, Gustafson KM, Mundy D, Yeast J, Georgieff MK, Markley LA, Kerling EH, Shaddy DJ. DHA supplementation and pregnancy outcomes. *Am J Clin Nutr*. 2013;97:808–815.

Carlson SE, Neuringer M. Polyunsaturated fatty acid status and neurodevelopment: A summary and critical analysis of the literature. *Lipids*. 1999;34:171–178.

Carlson SE, Rhodes PG, Ferguson MG. Docosahexaenoic acid status of preterm infants at birth and following feeding with human milk or formula. *Am J Clin Nutr*. 1986;44:798–804.

Carlson SE, Werkman SH. A randomized trial of visual attention of preterm infants fed docosahexaenoic acid until two months. *Lipids*. 1996;31:85–90.

Carrié I, Smirnova M, Clément M, DE JD, Francès H, Bourre JM. Docosahexaenoic acid-rich phospholipid supplementation: Effect on behavior, learning ability, and retinal function in control and n − 3 polyunsaturated fatty acid deficient old mice. *Nutr Neurosci*. 2002;5:43–52.

Carver JD, Benford VJ, Han B, Cantor AB. The relationship between age and the fatty acid composition of cerebral cortex and erythrocytes in human subjects. *Brain Res Bull*. 2001;56:79–85.

Castellanos FX, Lee PP, Sharp W, Jeffries NO, Greenstein DK, Clasen LS, Blumenthal JD et al. Developmental trajectories of brain volume abnormalities in children and adolescents with attention-deficit/hyperactivity disorder. *JAMA*. 2002;288:1740–1748.

Cetin I, Giovannini N, Alvino G, Agostoni C, Riva E, Giovannini M, Pardi G. Intrauterine growth restriction is associated with changes in polyunsaturated fatty acid fetal-maternal relationships. *Pediatr Res*. 2002;52:750–755.

Chalon S. Omega-3 fatty acids and monoamine neurotransmission. *Prostaglandins Leukot Essent Fatty Acids*. 2006;75:259–269.

Chalon S, Delion-Vancassel S, Belzung C, Guilloteau D, Leguisquet AM, Besnard JC, Durand G. Dietary fish oil affects monoaminergic neurotransmission and behavior in rats. *J Nutr*. 1998;128:2512–2519.

Cheatham CL, Nerhammer AS, Asserhøj M, Michaelsen KF, Lauritzen L. Fish oil supplementation during lactation: Effects on cognition and behavior at 7 years of age. *Lipids*. 2011;46:637–645.

Chen CT, Domenichiello AF, Trépanier MO, Liu Z, Masoodi M, Bazinet RP. The low levels of eicosapentaenoic acid in rat brain phospholipids are maintained via multiple redundant mechanisms. *J Lipid Res*. 2013;54:2410–2422.

Chen JR, Hsu SF, Hsu CD, Hwang LH, Yang SC. Dietary patterns and blood fatty acid composition in children with attention-deficit hyperactivity disorder in Taiwan. *J Nutr Biochem*. 2004;15:467–472.

Cherkes-Julkowski M. Learning disability, attention-deficit disorder, and language impairment as outcomes of prematurity: A longitudinal descriptive study. *J Learn Disabil.* 1998;31:294–306.

Cheruku SR, Montgomery-Downs HE, Farkas SL, Thoman EB, Lammi-Keefe CJ. Higher maternal plasma docosahexaenoic acid during pregnancy is associated with more mature neonatal sleep-state patterning. *Am J Clin Nutr.* 2002;76:608–613.

Childs CE, Romeu-Nadal M, Burdge GC, Calder PC. Gender differences in the $n-3$ fatty acid content of tissues. *Proc Nutr Soc.* 2008;67:19–27.

Chuang TC, Wu MT, Huang SP, Weng MJ, Yang P. Diffusion tensor imaging study of white matter fiber tracts in adolescent attention-deficit/hyperactivity disorder. *Psychiatry Res.* 2013;211:186–187.

Church MW, Jen KL, Dowhan LM, Adams BR, Hotra JW. Excess and deficient omega-3 fatty acid during pregnancy and lactation cause impaired neural transmission in rat pups. *Neurotoxicol Teratol.* 2008;30:107–117.

Church MW, Jen KL, Jackson DA, Adams BR, Hotra JW. Abnormal neurological responses in young adult offspring caused by excess omega-3 fatty acid (fish oil) consumption by the mother during pregnancy and lactation. *Neurotoxicol Teratol.* 2009;31:26–33.

Clandinin MT, Chappell JE, Leong S, Heim T, Swyer PR, Chance GW. Intrauterine fatty acid accretion rates in human brain: Implications for fatty acid requirements. *Early Hum Dev.* 1980a;4:121–129.

Clandinin MT, Chappell JE, Leong S, Heim T, Swyer PR, Chance GW. Extrauterine fatty acid accretion in infant brain: Implications for fatty acid requirements. *Early Hum Dev.* 1980b;4:131–138.

Clandinin MT, Van Aerde JE, Merkel KL, Harris CL, Springer MA, Hansen JW, Diersen-Schade DA. Growth and development of preterm infants fed infant formulas containing docosahexaenoic acid and arachidonic acid. *J Pediatr.* 2005;146:461–468.

Clayton EH, Hanstock TL, Hirneth SJ, Kable CJ, Garg ML, Hazell PL. Long-chain omega-3 polyunsaturated fatty acids in the blood of children and adolescents with juvenile bipolar disorder. *Lipids.* 2008;43:1031–1038.

Clayton EH, Hanstock TL, Hirneth SJ, Kable CJ, Garg ML, Hazell PL. Reduced mania and depression in juvenile bipolar disorder associated with long-chain omega-3 polyunsaturated fatty acid supplementation. *Eur J Clin Nutr.* 2009b;63:1037–1040.

Clayton EH, Hanstock TL, Watson JF. Estimated intakes of meat and fish by children and adolescents in Australia and comparison with recommendations. *Br J Nutr.* 2009a;101:1731–1735.

Coccaro EF, Kavoussi RJ, Trestman RL, Gabriel SM, Cooper TB, Siever LJ. Serotonin function in human subjects: Intercorrelations among central 5-HT indices and aggressiveness. *Psychiatry Res.* 1997;73:1–14.

Colombo J, Kannass KN, Shaddy DJ, Kundurthi S, Maikranz JM, Anderson CJ, Blaga OM, Carlson SE. Maternal DHA and the development of attention in infancy and toddlerhood. *Child Dev.* 2004;75:1254–1267.

Conklin HM, Luciana M, Hooper CJ, Yarger RS. Working memory performance in typically developing children and adolescents: Behavioral evidence of protracted frontal lobe development. *Dev Neuropsychol.* 2007;31:103–128.

Conklin SM, Runyan CA, Leonard S, Reddy RD, Muldoon MF, Yao JK. Age-related changes of $n-3$ and $n-6$ polyunsaturated fatty acids in the anterior cingulate cortex of individuals with major depressive disorder. *Prostaglandins Leukot Essent Fatty Acids.* 2010;82:111–119.

Connor WE, Neuringer M, Lin DS. Dietary effects on brain fatty acid composition: The reversibility of $n-3$ fatty acid deficiency and turnover of docosahexaenoic acid in the brain, erythrocytes, and plasma of rhesus monkeys. *J Lipid Res.* 1990;31:237–247.

Constable RT, Ment LR, Vohr BR, Kesler SR, Fulbright RK, Lacadie C, Delancy S et al. Prematurely born children demonstrate white matter microstructural differences at 12 years of age, relative to term control subjects: An investigation of group and gender effects. *Pediatrics*. 2008;121:306–316.

Cooke RW, Foulder-Hughes L. Growth impairment in the very preterm and cognitive and motor performance at 7 years. *Arch Dis Child*. 2003;88:482–487.

Coti Bertrand P, O'Kusky JR, Innis SM. Maternal dietary ($n − 3$) fatty acid deficiency alters neurogenesis in the embryonic rat brain. *J Nutr*. 2006;136:1570–1575.

Cressman VL, Balaban J, Steinfeld S, Shemyakin A, Graham P, Parisot N, Moore H. Prefrontal cortical inputs to the basal amygdala undergo pruning during late adolescence in the rat. *J Comp Neurol*. 2010;518:2693–2709.

Dangardt F, Osika W, Chen Y, Nilsson U, Gan LM, Gronowitz E, Strandvik B, Friberg P. Omega-3 fatty acid supplementation improves vascular function and reduces inflammation in obese adolescents. *Atherosclerosis*. 2010;212:580–585.

Delion S, Chalon S, Guilloteau D, Besnard JC, Durand G. alpha-Linolenic acid dietary deficiency alters age-related changes of dopaminergic and serotoninergic neurotransmission in the rat frontal cortex. *J Neurochem*. 1996;66:1582–1591.

DeMar JC Jr, Ma K, Bell JM, Igarashi M, Greenstein D, Rapoport SI. One generation of n − 3 polyunsaturated fatty acid deprivation increases depression and aggression test scores in rats. *J Lipid Res*. 2006;47:172–180.

Diau GY, Hsieh AT, Sarkadi-Nagy EA, Wijendran V, Nathanielsz PW, Brenna JT. The influence of long chain polyunsaturate supplementation on docosahexaenoic acid and arachidonic acid in baboon neonate central nervous system. *BMC Med*. 2005;3:11.

Diau GY, Loew ER, Wijendran V, Sarkadi-Nagy E, Nathanielsz PW, Brenna JT. Docosahexaenoic and arachidonic acid influence on preterm baboon retinal composition and function. *Invest Ophthalmol Vis Sci*. 2003;44:4559–4566.

Dickstein DP, Gorrostieta C, Ombao H, Goldberg LD, Brazel AC, Gable CJ, Kelly C et al. Fronto-temporal spontaneous resting state functional connectivity in pediatric bipolar disorder. *Biol Psychiatry*. 2010;68:839–846.

Dobbing J, Sands J. Quantitative growth and development of human brain. *Arch Dis Child*. 1973;48:757–767.

Ducharme S, Hudziak JJ, Botteron KN, Albaugh MD, Nguyen TV, Karama S, Evans AC; Brain Development Cooperative Group. Decreased regional cortical thickness and thinning rate are associated with inattention symptoms in healthy children. *J Am Acad Child Adolesc Psychiatry*. 2012;51:18–27.

Dutta-Roy AK. Transport mechanisms for long-chain polyunsaturated fatty acids in the human placenta. *Am J Clin Nutr*. 2000;71:315S–322S.

Dyall SC, Michael GJ, Whelpton R, Scott AG, Michael-Titus AT. Dietary enrichment with omega-3 polyunsaturated fatty acids reverses age-related decreases in the GluR2 and NR2B glutamate receptor subunits in rat forebrain. *Neurobiol Aging*. 2007;28:424–439.

Ernst M, Zametkin AJ, Matochik JA, Jons PH, Cohen RM. DOPA decarboxylase activity in attention deficit hyperactivity disorder adults. A [fluorine-18]fluorodopa positron emission tomographic study. *J Neurosci*. 1998;18:5901–5907.

Everitt BJ, Robbins TW. Central cholinergic systems and cognition. *Annu Rev Psychol*. 1997;48:649–684.

Farquharson J, Cockburn F, Patrick WA, Jamieson EC, Logan RW. Infant cerebral cortex phospholipid fatty-acid composition and diet. *Lancet*. 1992;340:810–813.

Farquharson J, Jamieson EC, Abbasi KA, Patrick WJ, Logan RW, Cockburn F. Effect of diet on the fatty acid composition of the major phospholipids of infant cerebral cortex. *Arch Dis Child*. 1995;72:198–203.

Favrelière S, Perault MC, Huguet F, DeJavel D, Bertrand N, Piriou A, Durand G. DHA-enriched phospholipid diets modulate age-related alterations in rat hippocampus. *Neurobiol Aging.* 2003;24:233–243.

Fedorova I, Alvheim AR, Hussein N, Salem N Jr. Deficit in prepulse inhibition in mice caused by dietary n – 3 fatty acid deficiency. *Behav Neurosci.* 2009;123:1218–1225.

Fedorova I, Hussein N, Baumann MH, Di Martino C, Salem N Jr. An n – 3 fatty acid deficiency impairs rat spatial learning in the Barnes maze. *Behav Neurosci.* 2009;123:196–205.

Ferrari D, Cysneiros RM, Scorza CA, Arida RM, Cavalheiro EA, deAlmeida AC, Scorza FA. Neuroprotective activity of omega-3 fatty acids against epilepsy-induced hippocampal damage: Quantification with immunohistochemical for calcium-binding proteins. *Epilepsy Behav.* 2008;13:36–42.

Flock MR, Skulas-Ray AC, Harris WS, Etherton TD, Fleming JA, Kris-Etherton PM. Determinants of erythrocyte omega-3 fatty acid content in response to fish oil supplementation: A dose-response randomized controlled trial. *J Am Heart Assoc.* 2013;2:e000513.

Foulder-Hughes LA, Cooke RW. Motor, cognitive, and behavioural disorders in children born very preterm. *Dev Med Child Neurol.* 2003;4:97–103.

Francois CA, Connor SL, Bolewicz LC, Connor WE. Supplementing lactating women with flaxseed oil does not increase docosahexaenoic acid in their milk. *Am J Clin Nutr.* 2003;77:226–233.

Freeman MP, Davis M, Sinha P, Wisner KL, Hibbeln JR, Gelenberg AJ. Omega-3 fatty acids and supportive psychotherapy for perinatal depression: A randomized placebo-controlled study. *J Affect Disord.* 2008;110:142–148.

Fujita S, Ikegaya Y, Nishikawa M, Nishiyama N, Matsuki N. Docosahexaenoic acid improves long-term potentiation attenuated by phospholipase A(2) inhibitor in rat hippocampal slices. *Br J Pharmacol.* 2001;132:1417–1422.

Gama CS, Canever L, Panizzutti B, Gubert C, Stertz L, Massuda R, Pedrini M et al. Effects of omega-3 dietary supplement in prevention of positive, negative and cognitive symptoms: A study in adolescent rats with ketamine-induced model of schizophrenia. *Schizophr Res.* 2012;141:162–167.

Gibson RA, Neumann MA, Makrides M. Effect of dietary docosahexaenoic acid on brain composition and neural function in term infants. *Lipids.* 1996;31:S177–S181.

Giedd JN, Blumenthal J, Jeffries NO, Castellanos FX, Liu H, Zijdenbos A, Paus T, Evans AC, Rapoport JL. Brain development during childhood and adolescence: A longitudinal MRI study. *Nat Neurosci.* 1999;2:861–863.

Giedd JN, Lalonde FM, Celano MJ, White SL, Wallace GL, Lee NR, Lenroot RK. Anatomical brain magnetic resonance imaging of typically developing children and adolescents. *J Am Acad Child Adolesc Psychiatry.* 2009;48:465–470.

Giltay EJ, Gooren LJ, Toorians AW, Katan MB, Zock PL. Docosahexaenoic acid concentrations are higher in women than in men because of estrogenic effects. *Am J Clin Nutr.* 2004;80:1167–1174.

Glantz LA, Gilmore JH, Hamer RM, Lieberman JA, Jarskog LF. Synaptophysin and postsynaptic density protein 95 in the human prefrontal cortex from mid-gestation into early adulthood. *Neuroscience.* 2007;149:582–591.

Gow RV, Sumich A, Vallee-Tourangeau F, Crawford MA, Ghebremeskel K, Bueno AA, Hibbeln JR, Taylor E, Wilson DA, Rubia K. Omega-3 fatty acids are related to abnormal emotion processing in adolescent boys with attention deficit hyperactivity disorder. *Prostaglandins Leukot Essent Fatty Acids.* 2013a;88:419–429.

Gow RV, Vallee-Tourangeau F, Crawford MA, Taylor E, Ghebremeskel K, Bueno AA, Hibbeln JR, Sumich A, Rubia K. Omega-3 fatty acids are inversely related to callous and unemotional traits in adolescent boys with attention deficit hyperactivity disorder. *Prostaglandins Leukot Essent Fatty Acids.* 2013b;88:411–418.

Gozzo Y, Vohr B, Lacadie C, Hampson M, Katz KH, Maller-Kesselman J, Schneider KC et al. Alterations in neural connectivity in preterm children at school age. *Neuroimage.* 2009;48:458–463.

Grayson DS, Kroenke CD, Neuringer M, Fair DA. Dietary omega-3 fatty acids modulate large-scale systems organization in the rhesus macaque brain. *J Neurosci.* 2014;34:2065–2074.

Green P, Gispan-Herman I, Yadid G. Increased arachidonic acid concentration in the brain of Flinders Sensitive Line rats, an animal model of depression. *J Lipid Res.* 2005;46:1093–1096.

Green P, Glozman S, Weiner L, Yavin E. Enhanced free radical scavenging and decreased lipid peroxidation in the rat fetal brain after treatment with ethyl docosahexaenoate. *Biochim Biophys Acta.* 2001;1532:203–212.

Green P, Yavin E. Fatty acid composition of late embryonic and early postnatal rat brain. *Lipids.* 1996;31:859–865.

Greiner RS, Moriguchi T, Hutton A, Slotnick BM, Salem N Jr. Rats with low levels of brain docosahexaenoic acid show impaired performance in olfactory-based and spatial learning tasks. *Lipids.* 1999;34 Suppl.:S239–S243.

Greiner RS, Moriguchi T, Slotnick BM, Hutton A, Salem N. Olfactory discrimination deficits in n − 3 fatty acid-deficient rats. *Physiol Behav.* 2001;72:379–385.

Grosso G, Pajak A, Marventano S, Castellano S, Galvano F, Bucolo C, Drago F, Caraci F. Role of omega-3 fatty acids in the treatment of depressive disorders: A comprehensive meta-analysis of randomized clinical trials. *PLoS One.* 2014;9:e96905.

Hamilton L, Greiner R, Salem N Jr, Kim HY. n − 3 fatty acid deficiency decreases phosphatidylserine accumulation selectively in neuronal tissues. *Lipids.* 2000;35:863–869.

Harel Z, Riggs S, Vaz R, White L, Menzies G. Omega-3 polyunsaturated fatty acids in adolescents: Knowledge and consumption. *J Adolesc Health.* 2001;28:10–15.

Hawkey E, Nigg JT. Omega-3 fatty acid and ADHD: Blood level analysis and meta-analytic extension of supplementation trials. *Clin Psychol Rev.* 2014;34(6):496–505.

Helland IB, Smith L, Blomén B, Saarem K, Saugstad OD, Drevon CA. Effect of supplementing pregnant and lactating mothers with n − 3 very-long-chain fatty acids on children's IQ and body mass index at 7 years of age. *Pediatrics.* 2008;122:472–479.

Helland IB, Smith L, Saarem K, Saugstad OD, Drevon CA. Maternal supplementation with very-long-chain n − 3 fatty acids during pregnancy and lactation augments children's IQ at 4 years of age. *Pediatrics.* 2003;111:e39–e44.

Hibbeln JR. Fish consumption and major depression. *Lancet.* 1998;351:1213.

Hibbeln JR. Seafood consumption, the DHA content of mothers' milk and prevalence rates of postpartum depression: A cross-national, ecological analysis. *J Affect Disord.* 2002;69:15–29.

Hibbeln JR, Davis JM, Steer C, Emmett P, Rogers I, Williams C, Golding J. Maternal seafood consumption in pregnancy and neurodevelopmental outcomes in childhood (ALSPAC study): An observational cohort study. *Lancet.* 2007;369:578–585.

Hichami A, Datiche F, Ullah S, Liénard F, Chardigny JM, Cattarelli M, Khan NA. Olfactory discrimination ability and brain expression of c-fos, Gir and Glut1 mRNA are altered in n − 3 fatty acid-depleted rats. *Behav Brain Res.* 2007;184:1–10.

Hill DE, Yeo RA, Campbell RA, Hart B, Vigil J, Brooks W. Magnetic resonance imaging correlates of attention-deficit/hyperactivity disorder in children. *Neuropsychology.* 2003;17:496–506.

Högyes E, Nyakas C, Kiliaan A, Farkas T, Penke B, Luiten PG. Neuroprotective effect of developmental docosahexaenoic acid supplement against excitotoxic brain damage in infant rats. *Neuroscience.* 2003;119:999–1012.

Hsieh AT, Anthony JC, Diersen-Schade DA, Rumsey SC, Lawrence P, Li C, Nathanielsz PW, Brenna JT. The influence of moderate and high dietary long chain polyunsaturated fatty acids (LCPUFA) on baboon neonate tissue fatty acids. *Pediatr Res.* 2007;61:537–545.

Huang SY, Yang HT, Chiu CC, Pariante CM, Su KP. Omega-3 fatty acids on the forced-swimming test. *J Psychiatr Res*. 2008;42:58–63.

Huttenlocher PR. Synaptic density in human frontal cortex–Developmental changes and effects of aging. *Brain Res*. 1979;163:195–205.

Igarashi M, Ma K, Gao F, Kim HW, Greenstein D, Rapoport SI, Rao JS. Brain lipid concentrations in bipolar disorder. *J Psychiatr Res*. 2010;44:177–182.

Ikemoto A, Kobayashi T, Watanabe S, Okuyama H. Membrane fatty acid modifications of PC12 cells by arachidonate or docosahaenoate affect neurite outgrowth but not norepinephrine release. *Neurochem Res*. 1997;22:671–678.

Ikemoto A, Nitta A, Furukawa S, Ohishi M, Nakamura A, Fujii Y, Okuyama H. Dietary n – 3 fatty acid deficiency decreases nerve growth factor content in rat hippocampus. *Neurosci Lett*. 2000;285:99–102.

Innis SM. Polyunsaturated fatty acids in human milk: An essential role in infant development. *Adv Exp Med Biol*. 2004;554:27–43.

Innis SM, de La Presa Owens S. Dietary fatty acid composition in pregnancy alters neurite membrane fatty acids and dopamine in newborn rat brain. *J Nutr*. 2001a;131:118–122.

Innis SM, Gilley J, Werker J. Are human milk long-chain polyunsaturated fatty acids related to visual and neural development in breast-fed term infants? *J Pediatr*. 2001b;139:532–538.

Itokazu N, Ikegaya Y, Nishikawa M, Matsuki N. Bidirectional actions of docosahexaenoic acid on hippocampal neurotransmissions in vivo. *Brain Res*. 2000;862:211–216.

Jacobson JL, Jacobson SW, Muckle G, Kaplan-Estrin M, Ayotte P, Dewailly E. Beneficial effects of a polyunsaturated fatty acid on infant development: Evidence from the inuit of arctic Quebec. *J Pediatr*. 2008;152:356–364.

Jacques C, Levy E, Muckle G, Jacobson SW, Bastien C, Dewailly E, Ayotte P, Jacobson JL, Saint-Amour D. Long-term effects of prenatal omega-3 fatty acid intake on visual function in school-age children. *J Pediatr*. 2011;158:83–90.

Jamieson EC, Farquharson J, Logan RW, Howatson AG, Patrick WJ, Weaver LT, Cockburn F. Infant cerebellar gray and white matter fatty acids in relation to age and diet. *Lipids*. 1999;34:1065–1071.

Jensen CL, Maude M, Anderson RE, Heird WC. Effect of docosahexaenoic acid supplementation of lactating women on the fatty acid composition of breast milk lipids and maternal and infant plasma phospholipids. *Am J Clin Nutr*. 2000;71:292S–299S.

Kadziela-Olech H, Piotrowska-Jastrzebska J. The duration of breastfeeding and attention deficit hyperactivity disorder. *Rocz Akad Med Bialymst*. 2005;50:302–306.

Kawakita E, Hashimoto M, Shido O. Docosahexaenoic acid promotes neurogenesis in vitro and in vivo. *Neuroscience*. 2006;139:991–997.

Keleshian VL, Kellom M, Kim HW, Taha AY, Cheon Y, Igarashi M, Rapoport SI, Rao JS. Neuropathological responses to chronic NMDA in rats are worsened by dietary n – 3 PUFA deprivation but are not ameliorated by fish oil supplementation. *PLoS One*. 2014;9:e95318.

Kesler SR, Reiss AL, Vohr B, Watson C, Schneider KC, Katz KH, Maller-Kesselman J et al. Brain volume reductions within multiple cognitive systems in male preterm children at age twelve. *J Pediatr*. 2008;152:513–520.

Kirby A, Woodward A, Jackson S, Wang Y, Crawford MA. A double-blind, placebo-controlled study investigating the effects of omega-3 supplementation in children aged 8–10 years from a mainstream school population. *Res Dev Disabil*. 2010;31:718–730.

Kodas E, Galineau L, Bodard S, Vancassel S, Guilloteau D, Besnard JC, Chalon S. Serotoninergic neurotransmission is affected by n – 3 polyunsaturated fatty acids in the rat. *J Neurochem*. 2004;89:695–702.

Kodas E, Page G, Zimmer L, Vancassel S, Guilloteau D, Durand G, Chalon S. Neither the density nor function of striatal dopamine transporters were influenced by chronic n − 3 polyunsaturated fatty acid deficiency in rodents. *Neurosci Lett.* 2002b;321:95–99.

Kodas E, Vancassel S, Lejeune B, Guilloteau D, Chalon S. Reversibility of n − 3 fatty acid deficiency-induced changes in dopaminergic neurotransmission in rats: Critical role of developmental stage. *J Lipid Res.* 2002a;43:1209–1219.

Koletzko B, Larqué E, Demmelmair H. Placental transfer of long-chain polyunsaturated fatty acids (LC-PUFA). *J Perinat Med.* 2007;35:S5–S11.

Kong W, Yen JH, Ganea D. Docosahexaenoic acid prevents dendritic cell maturation, inhibits antigen-specific Th1/Th17 differentiation and suppresses experimental autoimmune encephalomyelitis. *Brain Behav Immun.* 2011;25:872–882.

Kuperstein F, Eilam R, Yavin E. Altered expression of key dopaminergic regulatory proteins in the postnatal brain following perinatal n − 3 fatty acid dietary deficiency. *J Neurochem.* 2008;106:662–671.

Laino CH, Fonseca C, Sterin-Speziale N, Slobodianik N, Reinés A. Potentiation of omega-3 fatty acid antidepressant-like effects with low non-antidepressant doses of fluoxetine and mirtazapine. *Eur J Pharmacol.* 2010;648:117–126.

Lakhwani L, Tongia SK, Pal VS, Agrawal RP, Nyati P, Phadnis P. Omega-3 fatty acids have antidepressant activity in forced swimming test in Wistar rats. *Acta Pol Pharm.* 2007;64:271–276.

Lalovic A, Levy E, Canetti L, Sequeira A, Montoudis A, Turecki G. Fatty acid composition in postmortem brains of people who completed suicide. *J Psychiatry Neurosci.* 2007;32:363–370.

Lauritzen L, Carlson SE. Maternal fatty acid status during pregnancy and lactation and relation to newborn and infant status. *Matern Child Nutr.* 2011;7 Suppl. 2:41–58.

Lauritzen L, Harsløf LB, Hellgren LI, Pedersen MH, Mølgaard C, Michaelsen KF. Fish intake, erythrocyte n − 3 fatty acid status and metabolic health in Danish adolescent girls and boys. *Br J Nutr.* 2012;107:697–704.

Lauritzen L, Jørgensen MH, Hansen HS, Michaelsen KF. Fluctuations in human milk long-chain PUFA levels in relation to dietary fish intake. *Lipids.* 2002;37:237–244.

Lawrence KE, Levitt JG, Loo SK, Ly R, Yee V, O'Neill J, Alger J, Narr KL. White matter microstructure in subjects with attention-deficit/hyperactivity disorder and their siblings. *J Am Acad Child Adolesc Psychiatry.* 2013;52:431–440.

Lawson KR, Ruff HA. Early focused attention predicts outcome for children born prematurely. *J Dev Behav Pediatr.* 2004;25:399–406.

Lee HC, Lin HC. Maternal bipolar disorder increased low birthweight and preterm births: A nationwide population-based study. *J Affect Disord.* 2010;121:100–105.

Levant B, Ozias MK, Carlson SE. Diet (n − 3) polyunsaturated fatty acid content and parity interact to alter maternal rat brain phospholipid fatty acid composition. *J Nutr.* 2006a;136:2236–22342.

Levant B, Radel JD, Carlson SE. Decreased brain docosahexaenoic acid during development alters dopamine-related behaviors in adult rats that are differentially affected by dietary remediation. *Behav Brain Res.* 2004;152:49–57.

Levant B, Radel JD, Carlson SE. Reduced brain DHA content after a single reproductive cycle in female rats fed a diet deficient in N − 3 polyunsaturated fatty acids. *Biol Psychiatry.* 2006b;60:987–990.

Lin PY, Huang SY, Su KP. A meta-analytic review of polyunsaturated fatty acid compositions in patients with depression. *Biol Psychiatry.* 2010;68:140–147.

Lubsen J, Vohr B, Myers E, Hampson M, Lacadie C, Schneider KC, Katz KH, Constable RT, Ment LR. Microstructural and functional connectivity in the developing preterm brain. *Semin Perinatol.* 2011;35:34–43.

Lyoo IK, Noam GG, Lee CK, Lee HK, Kennedy BP, Renshaw PF. The corpus callosum and lateral ventricles in children with attention-deficit hyperactivity disorder: A brain magnetic resonance imaging study. *Biol Psychiatry*. 1996;40:1060–1063.

Makrides M, Gibson RA, McPhee AJ, Yelland L, Quinlivan J, Ryan P; DOMInO Investigative Team. Effect of DHA supplementation during pregnancy on maternal depression and neurodevelopment of young children: A randomized controlled trial. *JAMA*. 2010;304:1675–1683.

Makrides M, Neumann MA, Byard RW, Simmer K, Gibson RA. Fatty acid composition of brain, retina, and erythrocytes in breast- and formula-fed infants. *Am J Clin Nutr*. 1994;60:189–194.

Mansbach RS, Geyer MA, Braff DL. Dopaminergic stimulation disrupts sensorimotor gating in the rat. *Psychopharmacology (Berl)*. 1988;94:507–514.

Markhus MW, Skotheim S, Graff IE, Frøyland L, Braarud HC, Stormark KM, Malde MK. Low omega-3 index in pregnancy is a possible biological risk factor for postpartum depression. *PLoS One*. 2013;8:e67617.

Martin DS, Spencer P, Horrobin DF, Lynch MA. Long-term potentiation in aged rats is restored when the age-related decrease in polyunsaturated fatty acid concentration is reversed. *Prostaglandins Leukot Essent Fatty Acids*. 2002;67:121–130.

Martin RE, Bazan NG. Changing fatty acid content of growth cone lipids prior to synaptogenesis. *J Neurochem*. 1992;59:318–325.

Martinez M. Tissue levels of polyunsaturated fatty acids during early human development. *J Pediatr*. 1992;120:S129–S138.

Martinez M. Polyunsaturated fatty acids in the developing human brain, erythrocytes and plasma in peroxisomal disease: Therapeutic implications. *J Inherit Metab Dis*. 1995;18:61–75.

Martinez M. Docosahexaenoic acid therapy in docosahexaenoic acid-deficient patients with disorders of peroxisomal biogenesis. *Lipids*. 1996;31:S145–S152.

Martínez M, Mougan I. Fatty acid composition of human brain phospholipids during normal development. *J Neurochem*. 1998;71:2528–2533.

Martinez M, Vazquez E. MRI evidence that docosahexaenoic acid ethyl ester improves myelination in generalized peroxisomal disorders. *Neurology*. 1998;51:26–32.

Martínez M, Vázquez E, García-Silva MT, Manzanares J, Bertran JM, Castelló F, Mougan I. Therapeutic effects of docosahexaenoic acid ethyl ester in patients with generalized peroxisomal disorders. *Am J Clin Nutr*. 2000;71:376S–385S.

McGahon BM, Martin DS, Horrobin DF, Lynch MA. Age-related changes in synaptic function: Analysis of the effect of dietary supplementation with omega-3 fatty acids. *Neuroscience*. 1999;94:305–314.

McNamara RK. Deciphering the role of docosahexaenoic acid in brain maturation and pathology with magnetic resonance imaging. *Prostaglandins Leukot Essent Fatty Acids*. 2013b;88:33–42.

McNamara RK. Developmental long-chain omega-3 fatty acid deficiency and prefrontal cortex pathology in psychiatric disorders. In: RO Collins and JL Adams (Eds.), *Prefrontal Cortex: Developmental Differences and Role in Neurological Disorders*. Nova Science Publishers, Inc., New York, pp. 1–38, 2013d.

McNamara RK, Able J, Jandacek R, Rider T, Tso P. Inbred C57BL/6J and DBA/2J mouse strains exhibit constitutive differences in regional brain fatty acid composition. *Lipids*. 2009c;44:1–8.

McNamara RK, Able JA, Jandacek R, Rider T, Tso P, Eliassen JC, Alfieri D et al. Docosahexaenoic acid supplementation increases prefrontal cortex activation during sustained attention in healthy boys: A placebo-controlled, dose-ranging, functional magnetic resonance imaging study. *Am J Clin Nutr*. 2010b;91:1060–1067.

McNamara RK, Able JA, Liu Y, Jandacek R, Rider T, Tso P. Gender differences in rat erythrocyte and brain docosahexaenoic acid composition: Role of ovarian hormones and dietary omega-3 fatty acid composition. *Psychoneuroendocrinology*. 2009b;34:532–539.

McNamara RK, Able JA, Liu Y, Jandacek R, Rider T, Tso P, Lipton JW. Omega-3 fatty acid deficiency during perinatal development increases serotonin turnover in the prefrontal cortex and decreases midbrain tryptophan hydroxylase-2 expression in adult female rats: Dissociation from estrogenic effects. *J Psychiatr Res*. 2009a;43:656–663.

McNamara RK, Able JA, Liu Y, Jandacek R, Rider T, Tso P, Lipton JW. Omega-3 fatty acid deficiency does not alter the effects of chronic fluoxetine treatment on central serotonin turnover or behavior in the forced swim test in female rats. *Pharmacol Biochem Behav*. 2013a;114:1–8.

McNamara RK, Adler C, Strawn J, Strimpfel J, Mills N, Wulsin L, Jandacek R et al. Adolescent bipolar I disorder patients exhibit erythrocyte long-chain omega-3 fatty acid deficits during acute mania and euthymia following pharmacotherapy: Support for a trait versus state feature. *Society of Biological Psychiatry Meeting*, San Francisco, CA, 2011;67:S127.

McNamara RK, Carlson SE. Role of omega-3 fatty acids in brain development and function: Potential implications for the pathogenesis and prevention of psychopathology. *Prostaglandins Leukot Essent Fatty Acids*. 2006;75:329–349.

McNamara RK, Hahn C-G, Jandacek R, Rider T, Tso P, Stanford K, Richtand NM. Selective deficits in the omega-3 fatty acid docosahexaenoic acid in the postmortem orbitofrontal cortex of patients with major depressive disorder. *Biol Psychiatry*. 2007;62:17–24.

McNamara RK, Jandacek R, Rider T, Tso P, Cole-Strauss A, Lipton JW. Omega-3 fatty acid deficiency increases constitutive pro-inflammatory cytokine production in rats: Relationship with central serotonin turnover. *Prostaglandins Leukot Essent Fatty Acids*. 2010a;83:185–191.

McNamara RK, Jandacek R, Rider T, Tso P, Dwivedi Y, Pandey GN. Selective deficits in erythrocyte docosahexaenoic acid composition in adult patients with bipolar disorder and major depressive disorder. *J Affect Disord*. 2010c;126:303–311.

McNamara RK, Jandacek R, Rider T, Tso P, Dwivedi Y, Roberts RC, Conley RR, Pandey GN. Fatty acid composition of the postmortem prefrontal cortex of male and female adolescent suicide victims. *Prostaglandins Leukot Essent Fatty Acids*. 2009c;80:19–26.

McNamara RK, Jandacek R, Rider T, Tso P, Stanford K, Hahn C-G, Richtand NM. Deficits in docosahexaenoic acid and associated elevations in the metabolism of arachidonic acid and saturated fatty acids in the postmortem orbitofrontal cortex of patients with bipolar disorder. *Psychiatry Res*. 2008d;160:285–299.

McNamara RK, Jandacek R, Tso P, Dwivedi Y, Ren X, Pandey GN. Lower docosahexaenoic acid concentrations in the postmortem prefrontal cortex of adult depressed suicide victims compared with controls without cardiovascular disease. *J Psychiatr Res*. 2013c;47:1187–1191.

McNamara RK, Liu Y, Jandacek R, Rider T, Tso P. The aging human orbitofrontal cortex: Decreasing polyunsaturated fatty acid composition and associated increases in lipogenic gene expression and stearoyl-CoA desaturase activity. *Prostaglandins Leukot Essent Fatty Acids*. 2008a;78:293–304.

McNamara RK, Ostrander M, Abplanalp W, Richtand NM, Benoit SC, Clegg DJ. Modulation of phosphoinositide-protein kinase C signal transduction by omega-3 fatty acids: Implications for the pathophysiology and treatment of recurrent neuropsychiatric illness. *Prostaglandins Leukot Essent Fatty Acids*. 2006;75:237–257.

McNamara RK, Strimpfel J, Jandacek R, Rider T, Tso P, Welge JA, Strawn JR, DelBello MP. Detection and treatment of long-chain omega-3 fatty acid deficiency in adolescents with SSRI-resistant major depressive disorder. *Pharma Nutrition*. 2014;2:38–46.

McNamara RK, Sullivan J, Richtand NM. Omega-3 fatty acid deficiency augments amphetamine-induced behavioral sensitization in adult mice: Prevention by chronic lithium treatment. *J Psychiatr Res.* 2008b;42:458–468.

McNamara RK, Sullivan J, Richtand NM, Jandacek R, Rider T, Tso P, Campbell N, Lipton J. Omega-3 fatty acid deficiency augments amphetamine-induced behavioral sensitization in adult DBA/2J mice: Relationship with ventral striatum dopamine concentrations. *Synapse.* 2008c;62:725–735.

Menon V. Large-scale brain networks and psychopathology: A unifying triple network model. *Trends Cogn Sci.* 2011;15:483–506.

Ment LR, Kesler S, Vohr B, Katz KH, Baumgartner H, Schneider KC, Delancy S et al. Longitudinal brain volume changes in preterm and term control subjects during late childhood and adolescence. *Pediatrics.* 2009;123:503–511.

Miller BJ, Murray L, Beckmann MM, Kent T, Macfarlane B. Dietary supplements for preventing postnatal depression. *Cochrane Database Syst Rev.* 2013;10:CD009104.

Milte CM, Parletta N, Buckley JD, Coates AM, Young RM, Howe PR. Eicosapentaenoic and docosahexaenoic acids, cognition, and behavior in children with attention-deficit/hyperactivity disorder: A randomized controlled trial. *Nutrition.* 2012;28:670–677.

Mirnikjoo B, Brown SE, Kim HF, Marangell LB, Sweatt JD, Weeber EJ. Protein kinase inhibition by omega-3 fatty acids. *J Biol Chem.* 2001;276:10888–10896.

Mitchell EA, Aman MG, Turbott SH, Manku M. Clinical characteristics and serum essential fatty acid levels in hyperactive children. *Clin Pediatr (Phila).* 1987;26:406–411.

Moltó-Puigmartí C, Plat J, Mensink RP, Müller A, Jansen E, Zeegers MP, Thijs C. FADS1 FADS2 gene variants modify the association between fish intake and the docosahexaenoic acid proportions in human milk. *Am J Clin Nutr.* 2010;91:1368–1376.

Moriguchi T, Greiner RS, Salem N Jr. Behavioral deficits associated with dietary induction of decreased brain docosahexaenoic acid concentration. *J Neurochem.* 2000;75:2563–2573.

Moriguchi T, Salem N Jr. Recovery of brain docosahexaenoate leads to recovery of spatial task performance. *J Neurochem.* 2003;87:297–309.

Morris RG. NMDA receptors and memory encoding. *Neuropharmacology.* 2013;74:32–40.

Mozaffarian D, Rimm EB. Fish intake, contaminants, and human health: Evaluating the risks and the benefits. *JAMA.* 2006;296:1885–1899.

Mullen KM, Vohr BR, Katz KH, Schneider KC, Lacadie C, Hampson M, Makuch RW, Reiss AL, Constable RT, Ment LR. Preterm birth results in alterations in neural connectivity at age 16 years. *Neuroimage.* 2011;54:2563–2570.

Murakami K, Miyake Y, Sasaki S, Tanaka K, Arakawa M. Fish and n − 3 polyunsaturated fatty acid intake and depressive symptoms: Ryukyus Child Health Study. *Pediatrics.* 2010;126:623–630.

Nagy Z, Westerberg H, Skare S, Andersson JL, Lilja A, Flodmark O, Fernell E et al. Preterm children have disturbances of white matter at 11 years of age as shown by diffusion tensor imaging. *Pediatr Res.* 2003;54:672–679.

Nemets H, Nemets B, Apter A, Bracha Z, Belmaker RH. Omega-3 treatment of childhood depression: A controlled, double-blind pilot study. *Am J Psychiatry.* 2006;163:1098–1100.

Nestler EJ, Carlezon WA Jr. The mesolimbic dopamine reward circuit in depression. *Biol Psychiatry.* 2006;59:1151–1159.

Neuringer M, Connor WE, Lin DS, Barstad L, Luck S. Biochemical and functional effects of prenatal and postnatal omega 3 fatty acid deficiency on retina and brain in rhesus monkeys. *Proc Natl Acad Sci USA.* 1986;83:4021–4025.

Nishikawa M, Kimura S, Akaike N. Facilitatory effect of docosahexaenoic acid on N-methyl-D-aspartate response in pyramidal neurones of rat cerebral cortex. *J Physiol.* 1994;475:83–93.

Noaghiul S, Hibbeln JR. Cross-national comparisons of seafood consumption and rates of bipolar disorders. *Am J Psychiatry.* 2003;160:2222–2227.

Noguer MT, Martinez M. Visual follow-up in peroxisomal-disorder patients treated with doco-sahexaenoic Acid ethyl ester. *Invest Ophthalmol Vis Sci.* 2010;51:2277–2285.

Nosarti C, Al-Asady MH, Frangou S, Stewart AL, Rifkin L, Murray RM. Adolescents who were born very preterm have decreased brain volumes. *Brain.* 2002;125:1616–1623.

Nosarti C, Reichenberg A, Murray RM, Cnattingius S, Lambe MP, Yin L, MacCabe J, Rifkin L, Hultman CM. Preterm birth and psychiatric disorders in young adult life. *Arch Gen Psychiatry.* 2012;69:E1–E8.

Oddy WH, Hickling S, Smith MA, O'Sullivan TA, Robinson M, de Klerk NH, Beilin LJ et al. Dietary intake of omega-3 fatty acids and risk of depressive symptoms in adolescents. *Depress Anxiety.* 2011;28:582–588.

Olsén P, Vainionpää L, Pääkkö E, Korkman M, Pyhtinen J, Järvelin MR. Psychological find-ings in preterm children related to neurologic status and magnetic resonance imaging. *Pediatrics.* 1998;102:329–336.

Olsen SF, Østerdal ML, Salvig JD, Weber T, Tabor A, Secher NJ. Duration of pregnancy in relation to fish oil supplementation and habitual fish intake: A randomised clinical trial with fish oil. *Eur J Clin Nutr.* 2007;61:976–985.

Olsen SF, Sørensen JD, Secher NJ, Hedegaard M, Henriksen TB, Hansen HS, Grant A. Randomised controlled trial of effect of fish-oil supplementation on pregnancy duration. *Lancet.* 1992;339(8800):1003–1007.

Orr SK, Palumbo S, Bosetti F, Mount HT, Kang JX, Greenwood CE, Ma DW, Serhan CN, Bazinet RP. Unesterified docosahexaenoic acid is protective in neuroinflammation. *J Neurochem.* 2013;127:378–393.

O'Sullivan TA, Ambrosini GL, Mori TA, Beilin LJ, Oddy WH. Omega-3 Index correlates with healthier food consumption in adolescents and with reduced cardiovascular disease risk factors in adolescent boys. *Lipids.* 2011;46:59–67.

Otto SJ, deGroot RH, Hornstra G. Increased risk of postpartum depressive symptoms is asso-ciated with slower normalization after pregnancy of the functional docosahexaenoic acid status. *Prostaglandins Leukot Essent Fatty Acids.* 2003;69:237–243.

Otto SJ, van Houwelingen AC, Badart-Smook A, Hornstra G. Changes in the maternal essen-tial fatty acid profile during early pregnancy and the relation of the profile to diet. *Am J Clin Nutr.* 2001;73:302–307.

Ozyurt B, Sarsilmaz M, Akpolat N, Ozyurt H, Akyol O, Herken H, Kus I. The protective effects of omega-3 fatty acids against MK-801-induced neurotoxicity in prefrontal cor-tex of rat. *Neurochem Int.* 2007;50:196–202.

Paus T, Zijdenbos A, Worsley K, Collins DL, Blumenthal J, Giedd JN, Rapoport JL, Evans AC. Structural maturation of neural pathways in children and adolescents: In vivo study. *Science.* 1999;283:1908–1911.

Petanjek Z, Judaš M, Šimic G, Rasin MR, Uylings HB, Rakic P, Kostovic I. Extraordinary neoteny of synaptic spines in the human prefrontal cortex. *Proc Natl Acad Sci USA.* 2011;108(32):13281–13286.

Peterson BS, Vohr B, Staib LH, Cannistraci CJ, Dolberg A, Schneider KC, Katz KH et al. Regional brain volume abnormalities and long-term cognitive outcome in preterm infants. *JAMA.* 2000;284:1939–1947.

Pottala JV, Talley JA, Churchill SW, Lynch DA, von Schacky C, Harris WS. Red blood cell fatty acids are associated with depression in a case-control study of adolescents. *Prostaglandins Leukot Essent Fatty Acids.* 2012;86:161–165.

Powers JM, Moser HW. Peroxisomal disorders: Genotype, phenotype, major neuropathologic lesions, and pathogenesis. *Brain Pathol.* 1998;8:101–120.

Putnam JC, Carlson SE, DeVoe PW, Barness LA. The effect of variations in dietary fatty acids on the fatty acid composition of erythrocyte phosphatidylcholine and phosphatidyletha-nolamine in human infants. *Am J Clin Nutr.* 1982;36:106–114.

Rao JS, Ertley RN, Lee HJ, DeMar JC Jr, Arnold JT, Rapoport SI, Bazinet RP. n – 3 polyunsaturated fatty acid deprivation in rats decreases frontal cortex BDNF via a p38 MAPK-dependent mechanism. *Mol Psychiatry.* 2007;12:36–46.

Reardon HT, Brenna JT. Microsomal biosynthesis of omega-3 fatty acids. In: RK McNamara (Ed.), *The Omega-3 Fatty Acid Deficiency Syndrome: Opportunities for Disease Prevention.* Nova Science Publishers, Inc., New York, 2013, pp. 3–17.

Reisbick S, Neuringer M, Gohl E, Wald R, Anderson GJ. Visual attention in infant monkeys: Effects of dietary fatty acids and age. *Dev Psychol.* 1997;33:387–395.

Reisbick S, Neuringer M, Hasnain R, Connor WE. Polydipsia in rhesus monkeys deficient in omega-3 fatty acids. *Physiol Behav.* 1990;47:315–323.

Reisbick S, Neuringer M, Hasnain R, Connor WE. Home cage behavior of rhesus monkeys with long-term deficiency of omega-3 fatty acids. *Physiol Behav.* 1994;55:231–239.

Richardson AJ, Burton JR, Sewell RP, Spreckelsen TF, Montgomery P. Docosahexaenoic acid for reading, cognition and behavior in children aged 7–9 years: A randomized, controlled trial (the DOLAB Study). *PLoS One.* 2012;7:e43909.

Robbins TW, McAlonan G, Muir JL, Everitt BJ. Cognitive enhancers in theory and practice: Studies of the cholinergic hypothesis of cognitive deficits in Alzheimer's disease. *Behav Brain Res.* 1997;83:15–23.

Rosa Neto P, Lou H, Cumming P, Pryds O, Gjedde A. Methylphenidate-evoked potentiation of extracellular dopamine in the brain of adolescents with premature birth: Correlation with attentional deficit. *Ann NY Acad Sci.* 2002;965:434–439.

Ryan AS, Astwood JD, Gautier S, Kuratko CN, Nelson EB, Salem N Jr. Effects of long-chain polyunsaturated fatty acid supplementation on neurodevelopment in childhood: A review of human studies. *Prostaglandins Leukot Essent Fatty Acids.* 2010;82:305–314.

Salem N Jr, Litman B, Kim HY, Gawrisch K. Mechanisms of action of docosahexaenoic acid in the nervous system. *Lipids.* 2001;36:945–959.

Salt A, Redshaw M. Neurodevelopmental follow-up after preterm birth: Follow up after two years. *Early Hum Dev.* 2006;82:185–197.

Salvig JD, Lamont RF. Evidence regarding an effect of marine n – 3 fatty acids on preterm birth: A systematic review and meta-analysis. *Acta Obstet Gynecol Scand.* 2011;90:825–838.

Sanders TA, Naismith DJ. A comparison of the influence of breast-feeding and bottle-feeding on the fatty acid composition of the erythrocytes. *Br J Nutr.* 1979;41:619–623.

Sands SA, Reid KJ, Windsor SL, Harris WS. The impact of age, body mass index, and fish intake on the EPA and DHA content of human erythrocytes. *Lipids.* 2005;40:343–347.

SanGiovanni JP, Parra-Cabrera S, Colditz GA, Berkey CS, Dwyer JT. Meta-analysis of dietary essential fatty acids and long-chain polyunsaturated fatty acids as they relate to visual resolution acuity in healthy preterm infants. *Pediatrics.* 2000;105:1292–1298.

Sarkadi-Nagy E, Wijendran V, Diau GY, Chao AC, Hsieh AT, Turpeinen A, Lawrence P, Nathanielsz PW, Brenna JT. Formula feeding potentiates docosahexaenoic and arachidonic acid biosynthesis in term and preterm baboon neonates. *J Lipid Res.* 2004;45:71–80.

Sarkadi-Nagy E, Wijendran V, Diau GY, Chao AC, Hsieh AT, Turpeinen A, Nathanielsz PW, Brenna JT. The influence of prematurity and long chain polyunsaturate supplementation in 4-week adjusted age baboon neonate brain and related tissues. *Pediatr Res.* 2003;54:244–252.

Sarter M, Bruno JP. Cortical cholinergic inputs mediating arousal, attentional processing and dreaming: Differential afferent regulation of the basal forebrain by telencephalic and brainstem afferents. *Neuroscience.* 2000;95:933–952.

Schafer RJ, Lacadie C, Vohr B, Kesler SR, Katz KH, Schneider KC, Pugh KR et al. Alterations in functional connectivity for language in prematurely born adolescents. *Brain.* 2009;132:661–670.

Scholtz SA, Colombo J, Carlson SE. Clinical overview of effects of dietary long-chain poly-unsaturated fatty acids during the perinatal period. *Nestle Nutr Inst Workshop Ser.* 2013;77:145–154.

Schothorst PF, van Engeland H. Long-term behavioral sequelae of prematurity. *J Am Acad Child Adolesc Psychiatry.* 1996;35:175–183.

Schulzke SM, Patole SK, Simmer K. Long-chain polyunsaturated fatty acid supplementation in preterm infants. *Cochrane Database Syst Rev.* 2011;(2):CD000375.

Sichert-Hellert W, Wicher M, Kersting M. Age and time trends in fish consumption pattern of children and adolescents, and consequences for the intake of long-chain n − 3 polyun-saturated fatty acids. *Eur J Clin Nutr.* 2009;63:1071–1075.

Singh MK, DelBello MP, Kowatch RA, Strakowski SM. Co-occurrence of bipolar and attention-deficit hyperactivity disorders in children. *Bipolar Disord.* 2006;8:710–720.

Smithers LG, Collins CT, Simmonds LA, Gibson RA, McPhee A, Makrides M. Feeding pre-term infants milk with a higher dose of docosahexaenoic acid than that used in current practice does not influence language or behavior in early childhood: A follow-up study of a randomized controlled trial. *Am J Clin Nutr.* 2010;91:628–634.

Smithers LG, Gibson RA, Makrides M. Maternal supplementation with docosahexaenoic acid during pregnancy does not affect early visual development in the infant: A randomized controlled trial. *Am J Clin Nutr.* 2011;93:1293–1299.

Smyser CD, Snyder AZ, Shimony JS, Blazey TM, Inder TE, Neil JJ. Effects of white mat-ter injury on resting state fMRI measures in prematurely born infants. *PLoS One.* 2013;8:e68098.

Sowell ER, Thompson PM, Holmes CJ, Batth R, Jernigan TL, Toga AW. Localizing age-related changes in brain structure between childhood and adolescence using statistical parametric mapping. *Neuroimage.* 1999;9:587–597.

Sowell ER, Thompson PM, Welcome SE, Henkenius AL, Toga AW, Peterson BS. Cortical abnormalities in children and adolescents with attention-deficit hyperactivity disorder. *Lancet.* 2003;362:1699–1707.

Stein DJ. Depression, anhedonia, and psychomotor symptoms: The role of dopaminergic neu-rocircuitry. *CNS Spectr.* 2008;13:561–565.

Stevens LJ, Zentall SS, Deck JL, Abate ML, Watkins BA, Lipp SR, Burgess JR. Essential fatty acid metabolism in boys with attention-deficit hyperactivity disorder. *Am J Clin Nutr.* 1995;62:761–768.

Stewart AL, Rifkin L, Amess PN, Kirkbride V, Townsend JP, Miller DH, Lewis SW et al.. Brain structure and neurocognitive and behavioural function in adolescents who were born very preterm. *Lancet.* 1999;353:1653–1657.

Strakowski SM, Adler CM, Almeida J, Altshuler LL, Blumberg HP, Chang KD, Del Bello MP et al. The functional neuroanatomy of bipolar disorder: A consensus model. *Bipolar Disord.* 2012;14:313–325.

Su HM, Bernardo L, Mirmiran M, Ma XH, Corso TN, Nathanielsz PW, Brenna JT. Bioequivalence of dietary alpha-linolenic and docosahexaenoic acids as sources of docosahexaenoate accretion in brain and associated organs of neonatal baboons. *Pediatr Res.* 1999;45:87–93.

Su HM, Bernardo L, Mirmiran M, Ma XH, Nathanielsz PW, Brenna JT. Dietary 18:3n − 3 and 22:6n − 3 as sources of 22:6n − 3 accretion in neonatal baboon brain and associated organs. *Lipids.* 1999;34:S347–S350.

Su KP, Huang SY, Chiu TH, Huang KC, Huang CL, Chang HC, Pariante CM. Omega-3 fatty acids for major depressive disorder during pregnancy: Results from a randomized, dou-ble-blind, placebo-controlled trial. *J Clin Psychiatry.* 2008;69:644–651.

Sun L, Cao Q, Long X, Sui M, Cao X, Zhu C, Zuo X et al. Abnormal functional connectivity between the anterior cingulate and the default mode network in drug-naïve boys with attention deficit hyperactivity disorder. *Psychiatry Res.* 2012;201:120–127.

Suzuki H, Manabe S, Wada O, Crawford MA. Rapid incorporation of docosahexaenoic acid from dietary sources into brain microsomal, synaptosomal and mitochondrial membranes in adult mice. *Int J Vitam Nutr Res.* 1997;67:272–278.

Swenne I, Rosling A, Tengblad S, Vessby B. Omega-3 polyunsaturated essential fatty acids are associated with depression in adolescents with eating disorders and weight loss. *Acta Paediatr.* 2011;100:1610–1615.

Tian L, Jiang T, Wang Y, Zang Y, He Y, Liang M, Sui M et al. Altered resting-state functional connectivity patterns of anterior cingulate cortex in adolescents with attention deficit hyperactivity disorder. *Neurosci Lett.* 2006;400:39–43.

Tisserand DJ, Pruessner JC, Sanz Arigita EJ, van Boxtel MP, Evans AC, Jolles J, Uylings HB. Regional frontal cortical volumes decrease differentially in aging: An MRI study to compare volumetric approaches and voxel-based morphometry. *Neuroimage.* 2002;17:657–669.

Tsukada H, Kakiuchi T, Fukumoto D, Nishiyama S, Koga K. Docosahexaenoic acid (DHA) improves the age-related impairment of the coupling mechanism between neuronal activation and functional cerebral blood flow response: A PET study in conscious monkeys. *Brain Res.* 2000;862:180–186.

Tuzun F, Kumral A, Dilek M, Ozbal S, Ergur B, Yesilirmak DC, Duman N, Yilmaz O, Ozkan H. Maternal omega-3 fatty acid supplementation protects against lipopolysaccharide-induced white matter injury in the neonatal rat brain. *J Matern Fetal Neonatal Med.* 2012;25:849–854.

Uauy R, Hoffman DR, Peirano P, Birch DG, Birch EE. Essential fatty acids in visual and brain development. *Lipids.* 2001;36:885–895.

Ulmann L, Mimouni V, Roux S, Porsolt R, Poisson JP. Brain and hippocampus fatty acid composition in phospholipid classes of aged-relative cognitive deficit rats. *Prostaglandins Leukot Essent Fatty Acids.* 2001;64:189–195.

Vaisman N, Pelled D. n − 3 phosphatidylserine attenuated scopolamine-induced amnesia in middle-aged rats. *Prog Neuropsychopharmacol Biol Psychiatry.* 2009;33:952–959.

Valentine CJ, Morrow G, Pennell M, Morrow AL, Hodge A, Haban-Bartz A, Collins K, Rogers LK. Randomized controlled trial of docosahexaenoic acid supplementation in midwestern U.S. human milk donors. *Breastfeed Med.* 2013;8:86–91.

van Wezel-Meijler G, vander Knaap MS, Huisman J, Jonkman EJ, Valk J, Lafeber HN. Dietary supplementation of long-chain polyunsaturated fatty acids in preterm infants: Effects on cerebral maturation. *Acta Paediatr.* 2002;91:942–950.

Vancassel S, Blondeau C, Lallemand S, Cador M, Linard A, Lavialle M, Dellu-Hagedorn F. Hyperactivity in the rat is associated with spontaneous low level of n − 3 polyunsaturated fatty acids in the frontal cortex. *Behav Brain Res.* 2007;180:119–126.

Vancassel S, Leman S, Hanonick L, Denis S, Roger J, Nollet M, Bodard S, Kousignian I, Belzung C, Chalon S. n − 3 polyunsaturated fatty acid supplementation reverses stress-induced modifications on brain monoamine levels in mice. *J Lipid Res.* 2008;49:340–348.

Vaswani M, Linda FK, Ramesh S. Role of selective serotonin reuptake inhibitors in psychiatric disorders: A comprehensive review. *Prog Neuropsychopharmacol Biol Psychiatry.* 2003;27:85–102.

Volkow ND, Wang GJ, Newcorn J, Fowler JS, Telang F, Solanto MV, Logan J et al. Brain dopamine transporter levels in treatment and drug naïve adults with ADHD. *Neuroimage.* 2007;34:1182–1190.

Wanders RJA. Peroxisomal biosynthesis of omega-3 fatty acids and human peroxisomal diseases In: RK McNamara (Ed.), *The Omega-3 Fatty Acid Deficiency Syndrome: Opportunities for Disease Prevention.* Nova Science Publishers, Inc., New York, 2013, pp. 19–30.

Wang F, Bobrow L, Liu J, Spencer L, Blumberg HP. Corticolimbic functional connectivity in adolescents with bipolar disorder. *PLoS One.* 2012;7:e50177.

Werkman SH, Carlson SE. A randomized trial of visual attention of preterm infants fed docosahexaenoic acid until nine months. *Lipids*. 1996;31:91–97.

White TP, Symington I, Castellanos NP, Brittain PJ, Froudist Walsh S, Nam KW, Sato JR et al. Dysconnectivity of neurocognitive networks at rest in very-preterm born adults. *Neuroimage Clin*. 2014;4:352–365.

Williams C, Birch EE, Emmett PM, Northstone K; Avon Longitudinal Study of Pregnancy and Childhood Study Team. Stereoacuity at age 3.5 y in children born full-term is associated with prenatal and postnatal dietary factors: A report from a population-based cohort study. *Am J Clin Nutr*. 2001;73:316–322.

Wozniak J, Biederman J, Mick E, Waxmonsky J, Hantsoo L, Best C, Cluette-Brown JE, Laposata M. Omega-3 fatty acid monotherapy for pediatric bipolar disorder: A prospective open-label trial. *Eur Neuropsychopharmacol*. 2007;17:440–447.

Wu A, Ying Z, Gomez-Pinilla F. Dietary omega-3 fatty acids normalize BDNF levels, reduce oxidative damage, and counteract learning disability after traumatic brain injury in rats. *J Neurotrauma*. 2004;21:1457–1467.

Xiao Y, Huang Y, Chen ZY. Distribution, depletion and recovery of docosahexaenoic acid are region-specific in rat brain. *Br J Nutr*. 2005;94:544–550.

Yavin E, Brand A, Green P. Docosahexaenoic acid abundance in the brain: A biodevice to combat oxidative stress. *Nutr Neurosci*. 2002;5:149–157.

Yavin E, Himovichi E, Eilam R. Delayed cell migration in the developing rat brain following maternal omega 3 alpha linolenic acid dietary deficiency. *Neuroscience*. 2009;162:1011–1122.

Yoshida S, Yasuda A, Kawazato H, Sakai K, Shimada T, Takeshita M, Yuasa S, Kobayashi T, Watanabe S, Okuyama H. Synaptic vesicle ultrastructural changes in the rat hippocampus induced by a combination of alpha-linolenate deficiency and a learning task. *J Neurochem*. 1997;68:1261–1268.

Zimmer L, Delion-Vancassel S, Durand G, Guilloteau D, Bodard S, Besnard JC, Chalon S. Modification of dopamine neurotransmission in the nucleus accumbens of rats deficient in n – 3 polyunsaturated fatty acids. *J Lipid Res*. 2000b;41:32–40.

Zimmer L, Delpal S, Guilloteau D, Aioun J, Dur and G Chalon S. Chronic n – 3 polyunsaturated fatty acid deficiency alters dopamine vesicle density in the rat frontal cortex. *Neurosci Lett*. 2000a;284:25–28.

Zimmer L, Hembert S, Dur and G, Breton P, Guilloteau D, Besnard JC, Chalon S. Chronic n – 3 polyunsaturated fatty acid diet-deficiency acts on dopamine metabolism in the rat frontal cortex: A microdialysis study. *Neurosci Lett*. 1998;240:177–181.

Zimmer L, Vancassel S, Cantagrel S, Breton P, Delamanche S, Guilloteau D, Durand G, Chalon S. The dopamine mesocorticolimbic pathway is affected by deficiency in n – 3 polyunsaturated fatty acids. *Am J Clin Nutr*. 2002;75:662–667.

Zugno AI, Chipindo HL, Volpato AM, Budni J, Steckert AV, de Oliveira MB, Heylmann AS et al. Omega-3 prevents behavior response and brain oxidative damage in the ketamine model of schizophrenia. *Neuroscience*. 2014;259:223–231.

# 8 Research on the Effects of Vitamins and Minerals on Cognitive Function in Older Adults

*Celeste A. De Jager and Samrah Ahmed*

## CONTENTS

## SUMMARY

This chapter focuses on brain health and cognition as affected by micronutrients, including vitamins and essential minerals. Vitamins are regarded as nutrients that are essential for life, and the term is derived from *vita*, meaning life and *amine*, as originally it was thought that all vitamins were derived from amines. An organic compound is considered a vitamin if a lack of that compound in the diet results in overt symptoms of deficiency (Bender, 2003). Vitamin deficiencies that affect cognitive function in older adults will be discussed in more detail than other effects of vitamin deficiency.

## 8.1 FUNDAMENTAL STUDIES ON VITAMINS AND COGNITION

This section covers the main vitamins related to cognitive function with basic functional detail, food sources and recommended daily intakes. Some epidemiological data on those at risk of deficiencies, effects of deficiencies on general health and cognition, with emphasis on older adults, are presented. Minerals will be mentioned only where relevant to older adults. Table 8.1 summarises the section. Vitamins known to be associated with cognitive function include the antioxidant vitamins, the B vitamins which have been most researched in the field of cognitive impairment and vitamin D, more recently researched.

### 8.1.1 ANTIOXIDANT VITAMINS

Antioxidants are substances that have the capacity to neutralise free radicals. Dietary sources include the vitamins A, C and E, beta-carotene and other carotenoids including lycopene.

Oxidative stress occurs as an increase in free radicals, or reactive oxygen species (ROS), where antioxidant defences are insufficient in the body (Touyz and Schiffrin, 2008). Free radicals increase with exposure to oxidants, such as cigarette smoke or pollution, but also increase cumulatively over the lifespan as a result of normal metabolic processes (Barja, 2004). A decreased capacity of cells to respond to oxidative

**TABLE 8.1**
**Summary of Characteristics of Major Vitamins Associated with Cognition**

| | Vitamin A | Vitamin B | Vitamin C | Vitamin D | Vitamin E |
|---|---|---|---|---|---|
| Active forms | Retinoids, retinol and derivatives; carotenoids, α- and β-carotene and lycopene | Cobalamin Folate Pyridoxine | Ascorbic acid | Circulating 25(OH)D Active 1,25(OH)2D $D_2$: ergocalciferol $D_3$: cholecalciferol | Four tocopherols and four tocotrienols; alpha-, beta-, gamma- and delta- |
| Food sources | Red meat, fish, eggs, milk Precursors/carotenoids in cod liver and other oils, yellow and orange vegetables and fruits (e.g. pumpkin, carrots, sweet potato, mango) and green vegetables such as spinach and broccoli | $B_{12}$: meat, fish, dairy products (milk, cheese) and eggs Folate: dark green, leafy vegetables, citrus fruits and juices, whole grains, poultry, liver and shellfish $B_6$: fish, white meat, potato skin, fortified cereal, bananas, nuts, green vegetables, legumes | Blackcurrants, oranges, other citrus fruits, strawberries, broccoli, Brussels sprouts, red and green peppers | $D_3$: oily fish, eggs, fish oils such as cod liver oil and liver, cheese Vegan sources such as lichen for $D_3$, mushrooms, alfalfa for $D_2$, fortified milk, milk products and flour | Green vegetables, nuts, seeds and grains, wheat germ, plant oils (e.g. olive), avocado, dairy and eggs |
| RDA | Women, 700 µg/day Men, 900 µg/day retinol equivalents | M and W: $B_{12}$, 6–10 µg/day $B_6$: M/W, 1.3 mg/day; >50 years, M, 1.7 mg/day and W, 1.5 mg/day | Women, 75 mg/day Men, 90 mg/day | Women, 15 mcg/day Men, 15 mcg/day | 15 mg/day for United States Women, 7 mg/day Men, 10 mg/day |
| Deficiency effects | Blindness, immunodeficiency, retinitis pigmentosa, a genetic disorder | Peripheral neuropathy, cognitive impairment, depression, neural tube defects | Scurvy, poor wound healing and lethargy | Rickets in children, osteoporosis, falls and fractures in adults, depression and SAD | Fat malabsorption syndromes, neurological symptoms, ataxia, peripheral neuropathy, myopathy, pigmented retinopathy |

*(Continued)*

**TABLE 8.1 (Continued)**

**Summary of Characteristics of Major Vitamins Associated with Cognition**

| | Vitamin A | Vitamin B | Vitamin C | Vitamin D | Vitamin E |
|---|---|---|---|---|---|
| Overdose effects | 3000 μg daily = upper limit Hypervitaminosis A from preformed vitamin A (retinol) in supplements, viz. retinyl palmitate and retinyl acetate | $B_6$: sensory neuropathy, over 500 mg/day, 100 mg/day upper limit | Water soluble, so excess excreted | Hypercalcaemia, kidney stones, renal failure | Impaired blood clotting, haemorrhage, may accelerate retinitis pigmentosa Upper limit, 1000 mg/day |
| Benefits | Eye health, growth and bone formation, immune function, cancer prevention, antioxidant | DNA repair | Antioxidant, cofactor for synthesis of catecholamines, modulation of neurotransmitter, pro-oxidant in atherosclerotic plaque, connective tissue maintenance, wound healing | Anti-ischaemic, anti-inflammatory and antioxidant roles, neuroprotective and vasoprotective, neurotransmitter metabolism | Antioxidant, scavenges lipid radicals, lipid preservation, neuroprotection |

*Source:* Food and Nutrition Board, Institute of Medicine, 1998. *Vitamin B12. Dietary Reference Intakes for Thiamin, Riboflavin, Niacin, Vitamin B6, Vitamin B12, Pantothenic Acid, Biotin, and Choline. Washington, DC,* National Academy Press, pp. 306–356.

stress can also lead to a detrimental imbalance (Davies, 2000). Consequences of oxidative stress include modification of gene expression; suspension of cell growth or apoptosis; lipid peroxidation, which can cause cell membranes to become rigid and reduce permeability; DNA oxidation, which can disrupt the replication process, causing mutation and cell death; and accumulation of oxidised proteins within cells which can disrupt cell function (Davies, 2000).

### 8.1.1.1   Vitamin A

Vitamin A includes retinol, retinal, retinoic acid and related compounds known as retinoids. Beta-carotene, lycopene and other carotenoids that can be converted by the body into retinol are referred to as provitamin A carotenoids. Vitamin A is important for eye health. Retinol is stored in the retinal pigment epithelial cells. When needed, it is oxidised and transported to rod cells where it binds to a protein, opsin, to form the visual pigment, rhodopsin (Ross et al., 1999). Inadequate retinol available to the retina results in impaired dark adaptation, known as *night blindness.* Vitamin A has a role in bone formation and growth, immune function and cancer prevention (Braun and Cohen, 2010). Vitamin A, thyroid hormone and vitamin D may interact to influence gene transcription (Semba RD, 1998): for more on interactions between genes and nutrients, see Chapter 3 by Ordovas. Thus, retinoic acid plays a role in cellular differentiation. Vitamin A also has free-radical scavenging capacity and in this respect may be important for cardiovascular and cognitive health.

Vitamin A requirements are expressed in μg retinol equivalents, because the different forms have differing biological activity. Due to the limited capacity of the body to eliminate excess vitamin A and potential toxicity, upper limits are also important and are set at 3000 μg daily for both women and men (NHMRC, 2006). The principal forms of preformed vitamin A (retinol) in supplements are retinyl palmitate and retinyl acetate. Beta-carotene is also a common source of vitamin A in supplements, and many supplements provide a combination of retinol and beta-carotene (Hendler and Rorvik, 2001). The only essential and known function of carotenoids (alpha-carotene, beta-carotene and beta-cryptoxanthin) in humans is to serve as a source of vitamin A. It is unclear whether the biological effects of carotenoids in humans are a result of their antioxidant activity or other non-antioxidant mechanisms.

Limited experimental data suggest that excess retinol may stimulate bone resorption (Rohde and DeLuca, 2003) or interfere with the ability of vitamin D to maintain calcium balance (Johansson and Melhus, 2001). This may increase the risk of osteoporotic fracture and decreased bone mineral density in older men and women. For this reason, some companies have reduced the retinol content in their multivitamin supplements to 750 mcg (2500 IU).

### 8.1.1.2   Vitamin C

Vitamin C (ascorbic acid) is a water-soluble vitamin that cannot be stored in the body. It has many functions including acting as a cofactor for several enzymatic actions. But its role as an antioxidant is of major importance (Bender, 2003; Braun and Cohen, 2010). It can also act as a pro-oxidant in the reduction of metal (e.g. iron, copper) ions (Bender, 2003). Vitamin C accumulates in the central nervous system, with neurons of the brain having especially high levels. Deficiency causes scurvy, a potentially fatal disease. However, in scurvy, vitamin C is retained by the brain for neuronal function, and eventual death from the disease is more likely due to lack of vitamin C for collagen synthesis. Scurvy is rare in developed countries since vitamin C is now known to prevent it, although marginal deficiency can sometimes be found (Braun and Cohen, 2010).

Vitamin C increases the bioavailability of iron from foods by enhancing intestinal absorption of non-heme iron (Combs and Gerald, 2012). Vitamin C deficiency may cause oxidative damage to macromolecules (lipids, proteins) in the brain (Lykkesfeldt and Poulsen, 2010). Even in small amounts, vitamin C can protect indispensable molecules in the body, such as proteins, lipids, carbohydrates and nucleic acids (DNA and RNA), from damage by free radicals and ROS. Vitamin C also participates in redox recycling of other important antioxidants, for example, regeneration of vitamin E from its oxidised form (Bruno et al., 2006). It is essential for connective tissue maintenance, cellular integrity and wound healing.

### 8.1.1.3   Vitamin E

Vitamin E includes eight different molecules, including four tocopherols and four tocotrienols which act as antioxidants (Bender, 2003). The form most utilised in the body is α-tocopherol (Azzi and Stocker, 2000), which is lipid soluble. Vitamin E scavenges lipid radicals and is considered the most important antioxidant for lipid preservation (Azzi and Stocker, 2000) and maintenance of cell membrane integrity. Vitamin E deficiency causes brain tissue lipid peroxidation and, if severe, may result in neurological symptoms such as ataxia (impaired muscle coordination), peripheral neuropathy, myopathy or retinitis pigmentosa (damage to the retina). Vitamin E is critical to infant neural development, as if deficiency is not treated rapidly, neurological symptoms will develop. However, in adults with malabsorption problems, neurological symptoms may not develop for up to 20 years, and none have been reported for healthy individuals with low vitamin E diets (Kontush and Schekatolina, 2004; Sano et al., 1997). The literature suggests an increased risk for cardiovascular disease with serum levels below 20 μmol/L (Ford and Sowell, 1999). Recent data from NHANES 2003–2006 indicate that the average dietary intake of alpha-tocopherol from food (including enriched and fortified sources) (based on 24 h recall) among Americans 2 years and older is 6.9 mg/day (Fulgoni et al., 2011). This intake is well below the current U.S. recommendation of 15 mg/day.

## 8.2   VITAMIN D

Vitamin D is known as the sunshine vitamin, as it is synthesised in the skin from 7-dehydrocholesterol in the presence of sunlight. The main circulating metabolite form of vitamin D is 25-hydroxyvitamin D (25(OH)D); this is processed mainly via the liver and kidneys to the active form, 1,25(OH)2D, which is water soluble. Extrarenal cells can also produce 1,25(OH)2D. Blood levels are controlled by the parathyroid hormone, growth factors, cytokines and calcium (Holick, 2007). Vitamin D is known for its role in strengthening bones through metabolic processing of calcium (Cranney et al., 2007). Deficiencies are linked to conditions such as rickets in children and osteoporosis, falls and fractures in older adults, as well as some psychiatric conditions such as depression and seasonal affective disorder (SAD)

(Anglin et al., 2013). Levels vary seasonally, although exposure to sunshine is not absolutely necessary, if dietary sources and supplements are sufficient.

Vitamin D deficiency is a major problem worldwide, with up to a third of the population in the Western world having deficient or insufficient levels of circulating 25-hydroxyvitamin D (Holick, 2007). Vitamin D is known to be important for normal brain development and function (McCann and Ames, 2008). Ageing is associated with a reduced capacity to synthesise vitamin D in the skin from sun exposure (Holick et al., 1989). Thus, older adults may be more vulnerable to vitamin D deficiency and the resulting effects on cognition, although variability may occur in migrant groups such as observant Muslims in the Northern Hemisphere. It has been suggested that the anti-ischaemic, anti-inflammatory and antioxidant roles of vitamin D are neuroprotective and vasoprotective (Briones and Darwish, 2012; Hooshmand et al., 2014).

## 8.3  B VITAMINS

B vitamins are water-soluble organic compounds that cannot be synthesised in sufficient quantities by the body and therefore need to be obtained from the diet. There are eight distinct types of B vitamin, three of which, $B_6$ (pyridoxine), $B_9$ (folate) and $B_{12}$ (cobalamin), have most consistently been associated with protective roles in cognitive function and in neuronal health. Other B vitamins include $B_1$ (thiamine), $B_2$ (riboflavin), $B_3$ (niacin), $B_5$ (pantothenic acid) and $B_7$ (biotin), all with minor roles in neural structure or function.

### 8.3.1  VITAMIN $B_6$

There are six vitamers of vitamin $B_6$; the principal active form is pyridoxal 5′-phosphate (PLP), whereas pyridoxine hydrochloride is the usual form used in supplements (NHMRC, 2006). PLP can be synthesised by the intestinal flora and is available from the diet. Deficiency is rare, but marginal deficiency does occur, reportedly with a prevalence of 10%–20% in developed countries (Bender, 2003). This is more relevant for older people. Bates et al. (1999) reported that $B_6$ levels were below the normal range in 48% of community living older people and in about 75% of those in residential institutions.

### 8.3.2  VITAMIN $B_9$ (FOLATE)

Folate includes folic acid and derivatives of tetrahydrofolate, the reduced form of folate. Free folic acid is more commonly used in food fortification and in supplements and has higher bioavailability. The various forms of folate are found in food. Folate deficiency was common in developed countries (8%–10%), but has almost been eradicated with fortification (reduced from 16% to 0.05% in the United States) (Pfeiffer, 2005). Fortification was introduced to prevent neural tube defects in babies born to mothers with folate deficiency and is often provided as a supplement to pregnant women. However, there is evidence to suggest that fortification may not be of benefit to older adults (Smith, 2008, to be discussed later).

### 8.3.3 Vitamin B$_{12}$

Vitamin B$_{12}$ (cobalamin) includes a group of cobalt-containing compounds (corrinoids). Cyanocobalamin and hydroxocobalamin are forms commonly used in supplement preparations. Derivatives of B$_{12}$ include methylmalonic acid (MMA) and holotranscobalamin which are more stable in the circulation than vitamin B$_{12}$ itself. It is not found in plants or vegetables as it is synthesised by bacteria. Deficiency is quite common due to impaired absorption or metabolism, especially in older adults (Joosten, 1993), depending on the lower limits set. In a U.K. study, the prevalence was 5% for those aged 65–74, doubling to 10% in people aged 75 and over (Clarke et al., 2004).

### 8.3.4 Other B Vitamins and B Vitamin Deficiencies

Severe thiamine (B$_1$) deficiency which is rare in developed countries, except in patients with chronic alcoholism, HIV/AIDS or gastrointestinal conditions that impair vitamin absorption (Butterworth, 2003), results in the condition called beriberi, with many forms that involve neurological symptoms. The dry and wet forms of beriberi involve peripheral neuropathy, whereas cerebral beriberi can lead to neuronal cell death and the clinical conditions of Wernicke's encephalopathy and Korsakoff's psychosis, especially in those who chronically abuse alcohol (Bates, 2006; Todd and Butterworth, 1999).

The niacin (vitamin B$_3$) and coenzymes, NAD and NADP, are needed for several redox and other reactions in the body. Severe niacin deficiency, known as pellagra, has been historically associated with poverty and consumption of a diet predominantly based on corn, which is low in bioavailable niacin (Gregory, 1998; Park et al., 2000). Neurologic symptoms of pellagra include headache, fatigue, apathy, depression, ataxia, poor concentration, delusions and hallucinations, which can lead to confusion, memory loss, dementia, psychosis and eventual death (Hegyi et al., 2004).

Pantothenic acid (B$_5$) is required as a component of coenzyme A (CoA), needed for the oxidative metabolism of glucose and fatty acids and for the biosynthesis of fatty acids, cholesterol, steroid hormones, the hormone melatonin and the neurotransmitter acetylcholine. Deficiencies are very rare.

Vitamin B$_6$ concentrations in the brain exceed levels in the blood by about 100 times; thus, vitamin B$_6$ deficiency has neurologic effects (Gibson and Blass, 1999). Severe deficiency of vitamin B$_6$ is uncommon, but alcoholics may be most at risk due to low dietary intakes and impaired metabolism of the vitamin.

Vitamin B$_{12}$: Haematological changes, including elevated blood levels of homocysteine (Hcy) and MMA, are diagnostic of vitamin B$_{12}$ deficiency; however, in approximately 25% of cases, neurological symptoms are the only clinical indicator of vitamin B$_{12}$ deficiency (Lindenbaum et al., 1988). Symptoms include numbness and tingling of the extremities, especially the legs, difficulty walking, concentration problems, memory loss, disorientation and dementia that may or may not be accompanied by mood changes (Healton et al., 1991). Vitamin deficiency is known to damage the myelin sheath covering cranial, spinal and peripheral nerves. The autoimmune syndrome of pernicious anaemia may also occur, resulting in destruction of cells in the stomach lining with decreased secretion of acid and enzymes required to release food-bound vitamin B$_{12}$.

## 8.4  HOMOCYSTEINE

Hcy is a sulphur-containing amino acid that is an intermediate in metabolism of another sulphur-containing amino acid, methionine, from protein; see Figure 8.1a and b. Choline is also involved in Hcy metabolism, while its metabolite, betaine, can provide a methyl group for the conversion of Hcy to methionine. The conversion of

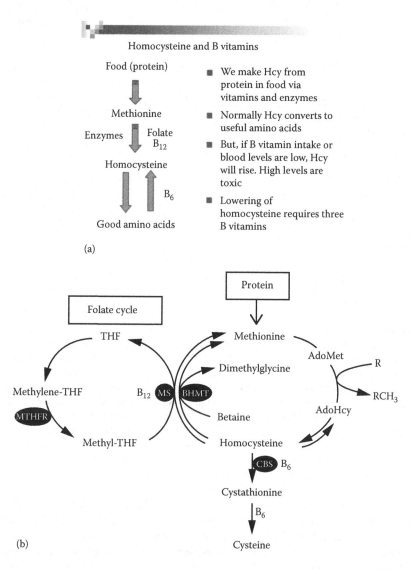

**FIGURE 8.1**  (a) Illustration of Hcy metabolism from protein. (b) Hcy metabolic cycles. Abbreviations: AdoHcy, S-adenosylhomocysteine; AdoMet, S-adenosylmethionine; $B_6$, vitamin $B_6$ (pyridoxal phosphate); $B_{12}$, vitamin $B_{12}$ (methylcobalamin); CBS, cystathionine $\beta$-synthase; MS, methionine synthase; MTHFR, methylenetetrahydrofolate reductase; THF, tetrahydrofolate. (Reprinted from Refsum, H. et al., *Annu. Rev. Med.*, 49, 31, 1998, doi: 10.1146/annurev.med.49.1.31.)

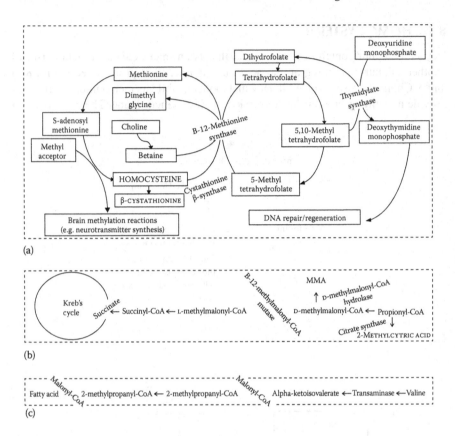

(a)

(b)

(c)

**FIGURE 8.2**  Diagram illustrating the biochemical rationale for associations among vitamin $B_{12}$, folate and cognitive function. (a) The roles of the two vitamins in Hcy remethylation, which result in the regeneration of the active form of folate, tetrahydrofolate, and the production of SAMe, the methyl donor for the central nervous system. Accumulation of Hcy and B-cystathionine indicates the loss of the cofactor and substrate functions of vitamin $B_{12}$ and folate in Hcy remethylation. (b) The role of vitamin $B_{12}$ as a cofactor to the enzyme methylmalonyl-CoA mutase. Build-up of MMA and 2-methylcitric indicates the loss of this vitamin $B_{12}$ function. (c) The role of malonyl-CoA in fatty acid synthesis. When vitamin $B_{12}$ is lacking, methylmalonyl-CoA builds up, perhaps substituting for malonyl-CoA, which might result in the accumulation of abnormal fatty acids in the membranes of neural tissues. (From Morris, M.S., *Adv. Nutr.*, 3(6), 801, 2012. Used with permission.)

Hcy to useful metabolites, S-adenosyl-methionine (SAMe) and glutathione, requires 3 B vitamins, methylfolate, vitamin $B_{12}$ and $B_6$ as cofactors (Morris, 2012a; Refsum et al., 2006). Hence, if the B vitamin supply through the diet is suboptimal, remethylation of Hcy via the enzyme methionine synthase is reduced, and plasma levels of Hcy rise. The importance of the remethylation process is the regeneration of the active form of folate, tetrahydrofolate, needed for thymidine synthesis, DNA replication and neurogenesis. SAMe is a methyl donor for the central nervous system and important to neurotransmitter synthesis. Vitamin $B_{12}$ is also important for fatty acid metabolism, acting as a cofactor for the enzyme methylmalonyl-CoA mutase and also promoting neural membrane formation. Build-up of MMA indicates the loss of this $B_{12}$ function. Disruption of any of these pathways is likely to contribute to neuronal atrophy and lead to loss of cognitive function; see Figure 8.2 for the functional role of B vitamins in the Hcy metabolism. Increased oxidative stress occurs in the brain when Hcy is elevated (Birch et al., 2009) and may increase the permeability of the blood–brain barrier. Hcy levels rise with age, possibly due to poor absorption of B vitamins from the diet. Deficiencies in $B_{12}$ and folate also increase with age.

## 8.5  ESSENTIAL MINERALS

Iron is essential for the formation of haemoglobin and certain other proteins, and copper acts as an essential cofactor in enzyme reactions among many other aspects of health. However, some studies have suggested that excessive iron and copper intake may contribute to cognitive problems for some individuals (Brewer, 2009; Squitti et al., 2014; Stankiewicz and Brass, 2009). In recent meta-analyses (Schrag et al., 2013; Squitti et al., 2013; Ventriglia et al., 2012), circulating non-protein-bound copper was associated with increased Alzheimer's disease (AD) risk.

Dietary zinc deficiency has been associated with memory impairment, but the mechanisms underlying this effect remain unclear. Detailed studies have revealed that $ZnT_3$ knockout mice exhibit impaired fear memory (Martel et al., 2010) as well as accelerated ageing-related decline of spatial memory (Adlard et al., 2010). Sindreu et al. (2011) have shown that zinc is required for spatial working memory and contextual discrimination memory in mice. Despite these advances, the functional role of zinc in learning and memory remains largely unsolved. Other minerals including manganese, calcium and magnesium may have benefits for cognition. Deficiencies of manganese may be associated with dizziness and convulsions, while magnesium deficiency can be related to irritability, insomnia and depression.

## 8.6  ROLES OF VITAMINS AND MINERALS IN THE BRAIN RELATED TO AGEING AND COGNITION

### 8.6.1  Oxidative Stress

Harman hypothesised that the ageing process was caused by free radical damage to DNA, lipids and proteins in 1956 (Harman, 1956). Further research since then has supported a role of oxidative stress in ageing (Ames et al., 1993). The brain is particularly sensitive to oxidative stress due to its high oxygen uptake (Halliwell, 2006). ROS can cause apoptosis in neurons and astrocytes (Barja, 2004) and may also disrupt the protective blood–brain barrier (Freeman and Keller, 2012). Oxidative stress directly damages cell components, resulting in damage to synapses and nerve cell death. Neural inflammation and oxidative stress are thought to be key mechanisms in AD and dementia with Lewy body (DLB) pathology, not merely a consequence of the disease process (Sayre et al., 2007); markers of protein, lipid and DNA oxidation are detected in patients with AD and DLB (Bennett et al., 2009). Antioxidants are thought to protect the brain against neurodegeneration by limiting the production of toxic substances and reducing free radical damage (Mao, 2013).

As there are relatively few antioxidant enzymes specifically associated with neuronal protection, antioxidant nutrients may have a more prominent role in older and ageing brains than in other organs or systems (Olanow, 1990).

Oxidative stress is observed in early stages of cognitive decline without dementia. Plasma markers of oxidative stress were associated with cognitive decline in the EVA study (Berr et al., 2004). Similarly, measures of free radicals in blood were inversely correlated with cognitive performance on the MMSE in elderly participants (Maugeri et al., 2004). $F_2\alpha$-isoprostanes and protein carbonyls were correlated with cognitive performance in healthy elderly, and these biomarkers were also lower in those with high fruit and vegetable intake (Polidori et al., 2009). Some studies have documented low levels of vitamin E in the cerebrospinal fluid of patients with AD (Kontush and Schekatolina, 2004). These findings have prompted investigation of ways to minimise oxidative damage to improve cognitive function.

### 8.6.2   ROLES OF ANTIOXIDANT VITAMINS IN COGNITION

The roles of vitamin C which may be relevant to cognition include acting as a cofactor in the synthesis of catecholamines (Harrison and May, 2009) and in the enzymatic reaction that synthesises the neurotransmitter norepinephrine from dopamine. It is essential for connective tissue maintenance, cellular integrity and wound healing. Ascorbic acid is protective against cold sore lesions caused by Herpes simplex virus (Yoon et al., 2000), which may be a risk factor for AD (Agostini et al., 2014).

### 8.6.3   ROLE OF VITAMIN D IN COGNITION

Recent research has shown links between vitamin $D_3$ deficiency (25(OH)D) and increases in the incidence of hypertension, hyperlipidaemia, diabetes, myocardial infarction and stroke (Schlögl and Holick, 2014). These conditions are associated with increased risk of neurodegenerative diseases such as vascular dementia, AD and Parkinson's disease. Cross-sectional and longitudinal observational studies used for a meta-analysis (Balion et al., 2012) showed associations of low 25(OH)D with cognitive impairment and decline in older adults. Generally, deficiency or low 25(OH)D was equated to serum levels below 20 ng/mL, while normal levels ranged between 20 and 50 ng/mL. Meta-analyses have confirmed significantly lower levels of vitamin D in AD patients and in those with mild cognitive impairment (MCI) compared to normal controls (Annweiler et al., 2013a).

A meta-analysis by van der Schaft et al. (2013) suggested a more than doubled risk of cognitive impairment in patients with vitamin D deficiency among 7688 participants. Sixty-seven percent (4/6) of the prospective studies showed a higher risk of cognitive decline after a follow-up period of 4–7 years in participants with lower 25(OH)D levels at baseline compared with participants with higher 25(OH)D levels. Depending on the cognitive status of those included in these studies, reverse causation limits the interpretability of the findings, as cognitive impairment may be the cause of poor nutritional status. Reduced risk of AD has been associated with higher vitamin D levels (Balion et al., 2012). Additionally, reduced risk of cognitive impairment, higher concentrations of CSF $A\beta_1$–42 and greater brain volumes (e.g. white matter, structures belonging to medial temporal lobe) were found in patients attending a memory clinic who had higher serum 25(OH)D (Hooshmand et al., 2014).

A biological rationale for the effect of vitamin D on cognitive performance is plausible. Vitamin D receptors have been located in many brain regions (including the hippocampus) (Eyles et al., 2005) associated with cognitive functions that decline with the development of dementia. Vitamin D correlates negatively with cerebral ventricle size, suggesting that it contributes to brain atrophy (Annweiler et al., 2013b). It has been suggested that the anti-ischaemic, anti-inflammatory and antioxidant roles of vitamin D are neuroprotective and vasoprotective (Briones, and Darwish, 2012; Hooshmand et al., 2014). In addition, various functions of vitamin D in neurotransmitter metabolism, particularly in the dopaminergic system, have been proposed (Eyles et al., 2005). Overexpression of the vitamin D receptor in the brain, or vitamin D treatment, may suppress amyloid precursor protein transcription (Wang et al., 2012).

### 8.6.4   ROLE OF B VITAMINS IN COGNITION

The human brain depends on a continual supply of glucose to meet its energy needs. Glucose oxidation requires cofactors including B vitamins thiamine, riboflavin, niacin and pantothenic acid (Haller, 2005). Additionally, essential minerals, magnesium, iron and manganese, are required as substrates for enzymes in glycolysis and the citric acid cycle (Voet and Voet, 1995a). Generation of cellular energy in the form of ATP requires riboflavin and niacin, iron and the endogenously synthesised compound coenzyme $Q_{10}$ (Voet and Voet, 1995b).

Together with various amino acids, vitamin $B_6$ (folate) and vitamin $B_{12}$ (thiamine), riboflavin and niacin are needed as cofactors for the synthesis of neurotransmitters. Choline is a precursor for the neurotransmitter acetylcholine (Gibson and Blass, 1999). There are two classes of neurotransmitters: small amino acids (e.g. gamma-aminobutyric acid [GABA], glutamate, aspartate and glycine) and amines (e.g. dopamine, epinephrine, norepinephrine, serotonin, histamine and acetylcholine) (von Bohlen et al., 2002). Folate and vitamin $B_{12}$ also have important roles in maintaining the integrity of the myelin sheath, while thiamine is needed for maintenance of neural membrane potential and proper nerve conductance (Haller, 2005). Iron has an important role in the development of oligodendrocytes, the cells in the brain that produce myelin (Todorich et al., 2009).

## 8.7   RECENT RESEARCH EVIDENCE FOR ASSOCIATIONS OF VITAMINS AND MINERALS WITH COGNITION

### 8.7.1   B VITAMINS AND HOMOCYSTEINE

#### 8.7.1.1   Epidemiological Studies

There have been a number of recent reviews on the association of B vitamins with cognition, both from epidemiological cohort studies and from randomised clinical trials (RCTs). The association between elevated plasma Hcy and cognitive impairment has been well established (Budge et al., 2002; McCaddon et al., 1998; Seshadri, 2006) and has been identified as a modifiable risk factor for cognitive impairment and dementia in 10 of 12 retrospective (Zhuo et al., 2011) cohort studies and further discussed in the ADI nutrition and dementia report (Prina and Albanese, 2014).

Of 21 good-quality cohort studies assessing the relationship between vitamin $B_{12}$ and $B_{12}$ biomarkers (MMA and holotranscobalamin, holoTC) reviewed by O'Leary et al. (2012), only seven reported significant associations between $B_{12}$ status and AD, dementia or cognitive decline. The authors concluded that this was insufficient evidence of a confirmed association of $B_{12}$ status and cognitive impairment. However, all the studies where the more specific $B_{12}$ biomarkers (MMA, holoTC) were included showed consistent associations. A similar lack of consistent evidence for associations of low folate and vitamin $B_6$ with cognitive impairment or dementia was reported. The inconsistencies may in part be due to methodological study issues, including a lack of baseline nutrient status of the populations studied (for more details, see Chapter 4 by Ahmed and de Jager). This is important especially with regard to folate, as many countries now have mandatory folic acid fortification.

### 8.7.2 RANDOMISED CONTROLLED TRIALS WITH B VITAMINS

There have been a number of RCTs which aimed to delay cognitive decline with B vitamins in participants with and without cognitive impairment and AD. Most reviews of these RCTs have shown little support for the efficacy of these interventions by meta-analysis of data (Clarke and Bennett, 2008; Malouf and Evans, 2008). In all 19 trials reviewed by Ford and Almeida (2012), B vitamin supplementation with combinations of $B_{12}$, folic acid and $B_6$, or singly, at various dosages reduced plasma levels of total Hcy in older adults with or without cognitive impairment. In sub-analyses selecting only studies over 6-month duration, those in countries without folic acid fortification, those that included folic acid and those with over 100 participants, there was still little efficacy shown for beneficial effects of supplementation on cognitive function in either group (Ford and Almeida, 2012). (See tables in Ford and Almeida for details of the trials included in the meta-analysis.)

A more recent meta-analysis by the B-Vitamin Treatment Trialists' Collaboration reported no significant effects, after approximately 5 years B vitamin treatment, on cognitive domain function in memory, executive function or global cognition in adults; however, they did not discount some effects on processing speed (Clarke et al., 2014). The analysis included 11 trials with a total of 22,000 participants with no previous diagnosis of cognitive impairment or dementia. The analysis controlled for baseline nutrient status and showed an overall reduction in biochemical levels of Hcy of approximately 25% across the trials, proving good compliance and absorption of the supplements.

However, there have been some successful trials. The FACIT trial (Durga et al., 2007) of folate treatment in those with tHcy levels above 13 μmol/L at baseline showed improvement in episodic memory and processing speed in cognitively healthy older people. The VITACOG trial showed that B vitamin supplements taken daily for 2 years reduced brain atrophy by 30%–53% in older adults with MCI (Smith et al., 2010). Rate of atrophy reduction was greatest in memory regions of the brain associated with AD (Douaud et al., 2013). It appears that there is a critical level of brain shrinkage, possibly mediated by elevated Hcy, which, when reached, results in cognitive decline, especially in episodic memory performance (de Jager, 2014). B vitamins also maintained verbal memory, semantic memory and global cognitive performance (assessed using MMSE) in those with higher baseline tHcy levels. Almost half of those with elevated tHcy reverted from MCI back to control status assessed with the Clinical Dementia Rating scale (de Jager et al., 2012).

### 8.7.3  Antioxidant Cohort Studies Related to Cognition

Much of the research on associations of antioxidants with cognition have focused on vitamin E. Longitudinal cohort studies have either used food frequency questionnaires as a measure of vitamin E status or blood levels. Lower levels of vitamin E intake have been shown to be associated with greater cognitive decline or incidence of dementia in most of these studies. However, the results from studies based on biomarker levels of individual tocopherols have been inconsistent. There is more consistency in reports of significant inverse associations between total tocopherols, cognitive decline and dementia incidence (Prina and Albanese, 2014).

In the Chicago Health and Aging Project, higher intakes of vitamin E from food sources were associated with reduced AD incidence (Morris et al., 2005). Similarly, in the Rotterdam study, high vitamin E intake was associated with reduced dementia incidence (Devore et al., 2010). The Nurses' Health Study data showed no significant associations of vitamin C or E intake (using a semi-quantitative food frequency questionnaire) with cognitive decline (Devore et al., 2013).

### 8.7.4  Antioxidant Supplement Trials

Supplementation studies with vitamin E were found to lack support for cognitive enhancement in a recent Cochrane review, based on 3 trials, one positive and two with negative results for slowing of cognitive decline or conversion from MCI to AD (ADI, 2013). A review by Mecocci and Polidori (2011) on MCI and AD antioxidant trials also found conflicting evidence, attributed possibly to low permeability for antioxidants by the blood–brain barrier. Thus, the role of vascular damage that contributes to oxidative stress needs to be considered when testing antioxidant treatments.

A recent RCT with multivitamin supplements containing beta-carotene, vitamin E (alpha-tocopherol) and ascorbic acid with 12-year follow-up for almost 6000 male physicians over 65 years of age showed no difference in mean cognitive function changes between intervention and placebo groups (Grodstein et al., 2013). However, the trial was not restricted to those with low baseline levels of the vitamins, and dosages may have been too low for detectable effects.

One double-blind RCT found no evidence that a daily antioxidant supplement containing 12 mg of beta-carotene, 500 mg of vitamin C and 400 mg of vitamin E, when taken for up to 12 months, improved mental performance in elderly people (Smith et al., 1999). Another placebo-controlled trial in older adults at high risk of dementia found that supplementation with vitamin C (200 mg/day) and vitamin E

(500 mg/day) for 12 weeks did not alter any of the measured cognitive functions despite nonsignificantly lowering levels of $F_2$-isoprostanes – biomarkers of lipid peroxidation, in vivo.

A large placebo-controlled intervention trial in individuals with moderate neurological impairment found that supplementation with 2000 IU (equivalent to 900 mg/day) of synthetic alpha-tocopherol daily for 2 years significantly slowed progression of AD (Sano et al., 1997). In contrast, a placebo-controlled trial in patients with MCI reported that the same dosage of vitamin E did not slow progression to AD over a 3-year period (Petersen et al., 2005).

### 8.7.5 MULTIVITAMIN AND MULTI-NUTRIENT SUPPLEMENT TRIALS

A broad range of nutrients such as amino acids, antioxidants, polyphenols, lipids and vitamins may be associated with cognitive decline (Manders et al., 2004). Thus, multi-arm and multivitamin supplement interventions have been proposed and trialled with various combinations of nutrients, not solely vitamin based.

The SU.VI.MAX trial in French adults was successful after long-term intervention with a multi-nutrient compound, and improvements in cognitive domains, particularly verbal memory and working memory, were maintained over 8 years of follow-up (Kesse-Guyot et al., 2011).

Most of the 21 studies with nutritional supplements reviewed by Manders et al. (2004) showed significant effects on cognitive functioning in selected groups of older adults, only a few with mild adverse side effects (guarana, inositol, acetyl-L-carnitine) including discomfort, insomnia and flatus. Treatment with a combined multivitamin, mineral and herbal supplement (Swisse Women's Ultivite® 50+) in older women (64–85 years) for 16 weeks showed efficacy for spatial working memory (Macpherson et al., 2012). A similar study in older men (50–74 years) for 8 weeks showed benefits for episodic memory (Harris et al., 2012).

### 8.7.6 MINERALS ASSOCIATED WITH COGNITION

The role of aluminium in AD remains controversial. Some researchers have called for caution, citing aluminium's known neurotoxic potential when entering the body in more than modest amounts (Kawahara and Kato-Negishi, 2011) and the fact that aluminium has been found/detected in the brains of individuals with AD (Crapper et al., 1973, 1976). Studies in the United Kingdom and France found increased Alzheimer's prevalence in areas where tap water contained higher aluminium concentrations (Martyn et al., 1989; Rondeau et al., 2009). However, because of the limited number of relevant studies, most experts regard current evidence as insufficient to indict aluminium as a contributor to AD risk.

## 8.8 DIETARY PATTERNS LIKELY TO BENEFIT COGNITION

A diet that provides simultaneously dietary intakes of antioxidants and other protective nutrients including vitamins B, C, D and E, carotenoids and polyphenols, EPA and DHA might be necessary to slow down neurodegeneration and the accompanying inflammatory and pro-oxidative phenomena (Barberger-Gateau et al., 2007). In this context, a dietary pattern approach considering the potential interactions between nutrients appears to be especially promising in observational studies.

The Mediterranean diet (MeDi) score, the French National Nutrition and Health Programme (Programme National Nutrition Sante) Guideline Score, the Recommended Food Score and Dietary Approaches to Stop Hypertension have all been associated with lower risks of cognitive impairment, cognitive decline and dementia or AD (Alles et al., 2012; see also Chapter 2 by Andreeva and Kesse-Guyot). However, a principal component analysis was not successful in identifying a healthy dietary pattern when combining results from studies on these scores. The authors contend that RCTs for dietary pattern may be impossible to do, given that the effects of diet on cognition are long term, spanning many years. Thus, epidemiological and observational studies may be more informative, and these are reviewed in Chapter 2 by Andreeva and Kesse-Guyot.

### 8.8.1   MEDITERRANEAN DIET

Evidence of the benefits of adherence to the Mediterranean style of diet (which includes high legume and whole grain intake) in the protection against overall mortality and incidence of non-communicable diseases including diabetes, cardiovascular disease and stroke and on cognitive impairment has been reported (Sofi et al., 2010; see also Chapter 2 by Andreeva and Kesse-Guyot). Meta-analysis of accrued data showed a 13% reduced risk of neurodegenerative disease incidence, 6% reduced risk of mortality or incidence of neoplastic disease and 10% reduced risk of incidence or mortality from cardiovascular disease associated with the MeDi. These results were obtained using an adherence score calculated from a list of key components of the diet but not on actual amounts or calories consumed. An important component of the MeDi is fatty acid intake. Long-chain polyunsaturated fatty acid intake was attributed mostly to fish intake, and the monounsaturated fatty acid (MUFA) to saturated fatty acid ratio was included (MUFA, based mostly on olive oil intake), while trans fats are not included in the diet, nor rated. The findings of the benefits of the Mediterranean-type diet are supported by studies assessing intake of fatty acids alone showing that fish intake, particularly of oily fish rich in omega-3, has benefits in maintaining cognitive function, as well as preventing cognitive decline in early stages, but not advanced stages of AD (Solfrizzi et al., 2011).

### 8.8.2   FATS AND CHOLESTEROL

In terms of fat intake, HDL versus LDL (or non-HDL) good cholesterol levels may be more important indicators than total cholesterol (Farnier, 2009). What is apparent is that certain fats are beneficial to both brain and body health. Sofi et al. (2012) recommend an increase in the consumption of fruits and vegetables up to the recommended five servings a day, with preference given to whole grains, saturated and trans fats to be replaced with unsaturated fats, consumption of sugar and sweetened beverages reduced and salt intake limited. 'Following the principles of the traditional Mediterranean diet, a substantial reduction of the risk of incidence and/or mortality from cardiovascular disease can be easily obtained'. These recommendations would apply to reduction of the risk of cognitive impairment as well, based on the review (Solfrizzi et al., 2011).

### 8.8.3 Low Glycaemic Index Diets

Carbohydrates are essential for energy, and glucose is necessary for brain energy metabolism; thus, very low carbohydrate intake can be detrimental (see Chapter 6 by Sunram-Lea). Low glycaemic index (GI) carbohydrates (e.g. from fresh fruits, such as berries, and vegetables) have been reported to be most beneficial as high GI carbohydrates are associated with insulin spikes, reduced insulin resistance and development of metabolic syndrome (Goff et al., 2013). Low GI diets have been recommended for the prevention of cognitive impairment and AD (Nilsson et al., 2009).

### 8.8.4 Dietary Recommendations for Prevention of Alzheimer's Disease

Barnard et al. (2014) have proposed a number of recommendations for the prevention of AD, based on current research on micronutrients and cognition presented at the *Conference on Nutrition and the Brain* (Washington DC, 2013).

The recommendations do not comprise a diet as such, but a set of dietary guidelines:

1. Minimise intake of saturated fats from dairy products, meats and oils (coconut, palm, corn, canola oil) and trans fats, present in many snack pastries and fried foods, labelled as partially hydrogenated oils. Olive and avocado oils with MUFA are recommended.
2. Vegetables, legumes (beans, peas and lentils), fruits and whole grains should replace meats and dairy products as primary staples of the diet. Vegetables, berries and whole grains provide healthful micronutrients important to the brain and have little or no saturated fat or trans fats. In both the Chicago Health and Aging Project and the Nurses' Health Study cohorts, high vegetable intakes were associated with reduced cognitive decline (Kang et al., 2005; Morris et al., 2006).
3. Vitamin E should come from foods, rather than supplements. Vitamin E from supplements has not been shown to reduce AD risk. Many common supplements provide only α-tocopherol, and most do not replicate the range of vitamin E forms found in foods. A high intake of α-tocopherol has been shown to reduce serum concentrations of g- and d-tocopherols (Huang and Appel, 2003). For non-vegetarians, three meals of fish or seafood per week were shown to provide adequate intake of vitamin E to benefit cognition (in addition to the omega-3 and B vitamins in fish that are likely to be beneficial to cognition).
4. A reliable source of vitamin $B_{12}$, such as fortified foods, or a supplement providing at least the recommended dietary allowance (2.4 mg/day for adults) should be part of the daily diet. Blood levels of vitamin $B_{12}$ (or Hcy, as a marker of B vitamin status) should be checked regularly as many factors,

including age, may impair absorption. $B_{12}$ is found in supplements and for-tified foods, such as some breakfast cereals or plant milks. Vitamin $B_{12}$ is also found in meats and dairy products, although absorption from these sources is limited in many individuals. The U.S. government recommends that vitamin $B_{12}$ from supplements or fortified foods be consumed by all individuals older than 50 years. Individuals on plant-based diets or with absorption problems should take vitamin $B_{12}$ supplements regardless of age. Some individuals require vitamin $B_{12}$ injections to maintain adequate levels.

5. If using multiple vitamins, those without iron and copper are preferable. Iron supplements should only be taken if tests show a deficiency due to anaemia or under direction from a physician.

6. Although aluminium's role in AD remains a matter of investigation, those who desire to minimise their exposure can avoid the use of cookware or products that contain aluminium. Aluminium is found in some brands of baking powder, antacids, certain food products and antiperspirants.

## 8.9   LIMITATIONS AND CAUTIONS

### 8.9.1   FOLIC ACID FORTIFICATION

Folic acid fortification of foods was introduced as a measure to prevent neural tube defects in the developing foetus and thus targeted at pregnant women. However, folic acid fortification is not always beneficial, especially for the elderly population (Smith et al., 2008) and to those suffering from pernicious anaemia, which is quite common (Morris, 2012b). The elevated folic acid will reduce Hcy levels but mask $B_{12}$ deficiency, which if not treated will result in peripheral neuropathy, tiredness, lack of energy and permanent cognitive deficits. A vitamin $B_{12}$ level below 150 pmol/L is considered deficient and a sign of anaemia. People with this condition are often treated with intramuscular $B_{12}$ injections (1000 µg) regularly to reverse the condition and improve memory performance. A combination of high-dose oral plus intramus-cular vitamin $B_{12}$ may improve haematological and neurological responses in vita-min $B_{12}$–deficient patients (Butler et al., 2006).

Studies of the effects of high folic acid supplementation have revealed deleteri-ous effects on cognition. The NHANES study showed that if both $B_{12}$ and folic acid are at normal levels, there is no deficit in cognition. With normal $B_{12}$ and high folate (>59 nmol/L), cognition improved and reduced the odds of anaemia by 0.5. However, low $B_{12}$ (<148 pmol/L) with normal folate increased the odds ratio for anaemia to 2:1 and for cognitive impairment to 1.7:1. But the most dramatic effects were seen with low $B_{12}$ and high folate where the odds ratio for anaemia and cog-nitive impairment rose to 5:1; see Table 8.2 for summary (Morris et al., 2007). Thus, fortification of food with folic acid is potentially harmful for those with $B_{12}$ deficiency. A similar effect on cognitive decline over 8 years for those with low $B_{12}$ levels who took folic acid supplements was shown in the Framingham study (Morris et al., 2012). There is a small risk of active cancers being stimulated by excess folic acid intake, so folate levels should be checked with one's physician before taking any supplements.

**TABLE 8.2**

**Summary of Evidence for Each Nutrient**

↓ signifies decreased risk with higher levels of nutrient, while ↑ signifies increased risk.

| Nutrient | Type of Association | Evidence for Cohort Studies | Evidence from Randomised Controlled Trials |
|---|---|---|---|
| Vitamin $B_6$, $B_{12}$, folate | ↓ | Insufficient conflicting evidence | Insufficient evidence (but encouraging for participants with high Hcy levels) |
| Hcy levels | ↑ | Good evidence | |
| Vitamin C | ↓ | Conflicting, insufficient evidence | Insufficient evidence |
| Vitamin E | ↓ | Conflicting evidence (good evidence using frequency questionnaire, but not with biochemical levels) | Insufficient evidence |
| Flavonoids | ↓ | Insufficient evidence | Insufficient evidence |
| Omega-3 | ↓ | Insufficient evidence | Insufficient evidence |
| MeDi | ↓ | Moderate evidence | Insufficient evidence |

Reprinted from the ADI report (Prina and Albanese, 2014).

### 8.9.2 Other Factors That Influence Vitamin Absorption

- Alcohol consumption depletes B and C vitamins; thus supplements may be needed to replace the loss after over the normal limit of consumption for men and women.
- $B_{12}$ supplements are a more reliable source than protein foods in vulnerable groups such as older adults, vegetarians, pregnant women and those with anaemia.
- Coffee may elevate Hcy levels which can be reduced with B vitamins.
- In some cases due to inflammatory factors and oxidative stress associated with elevated Hcy, particular forms of vitamin $B_{12}$ supplements such as glutathionylcobalamin may be more beneficial than others such as cyano-cobalamin in combination with N-acetyl-L-cysteine (Birch et al., 2009).
- Aspirin use appears to negate the beneficial effect of B vitamins on cardiovascular disease (Hankey et al., 2012) and on brain atrophy (Smith et al., 2010).

## 8.10  STUDY DESIGN ISSUES

There may be a certain window of opportunity to capture and reverse cognitive decline. B vitamin trials in those with more advanced AD pathology may have been unsuccessful due to the severity of brain atrophy already reached. For example, in Aisen et al.'s study (2008), a significant slowing of cognitive decline was found only for patients with mild AD. Thus, early intervention is indicated. Further support for this concept comes from a clinical trial (Eastley et al., 2000) showing that 66 patients with dementia and low $B_{12}$ did not improve their cognitive scores after 7 months of B vitamin treatment. However, 21 patients with early cognitive impairment and low $B_{12}$ did improve their verbal fluency scores after 9 months of treatment.

Ford and Almeida (2012) tested studies with longer intervention, larger sample size and inclusion of folic acid supplementation in the subgroup analyses they performed, as these factors should have improved the likelihood of showing treatment effects of B vitamins. However, there were other issues that may have limited the findings. These included analyses of studies with normal participants combined with those with hypertension, CVD, low baseline B vitamin status or normal baseline Hcy status. Aspirin is known to negate the effects of B vitamins; thus, inclusion of patients on aspirin for these conditions may have reduced the treatment effect of B vitamins. Analyses with cognitively impaired participants included both those with mild impairment and those with moderate AD. Some trials used insensitive cognitive outcomes such as the MMSE (see Chapter 4 by Ahmed and de Jager). The Clarke meta-analysis included 8 trials with only the MMSE or TICS-M as outcomes. Three of the trials only had endpoint scores; therefore, baseline scores were imputed to calculate change scores. Decline in cognitively normal older adults on the MMSE is only ~0.1 points per year (Starr et al., 1997); thus, the placebo groups in these trials would have shown negligible decline. Thus, to show any difference in change scores due to B vitamin treatment would require extremely large study samples. The conclusion of the meta-analysis that there is no evidence that B vitamins can prevent AD is not one the authors can rightly make, as they only included studies with participants without dementia or AD, using trials mostly not designed to test effects of B vitamins on cognition.

The few RCTs with positive results of B vitamin treatment used selective inclusion criteria (e.g. high baseline Hcy, participants with only MCI or only mild AD), had large sample sizes and long-term intervention ( $\geq$ 2 years), but also used sensitive domain-specific cognitive outcome measures for episodic memory, processing speed and executive function (de Jager et al., 2012; Durga et al., 2007). The VITACOG trial used a novel biomarker outcome, namely, subtraction MRI for detecting rate of brain shrinkage as the primary outcome for treatment efficacy (Smith et al., 2010).

The B-Vitamin Treatment Trialists' Collaboration meta-analysis included sub-analyses for a number of risk factors for cognitive ageing and decline (Clarke et al., 2014). However, the subgroup analysis was only done for the trials using global cognition tests, and not domain-sensitive tests. These analyses showed no effects of B vitamin treatment versus placebo on z-score differences for those in various subgroups, although there were some trends. The biggest differences in the comparison groups were for smoking (z = 0.07 between never and current), cognitive impairment (z = 0.04, yes vs. no) and baseline Hcy (z = 0.04, 15+mcg/L vs. 11–14 and <11.0 mcg/L). These trends suggest that B vitamin supplements may be more effective for smokers, those with elevated Hcy and those with early or MCI. The latter two factors were confirmed in the VITACOG trial, where effects on cognition were significant for those with MCI and above the median level of Hcy at baseline (de Jager et al., 2012). The VITACOG trial also showed greater efficacy of B vitamins for those with than without stroke history.

Another important factor to consider controlling for would be the *APOE4* status, as this is a known risk factor for AD, including the age of onset and trajectory of cognitive decline (see Chapter 3 by Ordovas for more on *APOE4*). Younger adults with *APOE4* are more likely to decline faster (Martins et al., 2005). Low B vitamin status and *APOE4* allele combined have been associated with greater cognitive deficits (Vogiatzoglou et al., 2013). Sub-analyses may provide some guidance for those planning RCTs with healthy older adults, as to where expected benefits of treatment may be likely, and thus provide some guidance on population sampling and which inclusion/exclusion criteria to apply.

Wide differences in study design in the 21 studies with nutritional supplements reviewed by Manders et al. (2004) meant that no clear pattern emerged to explain the observed positive effects. In studies where cognitive function was tested with general cognitive tests, effects were not found for multi-nutrients. But when domain-specific tests were used, positive results were obtained, especially for fluid ability tests such as information processing (e.g. with B vitamins) rather than crystallised abilities. Manders et al. suggest that fluid abilities are more vulnerable to changes in nutritional status, and effects are subtle. Thus, dose and duration of intervention are critical to the effect size of the outcome. They conclude that the best way to improve cognitive functioning is to combine all positive effects of different nutrients to provide an adequate overall supply of nutrients, rather than relying on a single component. The duration of intervention should be long enough to counteract reversible damage processes to the brain and target people in specific age ranges at milder stages of cognitive decline, at least 1 year before onset of clinical symptoms. Ideally one standard neuropsychological battery of sensitive tests should be used by different researchers to enable comparison of results (see Chapter 4 by Ahmed and de Jager for more coverage of this issue).

## 8.11  COGNITIVE TESTS IN VITAMIN INTERVENTION TRIALS

Dangour et al. (2010) reported that available RCTs have utilised a plethora of cognitive tests to study the effects of micronutrient supplementation. A recent systematic review of 39 RCTs using supplemental micronutrients or phytochemicals found that the trials utilised 121 different cognitive tasks, thereby making it difficult for comparison among studies and for overall data interpretation (Macready et al., 2010). The Hoyland systematic review of the effects of macronutrients on mental performance reported 132 cognitive outcomes with 69 showing significant effects of macronutrients (Hoyland et al., 2008; see de Jager et al., 2014, Table 8.2 for tests used in RCTs with and without significant change due to nutrient interventions). It is notable that RCTs with cognitively healthy participants are more likely to have included sensitive neuropsychological tests as outcomes than RCTs with cognitively impaired participants. However, the field would benefit from more standardised and systematic approaches to study the effect of micronutrient supplementation on cognitive functions. Many of the paper and pencil questionnaires employed to assess cognitive abilities may not be sensitive enough to detect small changes that result from short-term interventions of micronutrient supplementation (Isaac and Oates, 2008; Schmitt et al., 2005). On the other hand, validated computer-based tests are becoming widely available; such tests ensure high sensitivity of measurement, both in terms of accuracy and speed of performance across various cognitive domains. Increased use of computerised cognitive assessments may aid in the ability to detect subtle changes that might result from micronutrient supplementation in healthy individuals.

## TOP 6 SUMMARY POINTS FROM THIS CHAPTER

- Certain vitamins and minerals from the diet are important for brain health. They can affect the neuronal structure, function and neural network connections, as well as the vasculature feeding into the brain.
- Vitamin deficiencies including B vitamins can affect neuronal integrity and result in detrimental effects on cognition.
- Certain minerals such as copper, aluminium and iron in excess can be neurotoxic, although iron is essential to brain development.
- Hcy metabolism is directly related to B vitamin intake and availability. Hcy will be neurotoxic if elevated, but levels can be reduced by intake of B vitamins.
- The balance of folate to vitamin $B_{12}$ is critical. High folate and low $B_{12}$ can impact negatively on cognition and risk of anaemia.
- Markers of $B_{12}$ including holotranscobalamin and MMA are better indicators of vitamin $B_{12}$ status than $B_{12}$ itself.

## WHAT'S UNDER DEBATE?

- Vitamin D: Is it beneficial to cognition in older adults? At what doses? There are some suggestions of harm when calcium levels are high.
- Vitamin $B_6$: Is it necessary in Hcy lowering trials? What role does it play in cognition/Hcy metabolism?
- Vitamin $B_{12}$ and folate: Can intervention prevent AD with better study design? Is treatment effective for cognitive efficacy?
- Are multivitamin products or combinations of vitamins and nutrients more beneficial to cognition than individual vitamins?
- Certain dietary factors are recommended for optimal brain function and cognitive performance. How can diet be monitored effectively to assess benefit?
- How can cognitive outcomes be standardised among trialists in this field?
- Will biomarkers provide better trial outcomes than cognitive tests?

**WHERE TO FROM HERE?**

- More research on mechanism of action of $B_6$, vitamin D, multi-nutrients, MeDi/other diets, tea/coffee, alcohol, sugar/glucose/ketones from high-protein diets
- More intervention research on vitamins B and omega-3, pre-dementia and post mild dementia
- More multi-arm intervention research, including nutrients plus other interventions for cognitive improvement in older adults
- More research of best study designs and outcome measures including cognitive, imaging and clinical

## REFERENCES

Adlard PA, Parncutt JM, Finkelstein DI, Bush AI. (2010). Cognitive loss in zinc transporter-3 knock-out mice: A phenocopy for the synaptic and memory deficits of Alzheimer's disease? *Journal of Neuroscience* 30:1631–1636.

Agostini S, Clerici M, Mancuso R. (2104). How plausible is a link between HSV-1infection and Alzheimer's disease? *Expert Review of Anti Infective Therapy* Mar;12(3):275–278. doi: 10.1586/14787210.2014.887442.

Aisen PS, Schneider LS, Sano M, Diaz-Arrastia R, van Dyck CH, Weiner MF, Bottiglieri T, Jin S, Stokes KT, Thomas RG, Thal LJ; Alzheimer Disease Cooperative Study. (2008). High-dose B vitamin supplementation and cognitive decline in Alzheimer disease: A randomized controlled trial. *JAMA* Oct 15;300(15):1774–1783. doi: 10.1001/jama.300.15.1774.

Allès B, Samieri C, Féart C, Jutand MA, Laurin D, Barberger-Gateau P. (2012). Dietary patterns: A novel approach to examine the link between nutrition and cognitive function in older individuals. *Nutrition Research Reviews* Dec;25(2):207–222. doi: 10.1017/S0954422412000133. Epub July 4, 2012. Review.

Ames BN, Shigenaga MK, Hagen TM. (1993). Oxidants, antioxidants, and the degenerative diseases of aging. *Proceedings of the National Academy of Sciences of the United States of America* 90(17):7915–7922.

Anglin RE, Samaan Z, Walter SD, McDonald SD. (2013). Vitamin D deficiency and depression in adults: Systematic review and meta-analysis. *British Journal of Psychiatry* Feb;202:100–107. Review. PubMed PMID: 23377209.

Annweiler C, Llewellyn DJ, Beauchet O. (2013a). Low serum vitamin D concentrations in Alzheimer's disease: A systematic review and meta-analysis. *Journal of Alzheimer's Disease* 33(3):659–674.

Annweiler C, Montero-Odasso M, Hachinski V, Seshadri S, Bartha R, Beauchet O. (2013b). Vitamin D concentration and lateral cerebral ventricle volume in older adults. *Molecular Nutrition and Food Research* 57(2):267–276.

Azzi A, Stocker A. (2000). Vitamin E: Non-antioxidant roles. *Progress in Lipid Research* 39(3):231–255.

Balion C, Griffith LE, Strifler L. et al. (2012). Vitamin D, cognition, and dementia: A systematic review and meta-analysis. *Neurology* 79(13):1397–1405. doi: 10.1159/000339702.

Barberger-Gateau P, Raffaitin C, Letenneur L. et al. (2007). Dietary patterns and risk of dementia: The Three-City cohort study. *Neurology* 69:1921–1930.

Barja G. (2004). Free radicals and aging. *Trends in Neurosciences* 27(10):595–600.

Barnard ND, Bush AI, Ceccarelli A, Cooper J, de Jager CA, Erickson KI, Fraser G, Kesler S, Levin SM, Lucey B, Morris MC, Squitti R. (2014). Dietary and lifestyle guidelines for the prevention of Alzheimer's disease. *Neurobiology of Aging* Sep;35(Suppl. 2):S74–S78. doi: 10.1016/j.neurobiolaging.2014.03.033. Epub May 14, 2014.

Bates CJ, Pentieva KD, Prentice A, Mansoor MA, Finch S. (1999). Plasma pyridoxal phosphate and pyridoxic acid and their relationship to plasma homocysteine in a representative sample of British men and women aged 65 years and over. *British Journal of Nutrition* 81(3):191–201.

Bates CJ. (2006). Thiamin. In: Bowman BA, Russell RM, eds. *Present Knowledge in Nutrition*, 9th edn. Vol. 1. Washington, DC: ILSI Press; pp. 242–249.

Bender DA. (2003). *Nutritional Biochemistry of the Vitamins*. New York: Cambridge University Press.

Bennett S, Grant MM, Aldred S. (2009). Oxidative stress in vascular dementia and Alzheimer's disease: a common pathology. *Journal of Alzheimer's Diseases* 17(2):245–257. doi: 10.3233/JAD-2009-1041. Review.

Berr C, Richard M-J, Gourlet V, Garrel C, Favier A. (2004). Enzymatic antioxidant balance and cognitive decline in aging – The EVA study. *European Journal of Epidemiology* 19(2):133–138.

Birch CS, Brasch NE, McCaddon A, Williams JH. (2009). A novel role for vitamin B(12): Cobalamins are intracellular antioxidants in vitro. *Free Radical Biology & Medicine* Jul 15;47(2):184–188. doi: 10.1016/j.freeradbiomed.2009.04.023.

Braun L, Cohen M. (2010). *Herbs & Natural Supplements: An Evidence Based Guide*, 3rd edn. Chatswood, New South Wales: Elsevier.

Brewer GJ. (2009). The risks of copper toxicity contributing to cognitive decline in the aging population and Alzheimer's disease. *Journal of the American College of Nutrition* 28:238–242.

Briones TL, Darwish H. (2012). Vitamin D mitigates age-related cognitive decline through the modulation of pro-inflammatory state and decrease in amyloid burden. *Journal of Neuroinflammation* 9:244. doi: 10.1186/1742-2094-9-244.

Bruno RS, Leonard SW, Atkinson J. et al. (2006). Faster plasma vitamin E disappearance in smokers is normalized by vitamin C supplementation. *Free Radical Biology & Medicine* 40(4):689–697.

Budge MM, de Jager C, Hogervorst E, Smith AD; Oxford Project To Investigate Memory and Ageing (OPTIMA). (2002). Total plasma homocysteine, age, systolic blood pressure, and cognitive performance in older people. *Journal of the American Geriatrics Society* Dec;50(12):2014–2018. PubMed PMID: 12473014.

Butler CC, Vidal-Aaball J, Cannings-John R, McCaddon A, Hood K, Papaioannou A, Mcdowell I, Goringe A. (2006). Oral vitamin B12 versus intramuscular vitamin B12 for vitamin B12 deficiency: A systematic review of randomized controlled trials. *Family Practice* Jun;23(3):279–285. Review. PubMed PMID: 16585128.

Butterworth RF. (2003). Thiamin deficiency and brain disorders. *Nutrition Research Reviews* 16(2):277–284.

Clarke R, Grimley Evans J, Schneede J. et al. (2004). Vitamin B12 and folate deficiency in later life. *Age and Ageing* Jan;33(1):34–41.

Clarke R, Bennett D, Parish S. et al. (2014). Effects of homocysteine lowering with B vitamins on cognitive aging: Meta-analysis of 11 trials with cognitive data on 22,000 individuals. *American Journal of Clinical Nutrition* Jun 25;100(2):657–666. [Epub ahead of print] PubMed PMID: 24965307.

Clarke RJ, Bennett DA. (2008). B vitamins for prevention of cognitive decline: Insufficient evidence to justify treatment. *JAMA* Oct 15;300(15):1819–1821.doi: 10.1001/jama.300.15.1819.

Combs J, Gerald F. (2012). *The Vitamins*, 4th edn. Burlington, MA: Elsevier Science.

Cranney A, Horsley T, O'Donnell S. et al. (2007). Effectiveness and safety of vitamin D in relation to bone health. *Evidence Report Technology Assessment* Aug;(158):1–235.

Crapper DR, Krishnan SS, Dalton AJ. (1973). Brain aluminum distribution in Alzheimer's disease and experimental neurofibrillary degeneration. *Transaction of the American Neurological Association* 98:17–20.

Crapper DR, Krishnan SS, Quittkat S. (1976). Aluminum, neurofibrillary degeneration and Alzheimer's disease. *Brain* 99:67–80.

Dangour AD, Allen E, Richards M, Whitehouse P, Uauy R. (2010). Design considerations in long-term intervention studies for the prevention of cognitive decline or dementia. *Nutrition Reviews* Nov;68 Suppl. 1:S16–21. doi:10.1111/j.1753-4887.2010.00330.x.

Davies KJ. (2000). Oxidative stress, antioxidant defenses, and damage removal, repair, and replacement systems. *IUBMB Life* 50(4–5), 279–289.

de Jager CA. (2014). Critical levels of brain atrophy associated with homocysteine and cognitive decline. *Neurobiology of Aging* Sep;35 Suppl. 2:S35–S39.doi: 10.1016/j.neurobiolaging.2014.03.040. Epub 2014 May 15. Review. PubMed PMID: 24927906.

de Jager CA, Dye L, de Bruin EA, Butler L, Fletcher J, Lamport DJ, Latulippe ME, Spencer JP, Wesnes K. (2014). Criteria for validation and selection of cognitive tests for investigating the effects of foods and nutrients. *Nutrition Reviews* Mar;72(3):162–79. PubMed PMID: 24697324.

de Jager CA, Oulhaj A, Jacoby R, Refsum H, Smith AD. (2012). Cognitive and clinical outcomes of lowering homocysteine-lowering B-vitamin treatment in mild cognitive impairment: A randomized controlled trial. *International Journal of Geriatric Psychiatry* 27:592–600.

Devore EE, Goldstein F, van Rooij FJ, Hofman A, Stampfer MF, Witteman JC, Breteler MM. (2010). Dietary antioxidants and long-term risk of dementia. *Archives of Neurology* 67:819–825.

Devore EE(1), Kang JH, Stampfer MJ, Grodstein F. (2013). The association of antioxidants and cognition in the Nurses' Health Study. *American Journal of Epidemiology* Jan 1;177(1):33–41. doi: 10.1093/aje/kws202.

Douaud G, Refsum H, de Jager CA, Jacoby R, Nichols TE, Smith SM, Smith A.D. (2013). Preventing Alzheimer's disease-related gray matter atrophy by B-vitamin treatment. *Proceedings of the National Academy of Sciences of the United States of America* 110:9523

Durga J, van Boxtel MP, Schouten EG. et al. (2007). Effect of 3-year folic acid supplementation on cognitive function in older adults in the FACIT trial: A randomised, double blind, controlled trial. *Lancet* 369(9557):208–216.

Eastley R, Wilcock GK, Bucks RS. (2000). Vitamin B12 deficiency in dementia and cognitive impairment: The effects of treatment on neuropsychological function. *International Journal of Geriatric Psychiatry* Mar;15(3):226–233. PubMed PMID: 10713580.

Eyles DW, Smith S, Kinobe R, Hewison M, McGrath JJ. (2005). Distribution of the vitamin D receptor and 1 alpha-hydroxylase in human brain. *Journal of Chemical Neuroanatomy* Jan;29(1):21–30. PMID: 15589699.

Farnier M. (2009). How to manage lipid profiles and their interpretation in patients with coronary heart disease? *Presse Med* 38:958–963.

Food and Nutrition Board, Institute of Medicine. (1998). *Vitamin B12. Dietary Reference Intakes for Thiamin, Riboflavin, Niacin, Vitamin B6, Vitamin B12, Pantothenic Acid, Biotin, and Choline*. Washington, DC: National Academy Press; pp. 306–356.

Ford AH, Almeida OP. (2012). Effect of homocysteine lowering treatment on cognitive function: A systematic review and meta-analysis of randomized controlled trials. *Journal of Alzheimer's Disease* 29(1):133–149.

Ford ES, Sowell A. (1999). Serum alpha-tocopherol status in the United States population: Findings from the Third National Health and Nutrition Examination Survey. *American Journal of Epidemiology* 150(3):290–300.

Freeman LR, Keller JN. (2012). Oxidative stress and cerebral endothelial cells: Regulation of the blood–brain-barrier and antioxidant based interventions. *Biochimica et Biophysica Acta (BBA) – Molecular Basis of Disease*, 1822(5):822–829.

Fulgoni VL 3rd, Keast DR, Bailey, Dwyer J. Foods, fortificants, and supplements: Where do Americans get their nutrients? *Journal of Nutrition* 2011;141(10):1847–1854.

Gibson GE, Blass JP. (1999). Nutrition and brain function. In: Siegel GJ, ed., *Basic Neurochemistry: Molecular, Cellular and Medical Aspects*. Philadelphia, PA: Lippincott Williams & Wilkins; pp. 692–709.

Goff LM, Cowland DE, Hooper L, Frost GS. (2013). Low glycaemic index diets and blood lipids: A systematic review and meta-analysis of randomised controlled trials. *Nutrition, Metabolism and Cardiovascular Diseases* 23:1–10.

Gregory JF, 3rd. (1998). Nutritional properties and significance of vitamin glycosides. *Annual Review of Nutrition* 18:277–296.

Grodstein F, O'Brien J, Kang JH. et al. (2013). Long-term multivitamin supplementation and cognitive function in men: A randomized trial. *Annals of Internal Medicine* Dec 17;159(12):806–814. PubMed PMID: 24490265.

Haller J. (2005). Vitamins and brain function. In: Lieberman HR, Kanarek RB, Prasad C, eds., *Nutritional Neuroscience*. Boca Raton, FL: CRC Press.

Halliwell, B. (2006). Oxidative stress and neurodegeneration: Where are we now? *Journal of Neurochemistry* 97(6):1634–1658.

Hankey GJ, Eikelboom JW, Yi Q. et al. (2012). Antiplatelet therapy and the effects of B vitamins in patients with previous stroke or transient ischaemic attack: A post-hoc subanalysis of VITATOPS, a randomised, placebo-controlled trial. *The Lancet Neurology* 11(6):512–520. doi: 10.1016/s1474-4422(12)70091-1.

Harman, D. (1956). Aging: A theory based on free radical and radiation chemistry. *Journal of Gerontology* 11(3):298–300.

Harris E, MacPherson H, Vitetta L, Kirk J, Sali A, Pipingas A. (2012). Effects of a multivitamin, mineral and herbal supplement on cognition and blood biomarkers in older men: A randomised, placebo-controlled trial. *Human Psychopharmacology* 27(4):370–377.

Harrison FE, May JM. (2009). Vitamin C function in the brain: Vital role of the ascorbate transporter SVCT2. *Free Radical Biology and Medicine* 46(6):719–730.

Healton EB, Savage DG, Brust JC, Garrett TJ, Lindenbaum J. (1991). Neurologic aspects of cobalamin deficiency. *Medicine (Baltimore)* Jul;70(4):229–245. PubMed PMID: 1648656.

Hegyi J, Schwartz RA, Hegyi V. (2004). Pellagra: Dermatitis, dementia, and diarrhea. *International Journal of Dermatology* 43(1):1–5.

Hendler SS, Rorvik DR, eds. (2001). *PDR for Nutritional Supplements*. Montvale, NJ: Medical Economics Company, Inc.

Holick MF. (2007). Vitamin D deficiency. *The New England Journal of Medicine* 357(3):266–281.

Holick MF, Matsuoka LY, Wortsman J. (1989). Age, vitamin D, and solar ultraviolet. *Lancet* 2(8671):1104–1105.

Hooshmand B, Lökk J, Solomon A. et al. (2014). Vitamin D in relation to cognitive impairment, cerebrospinal fluid biomarkers, and brain volumes. *The Journals of Gerontology Series A: Biological Sciences and Medical Sciences* Sep;69(9):1132–1138. [Epub ahead of print] PubMed PMID: 24568931.

Hoyland A, Lawton C, Dye L. (2008). Acute effects of macronutrient manipulations on cognitive test performance in healthy young adults: A systematic research review. *Neuroscience & Biobehavioral Reviews* 32:72–85.

Huang HY, Appel LJ. (2003). Supplementation of diets with α-tocopherol reduces serum concentrations of γ- and δ-tocopherol in humans. *Journal of Nutrition* 133:3137–3140.

Isaacs E, Oates J. (2008). Nutrition and cognition: Assessing cognitive abilities in children and young people. *European Journal of Nutrition* 47 (Suppl. 3):4–24.

Johansson S, Melhus H. (2001). Vitamin A antagonizes calcium response to vitamin D in man. *Journal of Bone and Miner Research* 16(10):1899–1905.

Joosten E, Van den Berg A, Riezler R, Naurath HJ, Lindenbaum J, Stabler SP, Allen RH. (1993). Metabolic evidence that deficiencies of vitamin B-12 (cobalamin), folate, and vitamin B-6 occur commonly in elderly people. *American Journal of Clinical Nutrition* 58(4):468–476.

Kang JH, Ascherio A, Grodstein F. (2005). Fruit and vegetable consumption and cognitive decline in aging women. *Annals of Neurology* 57:713–720.

Kawahara M, Kato-Negishi M. (2011). Link between aluminum and the pathogenesis of Alzheimer's disease: The integration of aluminum and amyloid cascade hypotheses. *International Journal of Alzheimer's Disease* 2011:276393.

Kesse-Guyot E, Amieva H, Castetbon K, Henegar A, Ferry M, Jeandel C, Hercberg S, Galan P; SU.VI.MAX 2 Research Group. (2011). Adherence to nutritional recommendations and subsequent cognitive performance: Findings from the prospective supplementation with antioxidant vitamins and minerals 2 (SU.VI.MAX 2) study. *American Journal of Clinical Nutrition* Jan;93(1):200–210. doi: 10.3945/ajcn.2010.29761. Epub Nov 24, 2010.

Kontush K, Schekatolina S. (2004). Vitamin E in neurodegenerative disorders: Alzheimer's disease. *Annals of the New York Academy of Sciences* 1031:249–262.

Lindenbaum J, Healton EB, Savage DG. et al. (1988). Neuropsychiatric disorders caused by cobalamin deficiency in the absence of anemia or macrocytosis. *The New England Journal of Medicine* 318(26):1720–1728.

Lykkesfeldt J, Poulsen HE. (2010). Is vitamin C supplementation beneficial? Lessons learned from randomised controlled trials. *British Journal of Nutrition* 103(9):1251–1259.

Macpherson H, Ellis KA, Sali A, Pipingas A. (March 2012). Memory improvements in elderly women following 16 weeks treatment with a combined multivitamin, mineral and herbal supplement: A randomized controlled trial. *Psychopharmacology (Berl)*. 220(2):351–65. doi: 10.1007/s00213-011-2481-3. Epub 2011 October 18.

Macready AL, Butler LT, Kennedy OB, Ellis JA, Williams CM, Spencer JP. 2010. Cognitive tests used in chronic adult human randomised controlled trial micronutrient and phytochemical intervention studies. *Nutrition Research Reviews* 23(2):200–229.

Malouf R, Evans JG. (2008). Folic acid with or without vitamin B12 for the prevention and treatment of healthy elderly and demented people. *Cochrane Database of Systematic Reviews* Oct 8;(4): CD004514.

Manders M, de Groot LC, van Staveren WA, Wouters-Wesseling W, Mulders AJ, Schols JM, Hoefnagels WH. (2004). Effectiveness of nutritional supplements on cognitive functioning in elderly persons: A systematic review. *The Journals of Gerontology Series A: Biological and Medical Sciences* Oct;59(10):1041–1049. Review. PubMed PMID: 15528776.

Mao P. (2013). Oxidative stress and its clinical applications in dementia. *Journal of Neurodegenerative Diseases* 2013:15.

Martel G, Hevi C, Friebely O, Baybutt T, Shumyatsky GP. (2010). Zinc transporter 3 is involved in learned fear and extinction, but not in innate fear. *Learning & Memory* 17:582–590.

Martins CA, Oulhaj A, de Jager CA, Williams JH. (2005). *APOE* alleles predict the rate of cognitive decline in Alzheimer disease: A nonlinear model. *Neurology* Dec 27;65(12):1888–1893.

Martyn CN, Osmond C, Edwardson JA, Barker DJP, Harris EC, Lacey RF. (1989). Geographical relation between Alzheimer's disease and aluminum in drinking water. *Lancet* 333:61–62.

Maugeri D, Santangelo A, Bonanno M, Testai M, Abbate S, Lo Giudice F, Panebianco P. (2004). Oxidative stress and aging: Studies on an East-Sicilian, ultraoctagenarian population living in institutes or at home. *Archives of Gerontology and Geriatrics* 38:271–277.

McCaddon A, Davies G, Hudson P, Tandy S, Cattell H. (1998). Total serum homocysteine in senile dementia of Alzheimer type. *Internation Journal of Geriatric Psychiatry* Apr;13(4):235–239. PubMed PMID: 9646150.

McCann JC, Ames BN. (2008). Is there convincing biological or behavioral evidence linking vitamin D deficiency to brain dysfunction? *FASEB Journal* 22(4):982–1001.

Mecocci P, Polidori MC. (2012). Antioxidant clinical trials in mild cognitive impairment and Alzheimer's disease. *Biochimica et Biophysica Acta* May;1822(5):631–638.

Morris MC. (2012a). Nutritional determinants of cognitive aging and dementia. *Proceedings of the Nutrition Society* Feb;71(1):1–13.

Morris MC, Evans DA, Tangney CC. et al. (2005). Relation of the tocopherol forms to incident Alzheimer disease and cognitive change. *American Journal of Clinical Nutrition* 81:508–514.

Morris MC, Evans DA, Tangney CC, Bienias JL, Wilson RS. (2006). Associations of vegetable and fruit consumption with age-related cognitive change. *Neurology* 67:1370–1376.

Morris MS. (2012b). The role of B vitamins in preventing and treating cognitive impairment and decline. *Advances in Nutrition* 3(6):801–812.

Morris MS, Jacques PF, Rosenberg IH, Selhub J. (2007). Folate and vitamin B-12 status in relation to anemia, macrocytosis, and cognitive impairment in older Americans in the age of folic acid fortification. *American Journal of Clinical Nutrition* Jan;85(1):193–200. PubMed PMID: 17209196; PubMed Central PMCID: PMC1828842.

Morris MS, Selhub J, Jacques PF. (2012). Vitamin B-12 and folate status in relation to decline in scores on the mini-mental state examination in the Framingham heart study. *Journal of the American Geriatric Society* Aug;60(8):1457–1464.

NHMRC. (2006). *Nutrient Reference Values for Australia and New Zealand Including Recommended Dietary Intakes.* Canberra, Australian Capital Territory, Australia: National Health and Medical Research Council, Australian Government Department of Health and Ageing.

Nilsson A, Radeborg K, Björck I. (2009). Effects of differences in postprandial glycaemia on cognitive functions in healthy middle-aged subjects. *European Journal of Clinical Nutrition* Jan;63(1):113–120. PubMed PMID: 17851459.

Olanow CW. (1990). Oxidation reactions in Parkinson's disease. *Neurology* Oct;40(10 Suppl. 3): suppl. 32–37; discussion 37–39.

O'Leary F, Allman-Farinelli M, Samman S. (2012). Vitamin B12 status, cognitive decline and dementia: A systematic review of prospective cohort studies. *British Journal of Nutrition* 108(11):1948–1961.

Park YK, Sempos CT, Barton CN, Vanderveen JE, Yetley EA. (2000). Effectiveness of food fortification in the United States: The case of pellagra. *American Journal of Public Health* 90(5):727–738.

Petersen RC, Thomas RG, Grundman M. et al. (2005). Vitamin E and donepezil for the treatment of mild cognitive impairment. *The New England Journal of Medicine* 352(23):2379–2388.

Pfeiffer CM, Caudill SP, Gunter EW, Osterloh J, Sampson EJ. (2005). Biochemical indicators of B vitamin status in the US population after folic acid fortification: Results from the National Health and Nutrition Examination Survey 1999–2000. *American Journal of Clinical Nutrition* 82(2):442–450.

Polidori MC, Praticó D, Mangialasche F. et al. (2009). High fruit and vegetable intake is positively correlated with antioxidant status and cognitive performance in healthy subjects. *Journal of Alzheimer's Disease* 17(4):921–927.

Prina M, Albanese E. (2014). Chapter 3. In: Prince M, Albanese E, Prina M, Guerchet M. eds., *Nutrition and Dementia – A Review of Available Research.* London, U.K.: Alzheimer's Disease International (ADI).

Refsum H, Nurk E, Smith AD, Ueland PM, Gjesdal CG, Bjelland I, Vollset SE. (2006). The Hordaland Homocysteine Study: A community-based study of homocysteine, its determinants, and associations with disease. *Journal of Nutrition* 136(6):1731S–1740S.

Refsum H, Ueland PM, Nygård O, Vollset SE. (1998). Homocysteine and cardiovascular disease. *Annual Review of Medicine* 49:31–62; doi: 10.1146/annurev.med.49.1.31.

Rohde CM, DeLuca H. (2003). Bone resorption activity of all-trans retinoic acid is independent of vitamin D in rats. *Journal of Nutrition* 133(3):777–783.

Rondeau V, Jacqmin-Gadda H, Commenges D, Helmer C, Dartigues J-F. (2009). Aluminum and silica in drinking water and the risk of Alzheimer's disease or cognitive decline: Findings from 15-year follow up of the PAQUID cohort. *American Journal of Epidemiology* 169:489–496.

Ross AC. (1999). Vitamin A and retinoids. In: Shils M, Olson JA, Shike M, Ross AC. eds., *Modern Nutrition in Health and Disease*, 9th edn. Baltimore, MD: Lippincott Williams & Wilkins; pp. 305–327.

Sano M, Ernesto C, Thomas RG. et al. (1997). A controlled trial of selegiline, alpha-tocopherol, or both as treatment for Alzheimer's disease. The Alzheimer's Disease Cooperative Study. *The New England Journal of Medicine* 336(17):1216–1222.

Sayre LM, Perry G, Smith MA. (2007). Oxidative stress and neurotoxicity. *Chemical Research in Toxicology* 21(1):172–188.

Schlögl M, Holick MF. (2014). Vitamin D and neurocognitive function. *Clinical Interventions in Aging* Apr 2;9:559–568.

Schmitt JA, Benton D, Kallus KW. (2005). General methodological considerations for the assessment of nutritional influences on human cognitive functions. *European Journal of Nutrition* 44(8):459–464.

Schrag M, Mueller C, Zabel M, Crofton A, Kirsch WM, Ghribi O, Squitti R, Perry G. (2013). Oxidative stress in blood in Alzheimer's disease and mild cognitive impairment: A meta-analysis. *Neurobiology of Disease* Nov;59:100–110. doi: 10.1016/j.nbd.2013.07.005. Review.

Semba RD. (1998). The role of vitamin A and related retinoids in immune function. *Nutrition Reviews* 56(1 Pt 2):S38–S48.

Seshadri S. (2006). Elevated plasma homocysteine levels: Risk factor or risk marker for the development of dementia and Alzheimer's disease? *Journal of Alzheimer's Disease* Aug;9(4):393–398. Review. PubMed PMID: 16917147.

Sindreu C, Palmiter RD, Storm DR. (2011). Zinc transporter ZnT-3 regulates presynaptic Erk1/2 signaling and hippocampus-dependent memory. *Proceedings of the National Academy of Sciences of the United States of America* 108:3366–3370.

Smith A, Clark R, Nutt D, Haller J, Hayward S, Perry K. (1999). Anti-oxidant vitamins and mental performance of the elderly. *Human Psychopharmacology* 14:459–471.

Smith AD, Kim YI, Refsum H. (2008). Is folic acid good for everyone? *American Journal of Clinical Nutrition* Mar;87(3):517–533. PubMed PMID: 18326588.

Smith AD, Smith SM, de Jager CA, Whitbread P, Johnston C, Agacinski G, Oulhaj A, Bradley KM, Jacoby R, Refsum H. (2010). Homocysteine-lowering by B vitamins slows the rate of accelerated brain atrophy in mild cognitive impairment: A randomized controlled trial. *PLoS One* Sep 8;5(9):e12244. doi: 10.1371/journal.pone.0012244.

Sofi F, Abbate R, Gensini GF, Casini A. (2012). Which diet for an effective cardiovascular prevention? *Monaldi Archives for Chest Disease* 78:60–65.

Sofi F, Macchi C, Abbate R. et al. (2010). Effectiveness of the Mediterranean diet: Can it help delay or prevent Alzheimer's disease? *Journal of Alzheimer's Disease* 20:795–801.

Solfrizzi V, Frisardi V, Seripa D. et al. (2011). Mediterranean diet in predementia and dementia syndromes. *Current Alzheimer Research* 8:520–542.

Squitti R, Hoogenraad T, Brewer G, Bush AI, Polimanti R. (2013). Copper status in Alzheimer's disease and other neurodegenerative disorders. *International Journal of Alzheimer's Disease* 2013:838274. doi: 10.1155/2013/838274. Epub 2013 Dec 19. PubMed PMID: 24455406; PubMed Central PMCID: PMC3880705.

Squitti R, Siotto M, Polimanti R. (September 2014). Low-copper diet as a preventive strategy for Alzheimer's disease. *Neurobiology of Aging.*, 35(Suppl 2):S40-S50. doi:10.1016/j.neurobiolaging.2014.02.031. Epub May 15, 2014.

Stankiewicz JM, Brass SD. (2009). Role of iron in neurotoxicity: A cause for concern in the elderly? *Current Opinion in Clinical Nutrition and Metabolic Care* 12:22–29.

Starr JM, Deary IJ, Inch S, Cross S, MacLennan WJ. (1997). Age-associated cognitive decline in healthy old people. *Age and Ageing* 26(4):295–300.

Todd K, Butterworth RF. (1998). Mechanisms of selective neuronal cell death due to thiamine deficiency. *Annals of the New York Academy of Sciences* 1999;893:404–411.

Todorich B, Pasquini JM, Garcia CI, Paez PM, Connor JR. (2009). Oligodendrocytes and myelination: The role of iron. *Glia* 57(5):467–478.

Touyz RM, Schiffrin EL. (2008). Oxidative stress and hypertension. In: Holtzman JL. ed., *Atherosclerosis and Oxidant Stress: A New Perspective*. Dordrecht, the Netherlands: Springer.

van der Schaft J, Koek HL, Dijkstra E, Verhaar HJ, van der Schouw YT, Emmelot-Vonk MH. (2013), The association between vitamin D and cognition: A systematic review. *Ageing Research Reviews* Sep;12(4):1013–1023. doi: 10.1016/j.arr.2013.05.004.

Ventriglia M, Bucossi S, Panetta V, Squitti R. (2012). Copper in Alzheimer's disease: A meta-analysis of serum, plasma, and cerebrospinal fluid studies. *Journal of Alzheimer's Disease* 30(4):981–984. doi: 10.3233/JAD-2012-120244. Review. PubMed PMID: 22475798.

Voet D, Voet JG. (1995a). *Biochemistry*, 2nd edn. New York: John Wiley & Sons, Inc.; pp. 538–598.

Voet D, Voet JG. Glycolysis. (1995b). *Biochemistry*, 2nd edn. New York: John Wiley & Sons, Inc.; pp. 443–483.

Vogiatzoglou A, Smith AD, Nurk E, Drevon CA, Ueland PM, Vollset SE, Nygaard HA, Engedal K, Tell GS, Refsum H. (2013). Cognitive function in an elderly population: Interaction between vitamin B12 status, depression, and apolipoprotein E ε4: The Hordaland Homocysteine Study. *Psychosomatic Medicine* Jan;75(1):20–29. doi: 10.1097/PSY.0b013e3182761b6c. Epub 2012 Dec 4.

von Bohlen und Halbach O, Dermietzel R. (2002). *Introduction. Neurotransmitters and Neuromodulators: Handbook of Receptors and Biological Effects*. Weinheim, Germany: Wiley-VCH; pp. 1–18.

Wang L, Song Y, Manson JE. et al. (2012). Circulating 25-hydroxy-vitamin D and risk of cardiovascular disease: A meta-analysis of prospective studies. *Circulation: Cardiovascular Quality and Outcomes* 5(6):819–829.

Yoon JC, Cho JJ, Yoo SM, Ha YM. (2000). Antiviral activity of ascorbic acid against herpes simplex virus. *Journal of the Korean Society for Microbiology* 35:1–8.

Zhuo JM, Wang H, Pratico D. (2011). Is hyperhomocysteinemia an Alzheimer's disease (AD) risk factor, an AD marker, or neither? *Trends Pharmacological Sciences* Sep;32(9):562–571.

# 9 Herbal Extracts and Nutraceuticals for Cognitive Performance

*Andrew Scholey, Matthew Pase, Andrew Pipingas, Con Stough, and David Alan Camfield*

## CONTENTS

## SUMMARY

There is growing evidence that certain plants have evolved to contain bioactive compounds that can modulate behaviour, including cognitive performance. This chapter briefly summarises the evidence pertaining to selected herbal extracts ginseng, *Ginkgo biloba*, *Salvia*, L-theanine, green tea catechins, *Bacopa* and guaraná. The focus is on evidence from well-controlled human trials examining the acute effects of supplementation in healthy adults. Although not discussed here, it should be noted that there is emerging evidence that some herbal extracts may also have chronic cognitive benefits in various clinical and non-clinical populations.

Certain botanical extracts have reliable cognition-enhancing properties in various populations. These appear to be similar in magnitude to the effects of pharmaceutical cognitive enhancers. In some cases, the mechanisms of action are reasonably well established, for example, pro-cholinergic (e.g. cholinesterase inhibiting) effects of sage. In most cases, multiple synergistic actions are likely to be involved. One constant challenge for the psychopharmacology of herbal extracts is the use of standardised extracts to allow rigorous and replicable evaluation of their behavioural properties.

## 9.1 INTRODUCTION

### 9.1.1 History of Use of Herbal Products for Neurocognition

Cognitive enhancement is increasing on the public agenda and has been the focus of intense research over the past two decades. Historically, cognition enhancement has been aimed at clinical populations and/or older individuals. More recently, however, there has been growing interest in the possibility of cognitive enhancement in healthy young adults. A survey by *Nature* in 2008 revealed that up to a quarter of the journal's readership took cognitive enhancers, including modafinil (Provigil™) and methylphenidate (Ritalin™), obtaining them largely through unregulated means (Maher, 2008). Improving mental performance is often cited as one of the key motivations to take herbal extracts amongst the so-called *baby boomer* generation, that is, those now in their fourth or fifth decade (Cardello & Schutz, 2006; Cox et al., 2004; Marinac et al., 2007).

The use of herbal extracts for cognition enhancement has a long history. Homer's Odyssey tells of Circe poisoning Odysseus and his men with a drug, which may have been *Datura stramonium*, a plant known variously as angel's trumpet, devil's weed and stinkweed (amongst other names). *D. stramonium* contains the anticholinergic agent atropine (Doaigey, 1991). Odysseus and his men take *a black root, but milk-like flower* as an antidote, which allows Odysseus to rescue his crew from Circe and to recover their memories. It has been suggested that this antidote may have been the snowdrop (*Galanthus nivalis*), the original source of the currently licensed anti-dementia drug and cholinesterase inhibitor (ChEI) galantamine (Reminyl®). In the late twentieth century, galantamine underwent clinical trial development to evaluate its potential to treat Alzheimer's disease (AD), a progressive disorder characterised by cognitive decline underpinned, in part (but by no means exclusively) by degeneration of the cholinergic system. Galantamine is a good illustration of *classical* drug development from a traditional neurocognitive use of a plant, involving the isolation and subsequent synthesis of an active agent followed by clinical trials.

Galantamine is one of many ancient cognitive enhancers. For example, the Greeks considered garden sage (*elelisphakon – Salvia officinalis*) to be good for helping *diminution of senses and loss of memory*, and Ayurvedic medicine recommends sage for promoting mental clarity and calmness. Unlike galantamine, the behavioural effects of sage do not seem to be the product of a single component of the plant, rather they rely on the synergistic interactions between various compounds. In other cases, the use of herbal extracts for enhancing cognition emerged from an understanding of their specific properties. For example, possibly the most widely researched botanical for brain function, *G. biloba*, was originally used for other, non-cognitive, purposes in traditional Chinese medicine, such as to treat respiratory disorders (Howes et al., 2003).

## 9.1.2 EVOLUTION OF PSYCHOACTIVES IN PLANTS

Why have plants evolved neuroactive compounds? There are several possibilities: one relates to the idea of *hormesis* – that is, that exposure to relatively low amounts of plant toxins can evoke adaptive responses, which are beneficial to the organism (note this refers to physiological levels and not the physiologically inactive trace dilutions in homoeopathy). Such effects are documented in the cancer literature where cancer prevention following exposure to low levels of potentially carcinogenic chemicals is fairly well established (Calabrese, 2005). Mattson and Cheng (2007) present a compelling argument for similar neurocognitive effects, where the same process has been referred to as *neurohormesis* (Mattson & Cheng, 2006). One example of neurohormesis relates to antioxidant effects in neuroprotection. Much has been made of the antioxidant properties of certain plant secondary metabolites. Many plant components, such as the flavonoids, exhibit antioxidant capacity at micromolar levels, which are physiologically unrealistic following oral ingestion. Thus, neuroprotective capacity may be attributable to neurohormesis-like effects (Mattson & Cheng, 2006).

Unlike the animal *fight-or-flight* response, plants cannot flee from danger and their *fight* capacity is more or less restricted to the production of noxious substances in leaves, roots and flowers. Over the course of millions of years, plants have evolved metabolic pathways that produce substances (often secondary metabolites) that are able to influence cellular targets in predators. These secondary metabolites include various bioactive compounds, including alkaloids, cardenolides, flavonoids, indoles and terpenoids (Koul, 2008). Some acute biological effects of herbal extracts are due to direct physiological actions of these compounds (Savelev et al., 2003).

## 9.1.3 MONOTHERAPY VERSUS POLYPHARMACOLOGY

Plant extracts may contain numerous potentially psychoactive components. While simple dose–response relationships are rare even in mainstream psychopharmacology, with herbal extracts, they can be even more complex. Mainstream drug development and, to some degree, traditional pharmacognosy (the study of medicines derived from natural sources) aims to isolate active principles from plant material. In some cases, this is highly effective, leading, for example, to the development of aspirin, opiate anaesthetics and more recently medicinal cannabinoids. In certain cases, however, attempts to isolate and refine active principles from plant extracts may be self-defeating since overall biological effects rely on synergistic interactions between plant components. For example, individual components of sage have far less cholinesterase-inhibiting properties than the whole extract (Savelev et al., 2003).

A more relevant issue might be the extent to which botanical extracts used in behavioural research can be standardised. Without standardisation, meaningful interpretation of findings across studies can be difficult at best and meaningless at worst, even when results appear consistent between studies. Even standardisation based on concentrations of one or several components does not guarantee that there is batch-to-batch consistency or *phytoequivalence* (physiological equivalence of extracts).

Herbal extracts may contain many active components, and whole plant extracts may exert multiple subtle effects. Individual plant components may have agonistic or antagonistic effects and may simultaneously affect multiple systems. For example, there are established effects of certain herbal extracts on neuronal systems (e.g. sage and lemon balm on cholinergic activity [Kennedy et al., 2005]); metabolic activity (e.g. ginseng on blood glucose [Reay et al., 2005], polyphenols on cerebral blood flow [Francis et al., 2006]), and hormonal systems (e.g. soy isoflavones on oestrogen [Setchell, 2001]). Since these same systems underpin behavioural processes, it is perhaps not surprising that certain herbal extracts can influence behaviour. The effects of herbal extracts may particularly depend upon complex interactions between them and physiological systems. Additionally, the interactions between active components in plant extracts may be synergistic, resulting in complex dose- and time-dependent effects. These factors are challenging for the cognitive science of nutrition and behaviour.

It is beyond the scope of this chapter to document the effects of all herbal extracts with cognition-enhancing properties. Instead, we will focus on selected herbal extracts and review the evidence for their efficacy as acute neurocognitive enhancers in healthy young adults.

## 9.2   GINSENG

Ginseng usually refers to species of the *Panax* genus of the Araliaceae plant family. Extracts of ginseng have been used for thousands of years in traditional Chinese medicine where these are typically taken as a *tonic* or *adaptogen* to provide energy and to aid convalescence in the ill and elderly (Fulder, 1990). It has been reported that the effects of ginseng became apparent when the energy demands of the organism are taxed and subsequently diminished (Brekhman & Dardymov, 1969). This role is supported by both anecdotal evidence, in users of the herb, and empirical evidence. The active components of ginseng are believed to be the ginsenosides (see in the following text), and individual ginsenosides have been shown to have multiple effects on physiological processes relevant to health, including anti-inflammatory effects in vivo (Matsuda et al., 1990) and anti-mutagenic and DNA-protective properties in vitro (Ong & Yong, 2000).

The constituents of the *Panax* genus. which are thought to contribute to its bioactivity, are the ginsenoside saponins. Ginsenosides can be classified into three groups on the basis of their chemical structure: the panaxadiol group (Rb1, Rb2, Rb3, Rc, etc.), panaxatriol group (Re, Rf, Rg1, Rg2, Rh1) and the oleanolic acid group (e.g. Ro) (Tachikawa et al., 1999). Standardised extracts of ginseng typically contain between 4% and 15% ginsenosides, with the proportion of individual ginsenosides varying depending on the specific species.

The ginsenosides have been reported to exert effects on the cholinergic system, which suggests that ginseng should exert effects on memory and attention. Isolated

Rb1 stimulates choline acetyltransferase activity (Salim et al., 1997) and acetylcholine release (Benishin et al., 1991) and is reported to capable of in vivo modulation of long-term potentiation, a putative analogue of memory formation, in rats (Abe et al., 1994).

As well as cholinergic activity, Rb1 (and ginsenoside Rg1) elicit marked alterations in brain serotonin concentrations, which may influence mood and sleep patterns. Other targets include nerve growth factor (Chu & Zhang, 2009). Other ginsenosides have also been reported to affect specific cognition-relevant mechanisms. For example, Rd influences corticosterone secretion (Hiai et al., 1983), and ginsenosides Rd and Re may increase levels of the neurotransmitters norepinephrine, dopamine, serotonin and GABA (Chu & Zhang, 2009; Tsang et al., 1985). The behavioural profile of ginseng is further complicated by variations in methods of assessment, age and dose effects (Kennedy & Scholey, 2003) (Table 9.1).

A series of double-blind, placebo-controlled studies have assessed the mood and cognitive effects of acute administration of ginseng in healthy young adults. These have found that enhancement by ginseng was observed largely for long-term memory, also called secondary memory. In the first study (Kennedy et al., 2001a), doses of 200, 400 and 600 mg of ginseng (G115) were administered to healthy young volunteers. Cognitive performance was measured using the cognitive drug research (CDR) computerised assessment system, which provides five composite scores relating to different aspects of memory and attention. Enhancement of *secondary memory* was found following 400 mg at four post-dose testing sessions. While the lower and higher dosage reduced performance for *speed of attention*, the speed at which participants completed a series of tasks assessing sustained attention. In a further study assessing combinations of ginseng and *Ginkgo* (ratio 100:60) at dosages of 320, 640, 960 mg, a similar pattern was observed (Kennedy et al., 2001b), with performance of secondary memory being improved by 960 mg, and performance on speed of attention reduced for the other doses (320 and 640 mg). A later study (Kennedy et al., 2002) replicated the finding that a 400 mg dosage improved *secondary memory*. A further study assessed the effect of 200, 400 and 600 mg ginseng on mental arithmetic performance, where cognitive demand was manipulated. Again this task was improved by a 400 mg dosage but only for the most demanding (serial sevens) task (Scholey & Kennedy, 2002).

Further work showed that 200 mg of G115 significantly shortened latency of the P300 component of auditory evoked potentials, an electrophysiological index of working memory (Kennedy et al., 2003). One further study reported faster responses on an attentional task 90 min following 400 mg G115 (Sünram-Lea et al., 2004). A more recent report found better performance on a deliberately demanding cognitive battery, coupled with reduced capillary blood glucose (Reay et al., 2005) suggesting that the effects may be modulated by processes involving cellular glucose uptake or disposal. However, a follow-up study did not find that the effect was further enhanced by co-administration of glucose with G115 (Reay et al., 2006). It appears to be the case that *Panax ginseng* or its constituents are capable of producing tangible cognitive-enhancing effects, and that for *P. ginseng,* a dose equivalent to 200 or 400 mg of a 4% ginsenoside extract may be the optimal dose for young healthy adults when administered acutely prior to a cognitive test.

**TABLE 9.1**

**Summary of Studies on Ginseng Administration**

| 1st Author/Year | Dose | Design | Sample | N | Results |
|---|---|---|---|---|---|
| Kennedy (2001a) | 200 mg<br>400 mg<br>600 mg of *Panax ginseng* (G115) | Ran<br>DB<br>PC<br>CO | Healthy young | 20 | Quality of memory was improved by 400 mg ginseng at 1, 2.5, 4 and 6 h post-dose. Quality of memory was improved by the 600 mg ginseng dose at 2.5 h. 200 mg of ginseng led to a decrement in speed of memory at 4 h post-dose. Speed of attention was impaired following both 200 and 600 mg of ginseng at 4 and 6 h post-dose. The 200 mg dose improved accuracy of attention at 6 h post-dose. The 600 mg dose improved a secondary memory sub-factor at 1, 2.5 and 4 h post-dose. The 400 mg dose improved secondary memory at each time points while the 200 mg dose improved secondary memory at 4 h. There were no differences in a working memory sub-factor. |
| Kennedy (2001b) | 230 mg<br>640 mg<br>960 mg of *P. ginseng* (G115)/*Gingko biloba* (GK501) combination | Ran<br>DB<br>PC<br>CO | Healthy young | 20 | The high dose improved both quality of memory performance and secondary memory at 1 and 6 h post-dose. Speed of attention was slowed for both the 230 and 640 mg doses at 4 h and for the 320 mg dose at 6 h. There were no effects on working memory, speed of memory, accuracy of attention or self-rated mood. |
| Kennedy (2002) | 360 mg *G. biloba* (GK501)<br>400 mg *P. Ginseng* (G115)<br>960 mg combination | Ran<br>DB<br>PC<br>CO | Healthy young | 20 | Ginseng: improved quality of memory at 4 h, secondary memory at 4 and 6 h, speed of memory at 4 h and quality of attention at 2.5 h post-dose.<br><br>Ginkgo: improved quality of memory at 6 h, secondary memory at 1 and 6 h, serial 3 error rate at 4 h and serial sevens response rate at 4 and 6 h. *Ginkgo* also increased alertness at each time points and contentedness at 1, 4 and 6 h post-dose.<br><br>Combination: improved quality of memory at 1, 2.5 and 4 h, secondary memory at 1 and 2.5 h, working memory at 1 and 6 h, speed of attention at 4 h post-dose, serial 3 response rate at 6 h and the serial sevens response rate at 4 h post-dose. The combination of *Ginkgo* and ginseng increased contentedness at 2.5, 4 and 6 h post-dose.<br>(*Continued*) |

**TABLE 9.1 (Continued)**
**Summary of Studies on Ginseng Administration**

| 1st Author/Year | Dose | Design | Sample | N | Results |
|---|---|---|---|---|---|
| Kennedy (2004) | 200 mg *P. ginseng* (G115) | Ran DB PC CO | Healthy young | 28 | Ginseng improved speed of attention 4 and 6 h post-dose and speed of memory at 1 h. Secondary memory was enhanced by ginseng at 2.5 h. Neither accuracy of attention nor working memory was affected by ginseng. Ginseng improved sentence verification speed at all post-dose time points. Ginseng results in more serial sevens subtractions at 1 and 6 h. Ginseng did not affect serial 3 performance. Ginseng had no effect on mood as measured by the Bond–Lader scales. |
| Kennedy (2007) | 200 mg *P. ginseng* | Ran DB PC CO | Healthy young | 18 | No acute effects were reported, including for the CDR computerised assessment system and the Bond–Lader mood scales. |
| Kennedy (2007) | 120 mg *G. biloba* | Ran DB PC CO | Healthy young | 28 | Cognitive measures, including CDR factor scores, serial sevens and serial threes, were unchanged by *G. biloba*. *G. biloba* increased self-rated calmness at 1 and 4 h post-dose. |
| Reay (2005) | 200 mg 400 mg of *P. ginseng* (G115) | Ran DB PC CO | Healthy young | 30 | The 200 mg dose increased the number of correct responses made during serial sevens subtraction during repetitions 2, 3, 4 and 6 of the cognitive demand battery. There were no effects on serial 3 or RVIP. The 200 mg dose attenuated mental fatigue experienced from the second through sixth completions of the demand battery, while the 400 mg dose attenuated mental fatigue experienced during the third repetition of the demand battery. |
| Reay (2006) | 200 mg *P. ginseng* (G115) | Ran DB PC CO | Healthy young | 27 | Ginseng increased the number of serial 3 subtractions at the third, fourth and sixth repetition of the cognitive demand battery. There were no effects on serial sevens performance. Ginseng reduced the number of false alarm errors on the sixth repetition of the RVIP. Ginseng reduced mental fatigue following the fifth and sixth repetition of the demand battery. |

*(Continued)*

**TABLE 9.1 (*Continued*)**

**Summary of Studies on Ginseng Administration**

| 1st Author/Year | Dose | Design | Sample | N | Results |
|---|---|---|---|---|---|
| Reay (2010) | 200 mg<br>400 mg of *P. ginseng* (G115) | Ran<br>DB<br>PC<br>CO | Healthy young | 30 | Both doses of ginseng increased self-rated calmness at 2.5 and 4 h. Although the 400 mg dose improved three-back reaction time performance at 2.5 h, the 200 mg dose slowed reaction time at 1, 2.5, and 4 h post-dose. The 400 mg dose improved three-back sensitivity index at 1, 2.5 and 4 h post-dose. |
| Scholey (2002)[a] | Study 1:<br>120 mg<br>240 mg<br>300 mg of *G. biloba* (GK501)<br>Study 2:<br>200 mg<br>400 mg<br>600 mg of *P. Ginseng* (G115)<br>Study 3:<br>320 mg<br>640 mg<br>960 mg of the combined extracts | Ran<br>DB<br>PC<br>CO | Healthy young | 20 | 200 mg ginseng alone impaired serial sevens speed, at 1, 2.5 and 6 h, and decreased serial sevens errors at 4 h. 200 mg decreased serial sevens errors at 4 and 6 h. In combination with 120 mg *Ginkgo*, 200 mg ginseng improved serial sevens at all time points. |

*(Continued)*

**TABLE 9.1 (Continued)**
**Summary of Studies on Ginseng Administration**

| 1st Author/Year | Dose | Design | Sample | N | Results |
|---|---|---|---|---|---|
| Scholey (2010) | 100 mg<br>200 mg<br>400 mg of *Panax quinquefolius* | Ran<br>DB<br>PC<br>CO | Healthy young | 32 | 200 mg of ginseng improved immediate word recall at each time point (1,3 and 6 h post-dose). Immediate free recall was also improved by the 100 mg dose at 6 h and the 400 mg dose at 1 h post-dose. The 100 mg dose improved choice reaction time accuracy at each time point. Choice reaction time accuracy also improved with 400 mg at 1 h and 200 mg at 6 h. The 200 mg dose improved numeric working memory at each time point. The 100 mg dose improved alphabetic working memory at each time point. Performance was similarly improved on this task at 1, 3 and 6 h by the 400 mg dose. The 100 mg dose improved corsi block performance at each time point, while the 200 and 400 mg doses improved corsi blocks at 1, 3 and 6 h, respectively. Calmness was improved with the 100 mg dose at 3 and 6 h. |

Ran, randomised; DB, double blind; PC, placebo controlled; CO, crossover; RVIP, rapid visual information processing.

[a] Study describes three studies, each separately examining the acute effects of ginseng and *Ginkgo*–ginseng in combination, respectively.

One recent study has examined the effects of a different species of ginseng – *Panax quinquefolius* or American ginseng (Scholey et al., 2010). This study found dose-specific enhancement on working memory functioning. *P. quinquefolius* has a different complement of ginsenosides, in particular, *P. quinquefolius* has higher expression of gensenoside Rb1.

## 9.3   GINKGO BILOBA

Like ginseng, *G. biloba* has been researched as a potential cognitive enhancer. Although the cognitive-enhancing effects of ginseng have been reviewed previously (Brown et al., 2010; Weinmann et al., 2010), such reviews typically focus on the potential of ginseng to treat age-related cognitive decline and dementia. This section focuses briefly on the acute cognitive effects of *Ginkgo*.

The *G. biloba* tree is believed to be one of the oldest surviving tree species on earth (McKenna et al., 2001). Extracts and infusions made from its leaves have been used in traditional Chinese medicine for millennia. There is extensive research into potential health benefits driven largely by the development of a standardised extract of *G. biloba* in the late 1960s (Schwabe extract EGb761). EGb761 is concentrated to a ratio of 1 part extract to 50 part dried leaves and is made up of 24% flavone glycosides (primarily quercetin, kaempferol and isorhamnetin) – all relatively powerful antioxidants and 6% terpene lactones (2.8%–3.4% ginkgolides A, B and C, and 2.6%–3.2% bilobalide). *G. biloba* extract (GBE) is prescribed in France and Germany for the treatment of conditions including problems with memory and concentration, confusion, depression, anxiety, dizziness, tinnitus and headache (Mahady, 2002; Smith & Luo, 2004). In the early 1990s, *Ginkgo* became one of the most popular supplements for memory enhancement in the United States (Smith & Luo, 2004). Currently, *Ginkgo* is marketed as a treatment for age-associated cognitive decline, as well as a treatment for slowing the progression of neurodegenerative diseases such as AD. However, despite relatively intense research on the cognitive effects of Ginkgo, there is still no conclusive evidence as to its efficacy in the treatment or prevention of dementia (Birks & Grimley Evans, 2009).

The peak plasma levels of various components of *Ginkgo* occur within the first 3 h following administration. For example, ginkgolide B peaks around 2.25 ± 0.45 h following oral administration with an elimination half-life (t½) of 4.31 ± 0.49 h (Drago et al., 2002). It follows that there may be acute benefits of *Ginkgo* administration (Elsabagh et al., 2005; Kennedy et al., 2000, 2002). An early well-controlled, double-blind, placebo-controlled, balanced crossover study involving 20 healthy young participants investigated the cognitive effects of single doses (120, 240, 360 mg) of standardised GBE over 6 h (Kennedy et al., 2000). There was a clear, linear, dose-dependent increase in *speed of attention* as measured by the CDR battery. This effect was significant for the two higher doses, with the lower 120 mg dose enhancing performance on a different measure, the *quality of memory* factor (comprising scores from six memory tasks). More recently, we published a reanalysis incorporating the data from that study and two others using similar methodology in which 120 mg *Ginkgo* was included as one arm (Kennedy et al., 2007). This revealed that the attentional effects may be fragile and indeed suggested that 120 mg may impair attentional speed. On the other hand, the memory effects appeared to be robust with 120 mg *Ginkgo* improving memory for 1–4 h following administration.

## 9.4  SALVIA

The *Salvia* genus consists of around 900 species. It owes its name to the Romans (from the Latin salvage meaning *to save*). The most common European members of the genus are *S. officinalis* (garden sage) and *Salvia lavandulaefolia* (Spanish sage). The proposed mechanisms of action for *S. officinalis* include acting acutely as a ChEI. Sage may also have longer term cognitive benefits in cognitive impairment and dementia (see Miroddi et al., 2014, for a recent review) possibly underpinned by antioxidant, anti-inflammatory and oestrogenic effects (Kennedy & Scholey, 2006; Perry et al., 1999).

Several randomised placebo-controlled trials have been conducted to assess the acute cognitive-enhancing effects of *S. officinalis* (see Table 9.2).

One of the first studies of the acute cognitive effects of sage used an essential oil of *S. lavandulaefolia*, a ChEI member of the sage family. A significant improvement in immediate and delayed word recall from the CDR battery was found following a 50 µL dose of the oil in 20 young healthy volunteers (Tildesley et al., 2003). Also using the CDR battery, a second study reported improvements in *speed of memory*, the speed at which the participants completed a group of memory tasks. These improvements were seen at 4 and 6 h post-dose associated with 50 µL of *S. lavandulaefolia*. Secondary memory performance was also improved at 1 h post-dose and *speed of memory* at 2.5 h post the 25 µL dose (Tildesley et al., 2005).

More recently, Kennedy et al. (2011) reported improved cognitive functioning from a terpenoid-rich extract of *S. lavandulaefolia* suggesting that this fraction may be responsible for the cognition-enhancing properties of sage. Another study by the same group examined the acute effects of *S. officinalis* on mood and cognition in 30 healthy participants, who completed a test battery at baseline then 1 and 4 h post dose on three separate testing occasions (Kennedy et al., 2005). On each occasion, they received placebo, 300 or 600 mg of dried sage leaf. The higher dose was found to be associated with improved performance on the stroop test as well as an aggregate score obtained from a simultaneously performed, multitasking battery of tests including tasks of mathematical processing and working memory at both post-dose time points.

The acute effects of *S. officinalis* have also been examined in an older cohort. Older volunteers (over 65 years) were administered 167, 333, 666 and 1332 mg of dried sage and underwent cognitive testing with the CDR battery at 1, 2, 5, 4 and 6 h post-dose (Scholey et al., 2008). Significant improvements in *secondary memory* performance were noted for the 333 mg dose in comparison to placebo at all post-dose time points. The extracts used in the study were subjected to in vitro analysis, confirming cholinesterase-inhibiting properties in comparison to an ethanol control sample

**TABLE 9.2**

**Summary of Studies on *Salvia* (Sage) Administration**

| 1st Author/Year | Dose | Design | Sample | N | Results |
|---|---|---|---|---|---|
| Kennedy (2006) | 300 mg<br>600 mg | Ran<br>DB<br>PC<br>CO | Healthy | 30 | Low dose impaired number tap performance at both 1 and 4 h time points and impaired the aggregate score at 4 h only. The high dose improved both the stroop and aggregate score at both time points. |
| Kennedy (2011) | 50 μL essential oil | Ran<br>DB<br>PC<br>CO | Healthy | 36 | Simple RT was faster with *Salvia* at both 1 and 4 h time points.<br>*Salvia* improved delayed word recall (number recalled) at 1 and 4 h.<br>*Salvia* improved delayed word recognition (number) after 1 and 4 h.<br>*Salvia* improved picture recognition (number) after 1 and 4 h. |
| Scholey (2008) | 167 mg<br>333 mg<br><br>666 mg<br><br>1332 mg | Ran<br>DB<br><br>PC<br><br>CO | Healthy, older | 20 | Secondary memory improved at all time points (1, 2.5, 4 and 6 h after 333 mg).<br>The 167 mg dose improved secondary memory at 2.5 and 4 h. The 1332 mg dose improved secondary memory at 4 h only.<br>Accuracy of attention was improved following 333 mg at 1, 4 and 6 h. Both the 666 and 1332 mg doses improved accuracy of attention at 4 h.<br>Working memory improved following 333 mg at 1 h. |
| Tildesley (2003) | 50, 100, 150 μL essential oil | Ran<br>DB<br>PC<br>CO | Undergraduate students | 20 | 50 μL improved immediate word recall (number recalled) at 1 and 2.5 h. 100 μL improved immediate word recall at 2.5 h.<br>50 μL improved the number improved delayed recall (number recalled) at 1 and 2.5 h. The 100 μL dose improved delayed word recall (number recalled) at 2.5 h (d = 0.46) |

*(Continued)*

**TABLE 9.2 (*Continued*)**
**Summary of Studies on *Salvia* (Sage) Administration**

| 1st Author/Year | Dose | Design | Sample | N | Results |
|---|---|---|---|---|---|
| Tildesley (2005) | 25, 50 μL essential oil | Ran<br><br>DB<br>PC<br>CO | Healthy | 24 | 50 μL improved immediate word recall (% correct) at 1 and 4 h note that this is reported in the 2003 paper.<br><br>The 25 μL dose improved quality of memory and secondary memory at 1 h.<br><br>Speed of memory was enhanced by the 25 μL condition at 2.5 h by 50 μL at 4 and 6 h.<br><br>50 μL improved serial 3 s speed of performance at 6 but increased errors at 2.5 and 4 h. The 25 μL dose also increased errors at 4 h.<br><br>Both the 25 and 50 μL doses were associated with more serial sevens subtractions at 6 h. 25 μL was also associated with more serial sevens subtractions at 4 h. Serial sevens errors were also reduced by 25 μL at 2.5 h. |

Ran, randomised; DB, double-blind; PC, placebo-controlled; PG, parallel groups; CO, cross-over.

(Scholey et al., 2008). Thus, it appears that the memory-enhancing effects of sage are robust, having been reported across species, extracts and different populations. While every extract examined has in vitro cholinesterase properties, we cannot rule out effects on other non-cholinergic processes contributing to the cognitive effects reported.

## 9.5 THEANINE

Constituents of tea have been evaluated for their potential to enhance cognitive function (see Camfield et al., 2014, for a recent systematic review and meta-analysis). Putative psychoactive agents in tea include caffeine (not covered in this chapter), the catechins, such as epigallocatechin gallate (EGCG), and L-theanine.

L-theanine (γ-glutamylethylamide) is one of the predominant amino acids found in green tea (*Camellia sinensis*). It is also present in other species of *Camellia* as well as in the edible bay boletes mushroom *Xerocomus badius*. Theanine is structurally similar to the amino acid neurotransmitter L-glutamate. It is water-soluble, readily absorbed and crosses the blood–brain barrier, reaching peak concentrations in mammals between 30 and 120 min (Unno et al., 1999; Yokogoshi et al., 1998). A recent study examined the human absorption of different L-theanine doses, both from tea and as an aqueous solution (van der Pijla et al., 2010). The study revealed dose-dependent increases in the levels of plasma theanine, with an administered range of ~25–100 mg producing roughly linear increases in plasma concentrations peaking at ~1–4 mg/L L-theanine.

The pharmacology of L-theanine is relatively unknown, however, animal studies have identified some neurochemical actions of L-theanine administration. These include direct effects on neurotransmitter systems including increased levels of dopamine in the striatum (Yokogoshi & Terashima, 2000), inhibition of glutamate reuptake (Sadzuka et al., 2002), increased GABA concentration (Kimura & Murata, 1971), decreased global brain serotonin with region-specific increases in the striatum, hippocampus and hypothalamus (Yokogoshi et al., 1998). Long-term intake of L-theanine is also thought to impart neuroprotective effects through the blockade of NMDA and AMPA receptors (Kakuda, 2011; Kakuda et al., 2002). A similar mechanism is potentially involved in the behavioural effects of L-theanine since increased glutamate activity has been associated with acute stress (Yuen et al., 2010). Effects on glutamate receptors appear to mediate the major central nervous system effects of L-theanine (Yamada et al., 2009).

In line with these mechanisms, L-theanine has historically been used as a relaxant. There is good evidence from studies recording brain bioelectrical activity and mixed evidence from behavioural studies to support this contention. Electroencephalography (EEG) uses electrodes attached to the scalp to record underlying brain activity, in microvolts over time (see Camfield and Scholey, Chapter 12). L-Theanine appears to have relaxing properties as inferred from its effects on human EEG activity (Juneja et al., 1999; Kobayashi et al., 1998). For example, Kobayashi et al. (1998) reported that administration of 200 mg L-theanine, but not 50 mg, led to increased α-wave activity in the occipital and parietal regions of the brain within 40 min of ingestion when administered to resting participants. (Studies evaluating these effects are presented in Table 9.3.)

**TABLE 9.3**

**Summary of Studies on Theanine Administration**

| Author/Year | Dosage | Design | Sample | N | Results |
|---|---|---|---|---|---|
| Higashiyama (2011) | 200 mg Suntheanine | Ran PC DB CO | Healthy young | 18 | Significant increased attention task score and reaction time found in high anxiety subjects; significant changes in EEG alpha band in high-anxiety group (suggesting beta–alpha transition). No differences in anxiety. |
| Gomez-Ramirez (2009) | 250 mg | NS | Healthy young | 13 | Data suggest L-theanine does not globally reduce tonic alpha power but exerts its influence more selectively over distinct brain regions; L-theanine may be associated with more difficult cognitive challenges. Study is not described as randomised. |
| Nobre (2008) | 50 mg | PG CB | Healthy young | 16/19 T/C | L-Theanine produced greater alpha activity than placebo in young adult participants. The effect is sustained, evident at 45 min in occipital regions and in occipital–parietal regions until at least 105 min post-ingestion. Study is not described as randomised. |
| Gomez-Ramirez (2007) | 250 mg | PC | Healthy young | 15 | Report significantly increased alpha activity in relation to the task being attended to and a decrease in background alpha activity, suggesting that L-theanine may have specific positive effects on focused attention. |
| Kimura (2007) | 200 mg | Ran PC DB CO | Healthy young | 20 | L-theanine reduced self-reported anxiety and physiological indices of stress under high-stress conditions compared with placebo. |

*(Continued)*

**TABLE 9.3 (*Continued*)**
**Summary of Studies on Theanine Administration**

| Author/Year | Dosage | Design | Sample | N | Results |
|---|---|---|---|---|---|
| Dimpfel (2007) | 500 mL drink with 9.2% LT, 4.6% theogallin, 0.1% caffeine | Ran PC DB CO | Healthy middle-aged | 12 | Significantly increased activity in frontal lobe region, suggesting cognitive benefits. |
| Lu (2004) | 200 mg (SunTheanine) | Ran PC DB CO | Healthy young | 16 | L-theanine did not produce statistically significant results for alleviation of acute anxiolytic effects (subjective anxiety) under conditions of increased anxiety in AA model. Compared L-theanine directly with the benzodiazepine Alprazolam (Xanax). |

Ran, randomised; DB, double-blind; PC, placebo-controlled; CO, crossover; PG, parallel groups; CB, counterbalanced; T/C, L-Theanine/Control.

Gomez-Ramirez et al. (2007) found a decrease in α activity following 250 mg L-theanine when measured during performance of an attention task (Gomez-Ramirez et al., 2007). While this may appear to be contradictory to the findings of Kobayashi et al. (1998), it may also be indicative of differing EEG effects of L-theanine when administered during attentional processing (requiring focus) as opposed to at rest. In particular, these data can be explained by the fact that, as well as the classic relaxation-associated *tonic* alpha, there is also a phasic alpha wave. This is believed to be associated with brain areas that are inhibited. In the experimental paradigm used by Gomez-Ramirez et al. (2007), subjects were presented with a cue indicating that they would need to process either visual or auditory stimuli, which were then presented a second later. During the second following the cue, there was a decrease in alpha activity in the parietal–occipital region. This area is known to be involved in attentional switching in the visual modality. Gomez-Ramirez et al. (2007) found that L-theanine facilitated this differential phasic α-wave switching in a way that would facilitate attentional performance. On the other hand, L-theanine was associated with a slowing of reaction time on the auditory attention task. A further study found that L-theanine again facilitated the EEG component of attentional switching, this time when the cue signalled a stimulus to the left or right visual field (Gomez-Ramirez et al., 2009). This latter study also confirmed an overall decrease in tonic alpha wave activity following L-theanine.

More recently, Higashiyama et al. (2011) reported that the administration of 200 mg L-theanine reduced heart rate and increased EEG alpha activity in high but not low anxiety–prone individuals (Higashiyama et al., 2011). Similarly, cognitive performance (attention and auditory choice reaction time) was improved following theanine, but only in those in the high-anxiety group. The failure to find cognitive-enhancing effects of theanine in the low-anxiety group may have been due to low statistical power, with only 8 and 10 subjects per cell in the high and low anxiety–prone groups, respectively.

Lu et al. (2004) have also reported evidence to suggest that L-theanine may have relaxing effects (Bond & Lader, 1974). The authors found that 200 mg of L-theanine improved relaxation during resting conditions as measured by the *tranquil-troubled* item of the Bond–Lader visual analogue scales (Lu et al., 2004). This finding was not replicated when participants were under conditions of increased anxiety, suggesting that L-theanine has differential effects depending on the arousal of the subject. Also supporting a calming effect of L-theanine, Kimura et al. (2007) reported that L-theanine reduced heart rate (using an index of sympathetic activity), secretory immunoglobulin A (s-IgA), subjective anxiety and perceived stress (Kimura et al., 2007).

With respect to cognitive performance, a randomised controlled trial has shown that L-theanine was associated with faster choice reaction times at both 30 and 90 min (Haskell et al., 2008). On the other hand, L-theanine slowed numeric working memory at 30 min and had a detrimental effect on performance of serial sevens at 90 min. Compared with placebo, L-theanine alone decreased ratings of mental fatigue at 30 min and increased ratings of calmness. This finding of increased calm ratings supports the findings of Lu et al. (2004) of improvements on the single *tranquil-troubled* subscale taken from the Bond–Lader visual analogue scales. These data also support those of Kobayashi et al. (1998) who suggest that L-theanine increases calmness without increasing drowsiness.

A study by Rogers et al. (2008) investigated the effects of 200 mg L-theanine, both alone and in combination with caffeine, on anxiety (Rogers et al., 2008). An attentional bias task was used to measure anxiety. The theory underlying this task is that faster reaction times to words associated with threat are underpinned by heightened anxiety. Rogers found that L-theanine slowed reaction times to *social threat* words, again supporting an anxiety-reducing effect.

## 9.6   THEANINE COMBINED WITH CAFFEINE

The combined effects of naturally concomitant psychoactives are complex and difficult to predict based on the effects of the individual components (Scholey et al., 2005). L-theanine and caffeine are often found together in tea drinks, and a number of studies have examined the effects of the two substances in combination (Table 9.4). In one study, the administration of 200 mg of L-theanine led to slower reaction time on a visual probe task, indicative of decreased anxiety, and was able to antagonise the increase in systolic and diastolic blood pressure seen following 200 mg of caffeine (Rogers et al., 2008). No such effect was seen on the increase in *alert* and *jittery* ratings as a result of caffeine administration. This study did not consider the effects of these treatments on cognition.

**TABLE 9.4**

**Summary of Studies on Caffeine–Theanine Administration**

| Author/Year | Dose | Design | Sample | N | Results |
|---|---|---|---|---|---|
| Einother (2010) | 97 mg Theanine/40 mg caffeine | Ran PC DB CO | Young adults | 29 | Improvement in attention on switch task; combo effect on attention not specific to visual modality – faster responses in both visual and auditory modality seen on intersensory task compared to placebo; improvements in attention as signified by behavioural tasks not associated with enhanced subjective alertness. |
| Rogers (2008) | 250 mg Caffeine/200 mg Theanine | Ran PC DB PG | Young adults | 48 | Theanine antagonised the effect on BP but did not significantly affect jitteriness, alertness or other aspects of mood. L-Theanine alone did have an effect on response time to heatening words, which was consistent with an anxiety-reducing effect. |
| Owen (2008) | 50 mg Caffeine/100 mg L-theanine | Ran PC DB CO | Young adults | 27 | Statistical significance in (1) word recognition (new words); (2) significant decrease in arousal from critical flicker fusion test; (3) attention switching task performance. Conclusion: L-theanine/caffeine combo appears to improve aspects of memory and attention to a greater extent than caffeine alone. |
| Kelly (2008) | 100 mg Theanine/50 mg caffeine and combined | Ran PC DB CO | Young adults | 16 | Significant decrease in tonic alpha for combined treatment but not L-theanine alone. Attentional biasing as indexed by alpha amplitude not affected, but cued biasing of attention between sensory modalities was affected. |
| Haskell (2008) | 250 mg Theanine, 150 mg caffeine and 250 mg Theanine | Ran DB PC CO | Young adults | 29 | Lack of effect of high dose LT on subjective calm or relaxation; however, no controls were in place for habitual caffeine intake amongst control subjects. |
| Giesbrecht (2010) | 97 mg Theanine/40 mg caffeine | Ran DB PC CO | Young adults | 44 | Treatment was associated with significantly improved attentional switching, increased alertness and reduced fatigue. |

Ran, randomised; DB, double-blind; PC, placebo-controlled; CO, crossover.

A randomised, placebo-controlled, double-blind, balanced crossover study investigated the cognitive and mood effects of administration L-theanine (250 mg) and caffeine (150 mg) both alone and in combination (Haskell et al., 2008). Haskell et al. (2008) found a number of measures that appeared to be differentially sensitive to an L-theanine-caffeine combination. In the case of simple reaction time, accuracy of rapid visual information processing and *alertness* ratings, the positive effects of treatment were numerically greater in the caffeine–L-theanine conditions. On the other hand, the caffeine effect on choice reaction time was attenuated by the addition of L-theanine. The addition of caffeine to L-theanine led to a reduction in *calm* ratings, which is an opposite effect to that seen with L-theanine alone. While the mechanisms underlying such effects are not known, they do suggest that there are psychopharmacological interactions between caffeine and L-theanine. This suggestion is further supported when examining several measures that were significantly affected by the combination treatment but not by the individual components. These mood effects contradict those of Kakuda et al. (2002) who reported an inhibitory effect of L-theanine on caffeine's stimulatory properties in rats all be it at substantially lower equivalent doses (Kakuda et al., 2002).

A recent meta-analysis of the effects of L-theanine and caffeine in combination suggested that the effects on alertness and the ability to switch attention are robust at 1 and 2 h post-administration (Camfield et al., 2014). In conclusion, there appears to be pharmacological interactions between caffeine and theanine. However, it is notable that most studies in this area use doses of both compounds that are much larger than what would be found in a standard serving of tea and at ratios that are opposite to those that occur naturally.

## 9.7   EPIGALLOCATECHIN GALLATE

In addition to theanine and caffeine, potential bioactive nutrients of green tea include the catechins, which typically account for 30%–42% of the dry weight of brewed green tea, (Sang et al., 2011). The four major tea catechins are (–)-EGCG, (–)-epigallocatechin, (–)-epicatechin gallate and (–)-epicatechin. EGCG is the most abundant, accounting for 50%–80% of total catechins (Graham, 1992). Two randomised controlled trials to date have focused on the potential for EGCG to acutely enhance mood and cognition, both including neuroimaging (Table 9.5). Scholey et al. (2012) showed that 300 mg of EGCG was associated with increased self-rated calmness and decreased stress as well as increased overall bioelectrical activity localised to the frontal lobes. Wightman et al. (2012) found no behavioural effects from either 135 mg or 270 mg of EGCG but did find decreases in frontal lobe blood flow between 45 and 88 min post-administration. These data suggest that EGCG is capable of modulating frontal lobe activity but that behavioural effects may be time specific, emerging after 90 min post-administration. It is worth noting that the plasma levels of EGCG as well as effects on vascular parameters peak at around 2 h post-administration.

**TABLE 9.5**
**Summary of Studies on Epigallocatechin Gallate Administration**

| 1st Author/ Year | Dose | Design | Sample | N | Results |
|---|---|---|---|---|---|
| Wightman (2012) | 135 mg 270 mg of EGCG | Ran DB PC CO | Healthy young | 27 | No differences were found for any of the cognitive or mood measures. The 135 mg dose reduced cerebral blood flow in the frontal cortex measured with near-infrared spectroscopy. |
| Scholey (2012) | 300 mg of EGCG | Ran DB PC CO | Healthy | 31 | Treatment increased calmness and reduced stress. Treatment was associated with a significant overall increase in alpha, beta and theta activity on EEG. |

Ran, randomised; DB, double-blind; PC, placebo-controlled; CO, crossover.

## 9.8 BACOPA MONNIERI

*Bacopa monniera* is a member of the Scrophulariaceae family. It has been referred to as *Brahmi* derived from the name of the Hindu *Brama* or creator (the brain is believed to be the creative centre in the Hindu religion). *Bacopa* has been used in Ayurvedic medicine for millennia as a sedative, analgesic, anti-inflammatory and anti-epileptic treatment and memory enhancer (Jain, 1994; Stough et al., 2001).

Saponins (specifically bacosides A and B) are the active ingredients that are believed to underlie the memory-enhancing effects of *Bacopa*. Suggested mechanisms of action include pro-cholinergic effects, GABA-ergic modulation, antioxidant effects, brain protein synthesis, serotonin agonism, modulation of brain stress hormones and reduction of $\beta$-amyloid (Calabrese et al., 2008).

Hota et al. (2009) investigated the effects of *Bacopa* on ameliorating the effects of hypobaric anoxia (reduced deliver of oxygen to brain tissue at altitude) on spatial memory function. *Bacopa* administration enhanced learning ability, increased memory retrieval and prevented dentritic atrophy following hypoxic exposure in rats. Further evidence was also provided for the role of glutamatergic transmission in the memory-enhancing effects of *Bacopa*, suggesting that it has an ability to modulate positive synaptic plasticity through augmentation of glutamatergic transmission, as well as the amelioration of cell death associated with glutamate-mediated excitotoxicity. *Bacopa* was also found to decrease oxidative stress, plasma corticosterone levels and neuronal degeneration, to increase cytochrome c oxidase activity and ATP levels. This suggests a positive effect of *Bacopa* on mitochondrial function and possibly brain energy metabolism.

*Bacopa* is a nutraceutical that holds great promise for the amelioration of age-related cognitive decline as well as cognitive enhancement in the young. A recent systematic review of the chronic cognitive effects of *Bacopa* administration concluded that free recall was preferentially enhanced (Pase et al., 2012).

**TABLE 9.6**
**Summary of Studies on *Bacopa* Administration**

| 1st Author/Year | Dose | Design | Sample | N | Results |
|---|---|---|---|---|---|
| Benson (2014) | 320 mg 640 mg CDRI08 | Ran DB PC CO | Healthy young | 17 | *Bacopa* improved letter search and stroop performance as part of a multitasking framework (at both 1 h post and 2 h post dose). *Bacopa* also reduced cortisol levels. |
| Downey (2013) | 320 mg 640 mg CDRI08 | Ran DB PC CO | Healthy young | 24 | The 320 mg dose improved performance on the 1st, 2nd, and 4th post-dose cycle of the CDB. There were no effect on cardiovascular function or task-induced stress or fatigue |
| Nathan (2001) | 300 mg CDRI08 | Ran DB PC PG | Healthy young | 18 | *Bacopa* had no effect on cognitive function 2 h post-dose. |

Ran, randomised; DB, double-blind; PC, placebo-controlled; CO, crossover; PG, parallel groups.

Three studies have examined the acute effects of *Bacopa* and shown mixed results (see Table 9.6). Nathan et al. (2001) reported no positive effects of 200 mg *Bacopa* on cognitive function, although there were only nine individuals per cell, suggesting that the study may have been underpowered. In a dose-ranging study, Downey and colleagues (2013) found improvements in attentional/working memory performance following 320 mg *Bacopa* during a cognitive demand battery. A recent study into the effects of *Bacopa* on multitasking (Benson et al., 2014) suggested that there may be increased performance following the active treatment and found treatment-related protection from cortisol rises, with indications of improved mood. Taken together these findings suggest that any acute effects of *Bacopa* become evident under more demanding and/or stressful conditions.

## 9.9 GUARANA

The plant species guaraná originates from the central Amazonian Basin, and has a long history of local usage, initially as a stimulant by indigenous tribes people (Henman, 1982) and more latterly as a ubiquitous ingredient in Brazilian soft drinks. An extensive range of products that include guaraná (*Paullinia cupana*) seed extracts as ingredients are commercially available. Examples include confections (e.g. chocolate products), fruit juice based drinks, *energy* drinks, dietary and herbal supplements, and, most controversially, natural weight loss products.

The putative stimulant properties are generally taken to reflect the presence of caffeine, which comprises 2.5%–5% of the extract's dry weight, although other purine alkaloids (theophylline and theobromine) are present in smaller quantities (Weckerle et al., 2003). The psychoactive properties of guaraná have also been attributed to a high content of both saponins and tannins (Espinola et al., 1997), the latter of which may well underlie the demonstrated antioxidant properties of the plant (Mattei et al., 1998).

Two studies in rodents have included behavioural measures. In one (Mattei et al., 1998), both acute and chronic administration of guaraná was found to have no toxic effects but also failed to modulate motor activity or pentobarbital-induced sleep parameters. In a further study, the chronic (9 months) administration of a lower (0.3 mg/mL) but not a higher (3.0 mg/mL) dose of guaraná improved swimming time in mice, and reversed memory deficits in rats on a passive avoidance task (Espinola et al., 1997). A similar effect was also found following acute administration of 3 mg/kg guaraná, 30 mg/kg guaraná and 1 mg/kg of caffeine (Espinola et al., 1997).

Few controlled studies have examined the neurocognitive effects of guaraná (Table 9.7). An early investigation into potential effects of guaraná in normal young volunteers failed to find any effects of guaraná using tests of digit span, free recall, digit symbol, cancellation tests and the mosaic test (Galduróz & Carlini, 1994). The same study also evaluated sleep interference and anxiety and again found no effects. The authors present possible explanations for their lack of positive results such as task insensitivity – they also failed to find effects of 25 mg caffeine in the same study, a dose twice that of the lowest known psychoactive dose (Smit & Rogers, 2000). In this first investigation in humans, 1000 mg guaraná was tested, containing only 2.1% caffeine; given the lack of data in this area, it is quite possible that any effects could have been missed simply as a result of inappropriate dose selection. Finally, the time course of testing may not have been sufficient, acute testing only being carried out at 1 h post-treatment and chronic testing following 3 days of treatment administration. In a follow-up study (Galduróz & Carlini, 1994), the same doses and tasks were used to assess chronic (5 months) effects in an elderly population. They found only one improvement, a significant effect of guaraná on mosaic performance at 5 months.

Several studies have examined acute behavioural effects associated with guaraná. In one randomised, double-blind, placebo-controlled, counterbalanced study, 75 g of a proprietary extract of guaraná (Pharmaton extract PC-102), ginseng and their combination were compared with placebo over the course of 6 h using a battery of computerised assessments (Kennedy et al., 2004). Guaraná speeded responses on attentional tasks and a heavily loaded serial subtraction task (serial sevens), although there was evidence of a speed–accuracy trade-off on the latter measure. There was also evidence of secondary memory improvements.

In another similarly controlled study from the same group, the cognitive and mood effects of different doses of guaraná were assessed. The doses used were 37.5, 75, 150 and 300 mg, and their effects were assessed using the same outcomes in 30 healthy participants. Testing took place pre-dose and at 1, 3 and 6 h thereafter with a 7-day *washout*. The data confirm the positive effects on secondary memory, which in this case was evident following 37.5 and 75 mg of extract. There was a significant positive effect on *alert* following the highest dose only and significant improvements of *content* ratings associated with all doses (Haskell et al., 2007).

**TABLE 9.7**

**Summary of Studies on Guaraná Administration**

| 1st Author/ Year | Dose | Design | Sample | N | Results |
|---|---|---|---|---|---|
| Kennedy (2004) | 75 mg extract guaraná | Ran DB PC CO | Healthy young | 28 | Guarana improved speed of attention at 1 and 6 h post-dose and secondary memory at 2.5 h post-dose. Guarana improved sentence verification speed at 2.5 and 4 h. Guarana reduced errors during serial 3s at 2.5 and 4 h. Gaurana increased the number of serial sevens subtractions at 1, 2.5 and 6 h. Guarana also decreased serial sevens accuracy at 4 h. There was no effect of mood. |
| Haskell (2007) | 37.5 mg 75 mg 150 mg 300 mg of Guaraná extract PC-102 | Ran DB PC CO | Healthy young | 26 | Secondary memory improved following the 37.5 and 75 mg doses. The 300 mg dose increased alertness, while all doses increased contentedness. |
| Kennedy (2008) | Vitamin/ mineral/ guaraná effervescent tablets (Berocca® Boost) in 200 mL water | Ran DB PC CO | Healthy young | 129 | Treatment improved speed on the RVIP task of the CDB at each post-dose repetition, excluding the fifth (note that cognitive tasks were completed 6 times as part of the cognitive demand battery). The treatment group was also more accurate on all post-dose repetitions of the RVIP. There was no treatment effect for serial 3s or 7s. Treatment reduced mental fatigue across the last four cycles of the cognitive battery. |
| Scholey (2013) | Berocca Performance (vitamin/ mineral) and Berocca Boost (vitamin/ mineral/ guaraná) | Ran DB PC CO | Healthy young | 20 | The multivitamin with guaraná treatment improved serial threes performance and self-rated contentment. Both treatments increased activation (on fMRI) in brain regions linked with working memory and attention, with greater effect observed following the multivitamin guaraná combination. |

Ran, randomised; DB, double-blind; PC, placebo-controlled; CO, crossover; RVIP, rapid visual information processing; CDB, cognitive demand battery; fMRI, functional magnetic resonance imaging.

Two studies have reported the effects of guaraná with multivitamins on cognitive function. The first reported acute improvements in working memory/vigilance performance and reduced mental fatigue following administration of a commercially available multivitamin and mineral preparation containing B vitamins and guaraná (Berocca Boost) (Kennedy et al., 2008). The second found improved working memory coupled with increased activation of a circuit known to underlie working memory performance (Scholey et al., 2013).

In conclusion, guaraná extracts appear to show positive effects on cognitive performance that may be robust in the secondary memory and working memory domains (though the latter need to be conformed using guaraná alone). These effects are probably not underpinned by caffeine alone and may be attributable to modulation of caffeine by other guaraná components or by direct effects of non-caffeine constituents. Examination of the behavioural effects of decaffeinated guaraná may resolve this issue. The effects of chronic guaraná administration are not known.

## 9.10  CONCLUSION AND FUTURE DIRECTIONS

There is good evidence that certain botanical extracts have robust and replicable cognition-enhancing properties. In the case of ginseng, the magnitude of the effect size is comparable with the pharmaceutical cognitive enhancer, modafinil (Neale et al., 2013). In some cases, the physiological and biochemical properties of the bioactive compounds likely to underlie the effects are well characterised.

The concentrations of the active components in herbal extracts and preparations vary from batch to batch, depending on a number of factors. These include the specific extraction method used and growth conditions (such as climate, soil composition, light levels and time of harvest). Contemporary agricultural techniques, including genetic modification of plant strains, and careful control of growing environments, offer the potential to grow *standardised* plants with enriched fractions of relevant bioactive nutrients that have benefits for cognition.

From both theoretical and methodological perspectives, the psychopharmacology of plant extracts offers unique and interesting challenges. It is important to perform replicable experiments using standardised extracts to allow meaningful comparison across studies (Scholey et al., 2005). It is also worth noting that one approach to addressing the role of individual components might be to compare the effects of extracts with differing profiles of bioactives. The example given earlier of the difference between American and Asian ginseng provides some insight into the roles of specific ginsenosides and their combinations. Another means of assessing the effects of individual components would be to assess the effects of the whole extract *without* the component of interest. As an example, one might assess the alerting effects of caffeine comparing caffeinated and decaffeinated coffee. This will require methodologically sophisticated research designs but does raise the possibility of *knockout psychopharmacology*.

## DEFINITIONS OF KEY TERMS

α-*wave* – Brain waves characterised by a frequency between 7.5 and 12.5 Hz
*Alkaloids* – Organic chemical compounds containing nitrogen bases
*Ayurvedic medicine* – Form of ancient traditional Hindu medicine
*Bacosides* – Saponins found within *Bacopa*
*Botanical* – Substances derived from plants
*Cardenolides* – Plant-derived steroids
*Catechins* – Type of flavanol found in green tea
*Electroencephalography* – Electrical activity recorded from the scalp
*Flavonoids* – Polyphenolic class of plant compounds
*Ginkgolides* – Compounds in *Ginkgo biloba*
*Ginsenosides* – Saponins found in ginseng
*Indoles* – Aromatic heterocyclic organic compound
*Pharmacognosy* – Study of medicines from natural sources
*Plant terpenoids* – Aromatic class of organic chemicals

# REFERENCES

Abe, K., Cho, S., Kitagawa, I., Nishiyama, N., & Saito, H. (1994). Differential effects of ginsenoside Rb1 and malonylginsenoside Rb1 on long-term potentiation in the dentate gyrus of rats. *Brain Research, 649*(1), 7–11.

Benishin, C., Lee, R., Wang, L., & Liu, H. (1991). Effects of ginsenoside Rbi on central cholinergic metabolism. *Pharmacology, 42*, 223–229.

Benson, S., Downey, L. A., Stough, C., Wetherell, M., Zangara, A., & Scholey, A. (2014). An acute, double-blind, placebo-controlled cross-over study of 320 mg and 640 mg doses of *Bacopa monnieri* (CDRI 08) on multitasking stress reactivity and mood. *Phytotherapy Research, 28*(4), 551–559.

Birks, J., & Grimley Evans, J. (2002). *Ginkgo biloba* for cognitive impairment and dementia. *Cochrane Database of Systematic Reviews 4*, Article No.: CD003120.

Bond, A., & Lader, M. (1974). The use of analogue scales in rating subjective feelings. *British Journal of Medical Psychology, 47*(3), 211–218.

Brekhman, I., & Dardymov, I. (1969). Pharmacological investigation of glycosides from Ginseng and Eleutherococcus. *Lloydia, 32*(1), 46.

Brown, L., Riby, L., & Reay, J. (2010). Supplementing cognitive aging: A selective review of the effects of *Ginkgo biloba* and a number of everyday nutritional substances. *Experimental Aging Research, 36*(1), 105–122.

Calabrese, C., Gregory, W. L., Leo, M., Kraemer, D., Bone, K., & Oken, B. (2008). Effects of a standardized *Bacopa monnieri* extract on cognitive performance, anxiety, and depression in the elderly: A randomized, double-blind, placebo-controlled trial. *Journal of Alternative and Complementary Medicine, 14*(6), 707–713.

Calabrese, E. (2005). Cancer biology and hormesis: Human tumor cell lines commonly display hormetic (biphasic) dose responses. *Critical Reviews in Toxicology, 35*(6), 463–582.

Camfield, D. A., Stough, C., Farrimond, J., & Scholey, A. (2014). Acute effects of tea constituents L-theanine, caffeine, and epigallocatechin gallate on cognitive function and mood: A systematic review and meta-analysis. *Nutrition Reviews, 72*(8), 507–522.

Cardello, A., & Schutz, H. (2006). The importance of taste and other product factors to consumer interest in nutraceutical products: Civilian and military comparisons. *Journal of Food Science, 68*(4), 1519–1524.

Chu, S., & Zhang, J. (2009). New achievements in ginseng research and its future prospects. *Chinese Journal of Integrative Medicine, 15*(6), 403–408.

Cox, D., Koster, A., & Russell, C. (2004). Predicting intentions to consume functional foods and supplements to offset memory loss using an adaptation of protection motivation theory. *Appetite, 43*(1), 55–64.

Doaigey, A. (1991). Occurrence, type, and location of calcium oxalate crystals in leaves and stems of 16 species of poisonous plants. *American Journal of Botany, 78*(12), 1608–1616.

Downey, L. A., Kean, J., Nemeh, F., Lau, A., Poll, A., Gregory, R., ... Pase, M. P. (2013). An acute, double-blind, placebo-controlled crossover study of 320 mg and 640 mg doses of a special extract of *Bacopa monnieri* (CDRI 08) on sustained cognitive performance. *Phytotherapy Research, 27*(9), 1407–1413.

Drago, F., Floriddia, M. L., Cro, M., & Giuffrida, S. (2002). Pharmacokinetics and bioavailability of a *Ginkgo biloba* extract. *Journal of Ocular Pharmacology and Therapeutics, 18*(2), 197–202.

Elsabagh, S., Hartley, D., Ali, O., Williamson, E., & File, S. (2005). Differential cognitive effects of *Ginkgo biloba* after acute and chronic treatment in healthy young volunteers. *Psychopharmacology, 179*(2), 437–446.

Espinola, E., Dias, R., Mattei, R., & Carlini, E. (1997). Pharmacological activity of Guarana (*Paullinia cupana* Mart.) in laboratory animals. *Journal of Ethnopharmacology, 55*(3), 223–229.

Francis, S. T., Head, K., Morris, P. G., & Macdonald, I. A. (2006). The effect of flavanol-rich cocoa on the fMRI response to a cognitive task in healthy young people. *Journal of Cardiovascular Pharmacology, 47*(Suppl. 2), S215–S220.

Fulder, S. (Ed.). (1990). *The book of ginseng.* Rochester, NY: Healing Arts Press.

Galduróz, J., & Carlini, E. (1994). Acute efects of the *Paulinia cupana*, 'Guaraná' on the cognition of normal volunteers. *Sao Paulo Medical Journal, 112*, 607–611.

Gomez-Ramirez, M., Higgins, B. A., Rycroft, J. A., Owen, G. N., Mahoney, J., Shpaner, M., & Foxe, J. J. (2007). The deployment of intersensory selective attention: A high-density electrical mapping study of the effects of theanine. *Clinical Neuropharmacology, 30*(1), 25.

Gomez-Ramirez, M., Kelly, S. P., Montesi, J. L., & Foxe, J. J. (2009). The effects of L-theanine on alpha-band oscillatory brain activity during a visuo-spatial attention task. *Brain Topography, 22*(1), 44–51.

Graham, H. N. (1992). Green tea composition, consumption, and polyphenol chemistry. *Preventive Medicine, 21*(3), 334–350. doi: 10.1016/0091–7435(92)90041-f

Haskell, C., Kennedy, D., Milne, A. L., Wesnes, K., & Scholey, A. (2008). The effects of L-theanine, caffeine and their combination on cognition and mood. *Biological Psychology, 77*(2), 113–122.

Haskell, C., Kennedy, D., Wesnes, K., Milne, A., & Scholey, A. (2007). *Journal of Psychopharmacology, 21*(1), 65–70.

Henman, A. (1982). Guarana (*Paullinia cupana* var. sorbilis): Ecological and social perspectives on an economic plant of the central Amazon basin. *Journal of Ethnopharmacology, 6*(3), 311–338.

Hiai, S., Yokoyama, H., Oura, H., & Kawashima, Y. (1983). Evaluation of corticosterone secretion-inducing activities of ginsenosides and their prosapogenins and sapogenins. *Chemical & Pharmaceutical Bulletin, 31*(1), 168.

Higashiyama, A., Htay, H. H., Ozeki, M., Juneja, L. R., & Kapoor, M. P. (2011). Effects of L-theanine on attention and reaction time response. *Journal of Functional Foods, 3*(3), 171–178.

Hota, S. K., Barhwal, K., Baitharu, I., Prasad, D., Singh, S. B., & Ilavazhagan, G. (2009). *Bacopa monniera* leaf extract ameliorates hypobaric hypoxia induced spatial memory impairment. *Neurobiology of Disease, 34*(1), 23–39.

Howes, M. J. R., Perry, N. S. L., & Houghton, P. J. (2003). Plants with traditional uses and activities, relevant to the management of Alzheimer's disease and other cognitive disorders. *Phytotherapy Research, 17*(1), 1–18.

Jain, S. K. (1994). Ethnobotany and research on medicinal plants in India. *Ciba Foundation Symposium, 185*, 153–164; discussion 164.

Juneja, L. R., Chu, D. C., Okubo, T., Nagato, Y., & Yokogoshi, H. (1999). L-theanine – A unique amino acid of green tea and its relaxation effect in humans. *Trends in Food Science & Technology, 10*(6–7), 199–204.

Kakuda, T. (2011). Neuroprotective effects of theanine and its preventive effects on cognitive dysfunction. *Pharmacological Research, 64*(2), 162–168.

Kakuda, T., Nozawa, A., Sugimoto, A., & Niino, H. (2002). Inhibition by theanine of binding of [3 H] AMPA,[3 H] kainate, and [3 H] MDL 105,519 to glutamate receptors. *Bioscience, Biotechnology, and Biochemistry, 66*(12), 2683–2686.

Kennedy, D., Dodd, F. L., Robertson, B. C., Okello, E. J., Reay, J. L., Scholey, A., & Haskell, C. F. (2011). Monoterpenoid extract of sage (*Salvia lavandulaefolia*) with cholinesterase inhibiting properties improves cognitive performance and mood in healthy adults. *Journal of Psychopharmacology, 25*(8), 1088–1100.

Kennedy, D., Haskell, C., Robertson, B., Reay, J., Brewster-Maund, C., Luedemann, J., … Scholey, A. (2008). Improved cognitive performance and mental fatigue following a multi-vitamin and mineral supplement with added guarana (*Paullinia cupana*). *Appetite, 50*(2–3), 506–513.

Kennedy, D., Haskell, C., Wesnes, K., & Scholey, A. (2004). Improved cognitive performance in human volunteers following administration of guarana (*Paullinia cupana*) extract: Comparison and interaction with *Panax ginseng. Pharmacology Biochemistry and Behavior, 79*(3), 401–411.

Kennedy, D., Jackson, P., Haskell, C., & Scholey, A. (2007). Modulation of cognitive performance following single doses of 120 mg *Ginkgo biloba* extract administered to healthy young volunteers. *Human Psychopharmacology: Clinical and Experimental, 22*(8), 559–566.

Kennedy, D., Pace, S., Haskell, C., Okello, E., Milne, A., & Scholey, A. (2005). Effects of cholinesterase inhibiting sage (*Salvia officinalis*) on mood, anxiety and performance on a psychological stressor battery. *Neuropsychopharmacology, 31*(4), 845–852.

Kennedy, D., & Scholey, A. (2003). Ginseng: Potential for the enhancement of cognitive performance and mood. *Pharmacology, Biochemistry, and Behavior, 75*(3), 687.

Kennedy, D., & Scholey, A. (2006). The psychopharmacology of European herbs with cognition-enhancing properties. *Current Pharmaceutical Design, 12*(35), 4613–4623.

Kennedy, D., Scholey, A., Drewery, L., Marsh, R., Moore, B., & Ashton, H. (2003). Topographic EEG effects of single doses of *Panax ginseng* and *Ginkgo biloba. Pharmacology, Biochemistry, and Behavior, 75*, 701–709.

Kennedy, D., Scholey, A., & Wesnes, K. (2000). The dose-dependent cognitive effects of acute administration of *Ginkgo biloba* to healthy young volunteers. *Psychopharmacology, 151*(4), 416–423.

Kennedy, D., Scholey, A., & Wesnes, K. (2001a). Dose dependent changes in cognitive performance and mood following acute administration of Ginseng to healthy young volunteers. *Nutritional Neuroscience, 4*, 295–310.

Kennedy, D., Scholey, A., & Wesnes, K. (2001b). Differential, dose dependent changes in cognitive performance following acute administration of a Ginkgo biloba/Panax ginseng combination to healthy young volunteers. *Nutritional Neuroscience, 4*(5), 399–412.

Kennedy, D., Scholey, A., & Wesnes, K. (2002). Modulation of cognition and mood following administration of single doses of *Ginkgo biloba*, ginseng, and a ginkgo/ginseng combination to healthy young adults. *Physiology and Behavior, 75*(5), 739–752.

Kimura, K., Ozeki, M., Juneja, L. R., & Ohira, H. (2007). L-Theanine reduces psychological and physiological stress responses. *Biological Psychology, 74*(1), 39–45.

Kimura, R., & Murata, T. (1971). Influence of alkylamides of glutamic acid and related compounds on the central nervous I. Central depressant effect of theanine. *Chemical and Pharmaceutical Bulletin, 19*, 1257–1261.

Kobayashi, K., Nagato, Y., Aoi, N., Juneja, L., Kim, M., Yamamoto, T., & Sugimoto, S. (1998). Effects of L-theanine on the release of α-brain waves in human volunteers. *Nippon Nōgei Kagakukaishi, 72*(2), 153–157.

Koul, O. (2008). Phytochemicals and insect control: An antifeedant approach. *Critical Reviews in Plant Sciences, 27*(1), 1–24.

Lu, K., Gray, M. A., Oliver, C., Liley, D. T., Harrison, B. J., Bartholomeusz, C. F., ... Nathan, P. J. (2004). The acute effects of L-theanine in comparison with alprazolam on anticipatory anxiety in humans. *Human Psychopharmacology: Clinical & Experimental, 19*(7), 457–465.

Mahady, G. B. (2002). *Ginkgo biloba* for the prevention and treatment of cardiovascular disease: A review of the literature. *The Journal of Cardiovascular Nursing, 16*(4), 21–32.

Maher, B. (2008). Poll results: Look who's doping. *Nature, 452*, 674–675.

Marinac, J., Buchinger, C., Godfrey, L., Wooten, J., Sun, C., & Willsie, S. (2007). Herbal products and dietary supplements: A survey of use, attitudes, and knowledge among older adults. *JAOA: Journal of the American Osteopathic Association, 107*(1), 13.

Matsuda, H., Samukawa, K., & Kubo, M. (1990). Anti-inflammatory activity of ginsenoside ro1. *Planta Medica, 56*(1), 19.

Mattei, R., Dias, R., Espínola, E., Carlini, E., & Barros, S. (1998). Guaraná (*Paullinia cupana*): Toxic behavioral effects in laboratory animals and antioxidant activity in vitro. *Journal of Ethnopharmacology, 60*(2), 111–116.

Mattson, M., & Cheng, A. (2006). Neurohormetic phytochemicals: Low-dose toxins that induce adaptive neuronal stress responses. *TRENDS in Neurosciences, 29*(11), 632–639.

McKenna, D. J., Jones, K., & Hughes, K. (2001). Efficacy, safety, and use of ginkgo biloga in clinical and preclinical applications. *Alternative Therapies in Health and Medicine, 7*(5), 70–90.

Miroddi, M., Navarra, M., Quattropani, M. C., Calapai, F., Gangemi, S., & Calapai, G. (2014). Systematic review of clinical trials assessing pharmacological properties of salvia species on memory, cognitive impairment and Alzheimer's disease. *CNS Neuroscience & Therapeutics, 20*(6), 485–495.

Nathan, P., Clarke, J., Lloyd, J., Hutchison, C., Downey, L., & Stough, C. (2001). The acute effects of an extract of *Bacopa monniera* (Brahmi) on cognitive function in healthy normal subjects. *Human Psychopharmacology: Clinical and Experimental, 16*(4), 345–351.

Neale, C., Camfield, D., Reay, J., Stough, C., & Scholey, A. (2013). Cognitive effects of two nutraceuticals Ginseng and Bacopa benchmarked against modafinil: A review and comparison of effect sizes. *British Journal of Clinical Pharmacology, 75*(3), 728–737.

Ong, Y., & Yong, E. (2000). Panax (ginseng)-panacea or placebo? Molecular and cellular basis of its pharmacological activity. *Annals-Academy of Medicine Singapore, 29*(1), 42–46.

Pase, M. P., Kean, J., Sarris, J., Neale, C., Scholey, A., & Stough, C. (2012). The cognitive-enhancing effects of *Bacopa monnieri*: A systematic review of randomized, controlled human clinical trials. *The Journal of Alternative and Complementary Medicine, 18*(7), 647–652.

Perry, E. K., Pickering, A. T., Wang, W. W., Houghton, P. J., & Perry, N. S. L. (1999). Medicinal plants and Alzheimer's disease: From ethnobotany to phytotherapy. *Journal of Pharmacy and Pharmacology, 51*(5), 527–534.

Reay, J., Kennedy, D., & Scholey, A. (2005). Single doses of *Panax ginseng* (G115) reduce blood glucose levels and improve cognitive performance during sustained mental activity. *Journal of Psychopharmacology, 19*(4), 357.

Reay, J., Kennedy, D., & Scholey, A. (2006). Effects of *Panax ginseng*, consumed with and without glucose, on blood glucose levels and cognitive performance during sustained 'mentally demanding' tasks. *Journal of Psychopharmacology, 20*(6), 771.

Rogers, P. J., Smith, J. E., Heatherley, S. V., & Pleydell-Pearce, C. (2008). Time for tea: Mood, blood pressure and cognitive performance effects of caffeine and theanine administered alone and together. *Psychopharmacology, 195*(4), 569–577.

Sadzuka, Y., Yamashita, Y., Kishimoto, S., Fukushima, S., Takeuchi, Y., & Sonobe, T. (2002). Glutamate transporter mediated increase of antitumor activity by theanine, an amino acid in green tea. *Yakugaku zasshi: Journal of the Pharmaceutical Society of Japan, 122*(11), 995.

Salim, K., McEwen, B., & Chao, H. (1997). Ginsenoside Rb1 regulates ChAT, NGF and trkA mRNA expression in the rat brain. *Molecular Brain Research, 47*(1–2), 177–182.

Sang, S., Lambert, J. D., Ho, C. T., & Yang, C. S. (2011). The chemistry and biotransformation of tea constituents. *Pharmacological Research, 64*(2), 87–99. doi: 10.1016/j. phrs.2011.02.007

Savelev, S., Okello, E., Perry, N., Wilkins, R., & Perry, E. (2003). Synergistic and antagonistic interactions of anticholinesterase terpenoids in *Salvia lavandulaefolia* essential oil. *Pharmacology, Biochemistry, and Behavior, 75*(3), 661.

Scholey, A., Bauer, I., Neale, C., Savage, K., Camfield, D., White, D., ... Hughes, M. (2013). Acute effects of different multivitamin mineral preparations with and without guaraná on mood, cognitive performance and functional brain activation. *Nutrients, 5*(9), 3589–3604.

Scholey, A., Downey, L. A., Ciorciari, J., Pipingas, A., Nolidin, K., Finn, M., ... Stough, C. (2012). Acute neurocognitive effects of epigallocatechin gallate (EGCG). *Appetite, 58*(2), 767–770. doi: 10.1016/j.appet.2011.11.016

Scholey, A., & Kennedy, D. (2002). Acute, dose-dependent cognitive effects of *Ginkgo biloba*, *Panax ginseng* and their combination in healthy young volunteers: Differential interactions with cognitive demand. *Human Psychopharmacology: Clinical and Experimental, 17*(1), 35–44.

Scholey, A., Kennedy, D., & Wesnes, K. (2005). The psychopharmacology of herbal extracts: Issues and challenges. *Psychopharmacology, 179*(3), 705–707.

Scholey, A., Ossoukhova, A., Owen, L., Ibarra, A., Pipingas, A., He, K., ... Stough, C. (2010). Effects of American ginseng (*Panax quinquefolius*) on neurocognitive function: An acute, randomised, double-blind, placebo-controlled, crossover study. *Psychopharmacology, 212*(3), 345–356.

Scholey, A., Tildesley, N., Ballard, C., Wesnes, K., Tasker, A., Perry, E., & Kennedy, D. (2008). An extract of Salvia (sage) with anticholinesterase properties improves memory and attention in healthy older volunteers. *Psychopharmacology, 198*(1), 127–139.

Setchell, K. D. R. (2001). Soy isoflavones – Benefits and risks from nature's selective estrogen receptor modulators (SERMs). *Journal of the American College of Nutrition, 20*(5 Suppl.), 354S–362S.

Smit, H., & Rogers, P. (2000). Effects of low doses of caffeine on cognitive performance, mood and thirst in low and higher caffeine consumers. *Psychopharmacology (Berlin), 152*(2), 167–173.

Smith, J., & Luo, Y. (2004). Studies on molecular mechanisms of *Ginkgo biloba* extract. *Applied Microbiology and Biotechnology, 64*(4), 465–472.

Stough, C., Lloyd, J., Clarke, J., Downey, L. A., Hutchison, C. W., Rodgers, T., & Nathan, P. J. (2001). The chronic effects of an extract of *Bacopa monniera* (Brahmi) on cognitive function in healthy human subjects. *Psychopharmacology, 156*(4), 481–484.

Sünram-Lea, S., Birchall, R., Wesnes, K., & Petrini, O. (2004). The effect of acute administration of 400 mg of *Panax ginseng* on cognitive performance and mood in healthy young volunteers. *Current Topics in Nutraceutical Research, 3*(1), 251–254.

Tachikawa, E., Kudo, K., Harada, K., Kashimoto, T., Miyate, Y., Kakizaki, A., & Takahashi, E. (1999). Effects of ginseng saponins on responses induced by various receptor stimuli. *European Journal of Pharmacology, 369*(1), 23–32.

Tildesley, N., Kennedy, D., Perry, E., Ballard, C., Savelev, S., Wesnes, K., & Scholey, A. (2003). *Salvia lavandulaefolia* (Spanish Sage) enhances memory in healthy young volunteers. *Pharmacology Biochemistry and Behavior, 75*(3), 669–674.

Tildesley, N., Kennedy, D., Perry, E., Ballard, C., Wesnes, K., & Scholey, A. (2005). Positive modulation of mood and cognitive performance following administration of acute doses of *Salvia lavandulaefolia* essential oil to healthy young volunteers. *Physiology & Behavior, 83*(5), 699–709.

Tsang, D., Yeung, H., Tso, W., & Peck, H. (1985). Ginseng saponins: Influence on neurotransmitter uptake in rat brain synaptosomes. *Planta Medica, 51*(3), 221.

Unno, T., Suzuki, Y., Kakuda, T., Hayakawa, T., & Tsuge, H. (1999). Metabolism of theanine, γ-glutamylethylamide, in rats. *Journal of Agricultural and Food Chemistry, 47*(4), 1593–1596.

van der Pijla, P., Chenb, L., & Muldera, T. (2010). Human disposition of L-theanine in tea or aqueous solution. *Journal of Functional Foods, 2*(4), 239–244.

Weckerle, C., Stutz, M., & Baumann, T. (2003). Purine alkaloids in Paullinia. *Phytochemistry, 64*(3), 735–742.

Weinmann, S., Roll, S., Schwarzbach, C., Vauth, C., & Willich, S. (2010). Effects of *Ginkgo biloba* in dementia: Systematic review and meta-analysis. *BMC Geriatrics, 10*(1), 14.

Wightman, E. L., Haskell, C., Forster, J. S., Veasey, R. C., & Kennedy, D. (2012). Epigallocatechin gallate, cerebral blood flow parameters, cognitive performance and mood in healthy humans: A double-blind, placebo-controlled, crossover investigation. *Human Psychopharmacology: Clinical and Experimental, 27*(2), 177–186.

Yamada, T., Terashima, T., Kawano, S., Furuno, R., Okubo, T., Juneja, L., & Yokogoshi, H. (2009). Theanine, γ-glutamylethylamide, a unique amino acid in tea leaves, modulates neurotransmitter concentrations in the brain striatum interstitium in conscious rats. *Amino Acids, 36*(1), 21–27.

Yokogoshi, H., Kobayashi, M., Mochizuki, M., & Terashima, T. (1998). Effect of theanine, r-glutamylethylamide, on brain monoamines and striatal dopamine release in conscious rats. *Neurochemical Research, 23*(5), 667–673.

Yokogoshi, H., & Terashima, T. (2000). Effect of theanine, r-glutamylethylamide, on brain monoamines, striatal dopamine release and some kinds of behavior in rats. *Nutrition, 16*(9), 776–777.

Yuen, E. Y., Liu, W., Karatsoreos, I. N., Ren, Y., Feng, J., McEwen, B. S., & Yan, Z. (2010). Mechanisms for acute stress-induced enhancement of glutamatergic transmission and working memory. *Molecular Psychiatry, 16*(2), 156–170.

# 10 Flavonoids and Cognitive Function

*Evidence and Recommendations from Acute and Chronic Interventions*

*Daniel J. Lamport and Rebecca J. Kean*

## CONTENTS

## SUMMARY

There is a great deal of interest in foods which can optimise or enhance cognitive performance. Research has identified that foods rich in flavonoids, such as red grapes, blueberries and cocoa, can provide benefits for the brain. This chapter critically evaluates the evidence from studies showing cognitive benefits in the acute postprandial period, for example, several hours post consumption and also following chronic consumption over several weeks. Overall, 18 of 26 intervention studies showed positive effects of consuming flavonoid-rich foods, indicating that flavonoids can exert benefits for the brain, particularly in older adults (60 years +). The mechanisms underlying these cognitive effects remain to be clearly identified; however, several proposed mechanisms are discussed including improvements in neuronal signalling pathways, protection against neuroinflammation and increased cerebral blood flow. Common methodological shortcomings in the literature are discussed and recommendations for good research practice when designing a human flavonoid intervention are presented. Future research in this field should examine the effects of flavonoids across the lifespan to include healthy young adults; the majority of studies to date focus on older adults. Gaining a clearer understanding of the mechanistic and physiological underpinnings of flavonoids on the brain is key for advancing this field.

## 10.1   AIMS OF THIS CHAPTER

Flavonoids are a group of naturally occurring substances which are found in fruits and plants. Flavonoids are a subcategory of polyphenols which is the family name for these types of phytochemicals. Other types of polyphenols include lignans, phenolic acids and stilbenes; however, the focus of this chapter is flavonoids because these are the group of polyphenols which are thought to have the strongest effects on health outcomes including cognitive function. Flavonoids can also be categorised into subclasses based upon their chemical structure (specifically the degree of oxidation of the heterocyclic ring) which include flavanols (found in, e.g. broccoli, leaks and onions), flavonols (e.g. cocoa, green/black tea and red wine), flavones (e.g. parsley and celery), flavanones (e.g. citrus fruits and tomatoes) and anthocyanins (e.g. red wine, grape juice and berries); see Figure 10.1 for a summary of dietary sources of flavonoids. Studies of the flavonoid subclass isoflavones are not discussed in this chapter due to their effects on hormonal function which confound any associations with cognitive function. Isoflavones have a very similar chemical structure to oestrogen and appear to act by affection oestrogen receptor processes in the brain (Lee et al. 2005). In the United Kingdom, we consume approximately 182 mg of flavonoids per day, 65% of which originate from fruits and vegetables that are high in anthocyanins and flavanols (Beking & Vieira, 2011). In recent years, epidemiological evidence has emerged supporting an association between increased flavonoid consumption and benefits for cognitive function (see Chapter 2), and as a result, a host of acute and chronic intervention studies have been conducted to test this association. The aims of this chapter are fourfold: (1) to provide an overview of these interventions, (2) to discuss potential mechanisms, (3) to highlight good and bad methodological practices within this field and (4) to propose future directions and

Dietary flavonoids

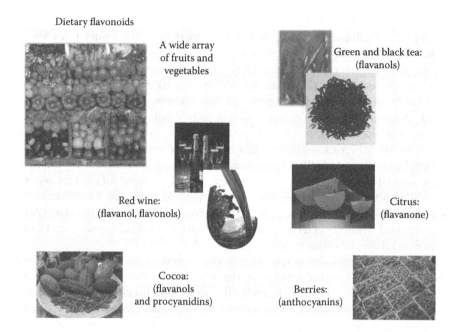

FIGURE 10.1   Dietary sources of flavonoids.

avenues of research. For clarity, the summary of the literature has been categorised according to the population studied and the food groups which have received most attention (berries and fruits, cocoa and extracts/supplements).

## 10.2   INTERVENTIONS IN HEALTHY ADULTS AND CHILDREN

### 10.2.1   BERRIES AND FRUITS

Intervention studies to date examining the effects of berries and fruits on cognition in younger adults have all employed acute designs examining effects in the immediate postprandial period. Using a randomised, double-blind, placebo-controlled crossover design, How and colleagues (How et al., 2008) administered a low-flavonoid (LF) placebo drink or a high-flavonoid (HF) milkshake containing 200 g of whole fresh blueberries mixed with 150 mL milk to young adults (18–30 years) and examined performance on a task of sustained attention (go–no go test). Change from baseline performance 5 h after ingestion was significantly better for the HF drink relative to the LF. Specifically, the HF drink improved the ability to detect the targets. Similarly, Watson et al. (2012) served HF powdered berry extract (521/mg polyphenols/60 kg body weight) and HF juiced extract (528 mg/60 kg body weight) or an LF placebo to 35 young adults following a randomised, double-blind design. After a 60 min absorption phase, attention was improved following the HF conditions relative to the placebo. Interestingly, slightly different benefits were observed between the two HF conditions; the powdered extract increased accuracy during a rapid visual information processing task, whilst the juiced extract improved reaction times during the digit vigilance task. This implies that cognitive effects may vary according to the flavonoid source, although an underlying mechanism for this has yet to be proposed (see Section 10.4).

Not all acute interventions in healthy adults have revealed significant effects. Hendrickson and Mattes (2008) served 1470 mg/day HF grape juice and a matched LF placebo to 35 young adults (mean age 26) according to a randomised, double-blind, placebo-controlled crossover design. No significant differences between drinks were reported for measures of implicit memory or mood, although baseline scores for the HF drink were significantly higher than placebo baseline scores for the implicit memory task. This is unfortunate as this may have masked any improvement associated with the HF drink. Moreover, participants were all smokers and it is unclear whether abstinence from smoking was required during the study procedures, which clearly could have implications for cognitive function. Bondonno et al. (2014) also reported no effects of a HF apple intervention on a range of cognitive and mood outcomes relative to a placebo in 30 healthy adults.

In contrast, findings from recent research in children are encouraging. Whyte and Williams (2014) served a blueberry-rich milkshake to 8–9-year-old children and reported improvement in delayed recall of the initial word list using the Rey Auditory Verbal Learning Task relative to a placebo; however, no benefits were observed using the go–no go or Stroop tests. This study is supported by Whyte and Williams (2012) whereby a group of 7–9-year-old children consumed an LF control, a medium-anthocyanin drink (126.5 mg) and a high-anthocyanin drink on separate days (253 mg), and cognitive performance was examined at 1.5, 3 and 6 h post ingestion. The children showed better verbal memory following both anthocyanin treatment groups when compared to the control, specifically for delayed word recognition, an effect which was sustained at each post-ingestive test point. Furthermore, benefits were also observed for the Stroop task; the high-anthocyanin drink was associated with improved accuracy on incongruent trials compared to the control drink. The findings indicate that flavonoid consumption may be particularly beneficial for the cognitive function of children in the immediate postprandial period.

## 10.2.2 COCOA

One of the first interventions examining the cognitive effects of cocoa flavanols was conducted by Francis et al. (2006). In this randomised, double-blind, placebo-controlled study, 16 females, aged 18–30, consumed either an HF cocoa drink (172 mg/day) or LF cocoa drink (13 mg/day) for 5 days. No significant differences in cognitive performance were found between the LF and HF drinks. However, in the same paper, the authors also reported on a small pilot study with a subset of the original participants (n = 4) examining the effects of an acute 450 mg cocoa flavanol dose on cerebral blood flow (CBF) in grey matter with an functional magnetic resonance imaging (fMRI) scan over 6 h. The HF drink was associated with a marked increase in blood oxygen level–dependent response compared to the LF drink whilst participants simultaneously performed a cognitive test (task switching) at 2 and 4 h post ingestion, although concomitant effects on task-switching performance were not observed. Whilst cognitive effects were not observed, these data indicate that the flavonoids found in cocoa have the potential to improve cognition via increased blood flow in the brain. In support, Scholey et al. (2010) reported significant improvements in working memory and attention in 30 healthy young adults using a randomised, double-blind, placebo-controlled, crossover, three-arm design (92 mg, 1040 mg and 1988 mg cocoa flavanols). Ninety minutes after ingestion, performance on the serial threes task was significantly higher following the two HF drink doses compared to the LF 92 mg control, in terms of both shorter reaction times and greater number of correct responses. Moreover, Field et al. (2011) reported improved spatial working memory and attention 120 min after consumption of a HF dark chocolate bar (773 mg) relative to an LF white chocolate bar control containing only trace amounts of flavanols.

Despite these positive findings, the effects of cocoa flavonoids have been largely inconsistent. Most recently, Pase et al. (2013) and Camfield et al. (2012) failed to find any effects on cognitive function or mood. Pase et al. (2013) examined cognitive performance and mood 1, 2.5 and 4 h post consumption of drinks containing 0 mg or 250 mg doses, whilst Camfield et al. (2012) examined chronic effects on spatial working memory after a 30-day daily consumption of drinks containing 0, 250 and 500 mg using a randomised, double-blind, parallel-group design. Interestingly, Camfield et al. (2012) also examined a measure of brain activation known as steady-state visually evoked potential (SSVEP; see Chapter 12 by Camfield for more details). The results showed that SSVEP amplitude and phase differences were significantly different in several posterior parietal and centro-frontal areas during memory encoding, working memory hold period and retrieval following the HF consumption compared to the LF condition. This indicates that neural efficiency was improved during performance of the spatial working memory task following chronic consumption of the cocoa flavonoid drink relative to the LF control. Despite an absence of acute effects, Pase et al. (2013) reported that a 30-day daily consumption of the HF cocoa drink (250 mg) was associated with significantly increased self-rated calmness and contentedness relative to placebo, yet there were no significant effects of the cocoa flavonoids on any of the cognitive test scores after 30 days.

## 10.2.3 EXTRACT AND SUPPLEMENTS

Rather than investigating specific food groups or items, several researchers have examined the effects of flavonoid-rich extracts such as *Ginkgo biloba* (which originates from pine bark) and pure flavonoids consumed in capsulated form. For example, Kennedy et al. (2000) studied the dose-dependent effects of 120 mg, 240 mg and 360 mg of standardised *G. biloba* extract (GK501, Pharmaton, SA) on cognitive performance at multiple time points (0, 1, 2.5, 4 and 6 h) in 20 young adults (19–24 years old) using a placebo-controlled, double-blind, crossover design. Compared with the placebo, the ingestion of Ginkgo produced a number of significant changes in cognitive performance. Most interestingly, a dose-dependent improvement of speed of attention was observed following the 240 and 360 mg doses at 2.5 and 6 h post ingestion. More recently, Mohamed et al. (2013) investigated the effects of catechin-rich palm oil leaf extract on cognition using a double-blind, randomised, placebo-controlled parallel-group design with 30 young Malaysian adults (22–24 years). The HF group consumed catechin-rich palm oil (*Elaeis guineensis*) leaf extract in capsules of 500 mg/day for 2 months and were tested using short-term memory, spatial visualisation, language skills and processing speed tasks. Benefits were observed for short-term memory in the HF group at 1 and 2 months relative to the placebo. For a more detailed discussion of the cognitive effects of Ginkgo, see Canter and Ernst (2007).

### 10.2.4 SUMMARY OF INTERVENTIONS IN HEALTHY ADULTS AND CHILDREN

Investigations into the effects of flavonoid-based interventions in young healthy adults show contrasting results. The data from the berry literature are encouraging; 2 studies in adults show acute improvements in sustained attention and visual vigilance (How et al., 2008; Watson et al., 2012), and further two studies in children report improvements in verbal memory and executive function (Whyte & Williams, 2012, 2014). The only study to report a null finding was conducted with grape juice (Hendrickson & Mattes, 2008), perhaps indicating that cognitive performance is more acutely sensitive to blueberry rather than grape-based interventions. The findings from the cocoa literature are more inconsistent. Two studies report improvements in acute attention and working memory (Field et al., 2011; Scholey et al., 2010), whereas two studies report null behavioural effects (Francis et al., 2006; Pase et al., 2013). Interestingly, some studies have reported significant physiological changes in the absence of any cognitive improvements. For example, Francis et al. (2006) observed a significant increase in CBF, whilst Camfield et al. (2012) reported improvements in neuronal activation in a 30-day chronic intervention. In fact, the only cognitive improvements reported chronically with cocoa supplementation are self-reported improvements in feelings of calmness and contentedness (Pase et al., 2013).

## 10.3 INTERVENTIONS IN OLDER AND COGNITIVELY IMPAIRED ADULTS

### 10.3.1 BERRIES AND FRUITS

Crews et al. (2005) were one of the first groups to investigate the chronic (6-week) effect of a berry-/fruit-based intervention. Participants in this study, 50 healthy older adults aged >60 years, consumed 32 oz/day of a drink containing either HF 27% cranberry juice per volume or LF placebo matched for smell, taste, vitamin C and appearance (both from Ocean Spray Cranberries, Inc.). The exact flavonoid content of these drinks was not reported. Participants completed a comprehensive battery of 8 cognitive tasks, yet no cognitive effects of the juice were observed when compared to the placebo in this parallel-group design. In contrast, Krikorian conducted two 12-week intervention studies with grape juice (2010a) and blueberry juice (2010b) in older adults diagnosed with mild cognitive impairment (MCI) and found benefits for immediate verbal and spatial memory following the HF drinks when compared with their matched placebos. It is important to note, however, that both of these parallel-group comparison studies had rather small sample sizes, with just 5 participants in the grape polyphenol condition (7 placebos) and 9 participants in the blueberry condition (7 placebos). Given these small sample sizes, it is entirely possible that the effects observed in these two studies might be explained by the differences in average age between the two groups. Those in the grape juice group (2010a) were, on average, 5 years younger (75 years) than those in the control group (80 years), and those in the blueberry group (2010b) were, on average, 4 years younger than their control group. This is important given that a 5-year age difference at the extreme ends of the lifespan can be related to considerable differences in cognitive ability (Letenneur et al., 2007). Moreover, the control group data for the blueberry study (2010b) were actually the control group data from the grape juice study (2010a), in which the group therefore consumed a grape juice control rather than a blueberry control. These shortcomings were addressed in a larger sample of adults with MCI (n = 21) who showed significant benefits for memory function following 16 weeks of grape juice consumption relative to a well-matched placebo (Krikorian et al., 2012).

Remington et al. (2010) supplemented 21 older adults diagnosed with moderate to late stage Alzheimer's disease (72–93 years old) with two daily 4 oz servings of apple juice for 1 month. There was no control group and the participants resided in a nursing home. No improvements were found in cognitive function using the Dementia Rating Scale; however, mood and behaviour were significantly improved following the intervention. This is the only published study to date which reports an apple-based intervention. This could be because citrus fruits provide a richer source of flavonoids. For example, Kean et al. (2014) reported that chronic daily consumption of flavanone-rich orange juice over 8 weeks was beneficial for executive function in healthy older adults (mean age 67). Specifically, the orange juice drink, containing 305 mg/day flavanones, was associated with a significant improvement in executive function and episodic memory relative to baseline, whereas no such improvements were observed for the LF (37 mg/day flavanones) orange squash drink.

### 10.3.2 COCOA

Saunders (PhD thesis, 2010) investigated the acute effects of cocoa flavonoid consumption in 63 healthy elderly adults (aged 62–75 years). In this double-blind crossover study, 63 healthy older adults consumed a high (494 mg total polyphenol) or low (23 mg total polyphenol) cocoa drink. The high-flavanol drink induced a significant improvement in executive function, episodic memory and blood pressure relative to the low-flavanol drink, with the high-flavanol drink leading to a reduction in diastolic blood pressure and the attenuation of a rise in systolic blood pressure 2 h post ingestion. A 6-week, parallel-group, placebo-controlled, randomised, double-blind intervention (Crews et al., 2008) administered 101 healthy elderly adults (mean age 60) flavonoid-rich dark chocolate bars and drinks. Specifically, one 37 g chocolate bar containing 397 mg proanthocyanidins and one 12 g cocoa drink containing 357 mg total proanthocyanidins were consumed daily for 6 weeks. The placebo cocoa bar and drink were matched for appearance, smell, taste and energy. However, no differences in cognitive performance between the high and LF groups were observed using an exhaustive cognitive battery. Interestingly, an increased heart rate was reported in HF group at 3 and 6 weeks. The authors proposed that this could be attributed to the methylxanthines (caffeine and theobromine) present in the HF cocoa products. This increase in pulse rate suggests that the HF cocoa was having some physiological effects, irrespective of the cognitive findings, replicating findings from other aforementioned studies in health young adults (e.g. Francis et al., 2006). More recently, Desideri et al. (2012) randomised 90 elderly Italians with MCI to one of three conditions: the HF group consumed 990 mg/day of cocoa flavanols, the intermediate-flavonoid (IF) group had 520 mg/day and the LF were given 45 mg/day for 8 weeks. No significant difference between groups in the mini mental state exam was apparent; however, participants in the HF and IF groups showed improvements in the Trail Making Test (a test of executive function and processing speed: see Chapter 4 for more details). Furthermore, at 8 weeks, change from baseline in verbal fluency performance (also a test of executive function) was significantly better in the HF group compared to the LF group. Interestingly, this study also reported that physiological changes including decreased insulin resistance, blood pressure and lipid peroxidation were observed in the HF and IF groups.

### 10.3.3 EXTRACTS AND SUPPLEMENTS

Two long-term intervention studies have reported cognitive benefits in older adults following 5-week ingestion of supplements comprising of approximately 768 mg of proanthocyanidins, flavonoid conjugates, phenolic acids and other water-soluble flavonoids (Pipingas et al., 2008) and 3-month ingestion of supplements containing 150 mg of the flavonoid antioxidant Pycnogenol® (Ryan et al., 2008). Specifically, the former study reported improvements in visuospatial recognition memory and in spatial working memory function, and the latter reported improvements using the cognitive drug research (CDR) test battery for quality of working memory and spatial working memory. Similar to the findings from studies in healthy younger adults, research in older adults with MCI or mild Alzheimer's disease has reported improvements in cognitive function following G. biloba extract (Le Bars et al., 2002; Mix & Crews, 2000). The former study examined the effects of an HF (180 mg) or placebo daily supplement in cognitive impaired adults (aged 55–86) for 6 weeks and reported a significant improvement in executive function in the HF group at follow-up. Likewise, Le Bars et al. (2002) investigated the effects of a 12-month supplementation of 120 mg/day (HF) compared to 0 mg/day (LF). Interestingly, this latter study examined the effect of treatment relative to severity of cognitive ability at baseline. Results indicated that overall, there was a significant cognitive benefit of the HF supplement compared to baseline regardless of the stage of dementia. Yet, the relative changes from baseline at the end of the 12 months depended greatly on the severity of cognitive impairment at baseline. In essence, those that were only mildly impaired (MMSE <24) showed improvement following the HF supplement at follow-up, whereas the more severe subgroup (MMSE <15) showed stabilisation or a slight attenuation of decline when compared with the LF group.

### 10.3.4 SUMMARY OF INTERVENTIONS IN OLDER ADULTS

In summary, research into the effects of fruit and berry interventions in older adults is limited and inconsistent. Crews et al. (2005) supplemented healthy older adults with cranberry juice for 5 weeks and reported no cognitive improvements, whereas

Kean et al. (2014) reported cognitive benefits following 8 weeks of flavanone-rich orange juice consumption. The most consistent findings have been reported from studies in adults with MCI; cognitive benefits were observed in three separate studies (Krikorian et al., 2010a,b, 2012), whereas the only study in institutionalised elderly adults reported null effects (Remington et al., 2010), although there was no control group. Summarising the cocoa data, one acute study reports better executive function and episodic memory in healthy older adults 2 h post ingestion of cocoa-rich flavonoids (Saunders et al., PhD thesis, 2010); however, two chronic interventions in older adults have failed to report cognitive effects (Crews et al., 2008; Desideri et al., 2012).

Research with flavonoid-rich supplements in older adults has varied notably in duration including 5 weeks in healthy older adults (Pipingas et al., 2008), 6 weeks in adults with MCI (Mix & Crews, 2000), 3 months in healthy volunteers (Ryan et al., 2008) and 12 months in adults with dementia (Le Bars et al., 2002). However, all of these studies report significant benefits for cognitive function, indicating clear potential for the development of flavonoid-rich supplements for attenuating cognitive decline.

## 10.4  MECHANISMS OF ACTION

The role of flavonoids in the brain is not well understood. There have been several proposed mechanisms by which consumption of flavonoids and flavonoid-rich foods may affect cognitive function (for review, see Spencer, 2009, 2010). It was originally/initially thought that the health benefits of flavonoids could be due to their antioxidant properties and their ability to exert antioxidant actions within the body and particularly within the brain. However, it is now widely accepted that flavonoids undergo extensive biotransformation following ingestion resulting in compounds with greatly reduced antioxidant properties (Halliwell, 2008). Moreover, flavonoids and their metabolites tend to be observed at much lower concentration in the brain than other antioxidant compounds (Manach et al., 2005). Therefore, it is unlikely that cognitive benefits are a direct result of antioxidant effects. Proposed alternative mechanisms can be broadly distinguished into three possibilities which, most likely, interact (1) improvements in neuronal signalling pathways, (2) protection against neuroinflammation and neurotoxins and (3) increased CBF and other cardiovascular effects such as improved blood pressure.

### 10.4.1  IMPROVEMENTS IN NEURONAL SIGNALLING PATHWAYS

There is evidence that flavonoids can cross the blood–brain barrier where they have the potential to affect the genetic expression of proteins in neurons (Shukitt-Hale et al., 2008). For example, various flavonoid binding sites on neuronal cell receptors have been identified including $GABA_A$ and opioid receptors which are understood to activate pathways that modulate activity-dependent plasticity and new synaptic protein synthesis. This can lead to morphological changes which may enhance the plasticity and efficiency of neurons and their signalling pathways. For example, in rodents, blueberry flavonoids have been shown to increase the expression of the protein brain-derived neurotrophic factor (BDNF) in the hippocampus (Rendeiro et al., 2013, 2014), an area of the brain which is strongly associated with memory. Increased expression of BDNF plays a crucial role in synaptic plasticity and promotes synaptic growth and increased neuronal density. These changes in neuronal morphology could lead to observable improvements in cognitive function. In support, concomitant improvements in spatial memory in rodents have been observed alongside increased BDNF expression in the hippocampus following a flavonoid-rich diet (Rendeiro et al., 2013, 2014; Williams et al., 2008). Despite this evidence, the exact site of the interaction between flavonoids and neuronal signalling pathways remains unresolved.

### 10.4.2 Neuroprotection

It is know that increased neuroinflammation plays an important role in the development of Alzheimer's disease and Parkinson's disease. A reduction in neuroinflammation may offer a mechanism to support the observation that flavonoids delay the onset and progression of cognitive decline. Flavonoids have been shown to reduce neuroinflammation by positively affecting signalling of the enzyme protein kinase and the associated pathways (Spencer, 2009). Kinase signalling pathways are associated with neuroinflammation and subsequent neurodegeneration. By affecting these pathways, flavonoids may reduce the rate of neuronal death which could provide a mechanism by which chronic flavonoid consumption may attenuate a decline in cognitive function, particularly in older adults. In addition, there is evidence that flavonoids may be able to counteract neuronal injury which is associated with neurodegeneration and cognitive decline. For example, flavonoid-rich G. biloba extract has been shown to protect hippocampal neurons against beta-amyloid-induced neurotoxicity (Luo et al., 2002). Further research in humans is required to identify the specific location and nature of the interaction between flavonoid metabolites and neuronal cell receptors and pathways, but there is good support from in vitro work and in vivo rodent research to support these mechanisms. Perhaps the most challenging aspect of this mechanistic jigsaw will be to show a direct relationship between flavonoid-induced improvement in neuronal signalling and a measurable improvement in human cognitive functions.

### 10.4.3 Cerebral and Peripheral Blood Flow

The mechanisms described earlier are most likely to be responsible for long-term chronic effects of flavonoids observed in epidemiological and longitudinal research where dietary patterns and cognitive performance have been analysed over several months and years. It is possible that some cognitive benefits observed from 12-week flavonoid interventions are explained by neuroprotective effects and improvements in neuronal signalling; however, such mechanisms cannot explain acute cognitive benefits in the immediate hours post flavonoid ingestion as reported in several studies (e.g. Field et al., 2011; Scholey et al., 2010). These effects are more likely to be mediated by peripheral vascular changes (Taubert et al., 2007), which may facilitate more efficient CBF, which is known to deteriorate with age, to be vital for optimal brain function and to be decreased in patients with dementia (Nagahama et al., 2003). There is support for this mechanism from studies with cocoa flavanols (for review see Scholey & Owen, 2013). Increases of approximately 10% have been observed in peripheral flow–mediated dilation (a measure of blood vessel and endothelial cell dilation) in humans 2 h after cocoa flavanol consumption (Schroeter et al., 2006). This time frame coincides with observations of improvement in cognitive function 2 h after consumption of cocoa flavanols (Field et al., 2011; Scholey et al., 2010). Increased CBF has also been reported with fMRI brain scans following cocoa flavanol consumption; however, concomitant improvements in cognitive function were not observed (Francis et al., 2006). Interestingly, these improvements in blood flow may extend beyond an acute time frame. Significantly improved flow velocity in the middle cerebral artery measured by Doppler ultrasound was reported at 1- and 2-week time points following daily cocoa flavanol consumption relative to a placebo (Sorond et al., 2008). Epidemiological studies show that long-term chronic consumption of flavonoid-rich foods and drinks such as tea and cocoa is associated with a reduction in cardiovascular disease risk factors and lower blood pressure (Vauzour et al., 2010), indicating that long-term benefits to health may also be achieved via this mechanism.

Improvements in blood flow to the brain may affect cognitive function in several ways. Most directly, increased oxygen supply could directly improve neuronal function. In support, increased activation of neurons during cognitive performance is strongly correlated with CBF. Second, the process of neurogenesis and neuronal growth tends to cluster around areas with optimum blood supply where new blood vessel growth occurs (angiogenesis) (Ohab et al., 2006). This indicates that blood vessel growth in the brain may be accompanied by neurogenesis. The mechanisms by which flavonoids induce vasodilation and angiogenesis are thought to be via increased nitric oxide production in the endothelium (Schroeter et al., 2006). Nitric oxide synthesis is a key regulator of angiogenesis, the dilation of cells and ultimately blood pressure. Therefore, it has been proposed that flavonoid-induced increases in the bioavailability of nitric oxide in the brain may lead to increases in blood vessel growth, subsequent neurogenesis and potential improvements in cognitive function. Nitric oxide is also released from neurons in response to neuronal activation since it is crucial for the coupling between increased blood supply and neuronal activity (Toda et al., 2009). Furthermore, increased blood flow in the brain is likely to stabilise the presence of neurons. It is interesting to note that these proposed flavonoid effects are similar to the impact of exercise; improved blood flow, reduced blood pressure and enhanced angiogenesis and vascular regeneration in the periphery and brain are induced by exercise. Exercise may also stimulate BDNF production, which is considered to be one possible mechanism by which flavonoids may benefit cognitive function. To summarise, it can be tentatively suggested that the association between improved cognitive performance and consumption of flavonoid-rich foods and drinks is mediated by nitric oxide–dependent vasodilation in the brain. An interesting recent study (Bondonno et al., 2014) investigated this hypothesis by examining cognitive function and circulating nitric oxide status following the consumption of flavonoid-rich apples and nitrate-rich spinach individually and in combination. Both the spinach and the flavonoids increased nitric oxide status; however, concomitant cognitive benefits were not observed. This supports a mechanism for flavonoids affecting nitric oxide status; however, direct observations between flavonoid-induced changes in nitric oxide synthesis and behavioural effects in humans have yet to be reported.

## 10.5 METHODOLOGICAL ISSUES

Thus far, we have seen that there is an accumulating body of literature which supports the hypothesis that consumption of flavonoids and flavonoid-rich foods is associated with benefits for cognitive function. However, there are clear inconsistencies in findings between studies. For example, a 12-week consumption of grape juice was beneficial for verbal memory in older adults with MCI (Krikorian et al., 2010a), but cognitive benefits were not observed in young adults following an acute dose of grape juice (Hendrickson and Mattes, 2008). In order to advance knowledge in the field, it is important to understand what is driving these inconsistencies. Careful evaluation of the literature indicates there is a great deal of methodological heterogeneity between studies, and it is likely that this is a significant contributor to the inconsistent findings. This section will outline recommendations for good methodological practice when investigating the effects of flavonoid-based interventions on cognitive function.

### 10.5.1 COGNITIVE TESTING

Selecting appropriate cognitive tests and following correct cognitive testing procedures are clearly of critical importance to any flavonoid intervention (see Chapter 4). There are a number of important considerations including the cognitive domains being assessed, the population and test sensitivity, all of which vary considerably between flavonoid interventions. The absence of consistency in cognitive testing procedures is beginning to be recognised as a severe limitation amongst researchers across the field, and there have been recent attempts to address this problem with the publication of guidelines for cognitive testing within nutritional interventions (de Jager et al., 2014). This is highlighted and discussed in more detail in Chapters 1 and 4. There is much contention regarding cognitive test selection, which is perhaps not surprising given that thousands of tests are available. For example, a 2009 review of the flavonoid/cognition literature reported the use of 55 different tests across 15 dietary interventions (Macready et al., 2009), and a broader review of the polyphenol/cognition literature reported 165 different cognitive tests across 28 studies (Lamport et al., 2012). The impact and recognition of the tests which are sensitive to the intervention can sometimes be lost amongst the vast majority of non-significant findings from the remainder of the cognitive battery. With respect to berry- and fruit-based flavonoids, the cognitive domains which appear to be most sensitive are verbal and spatial memory, as discussed earlier in this chapter (for review see Lamport et al., 2012; Macready et al., 2009). This is also supported by research in rodents which consistently demonstrates improvement in spatial learning following flavonoid-rich berry diets (Rendeiro et al., 2013; Williams et al., 2008). Presently, the mechanistic pathways which underlie cognitive benefits following flavonoid consumption in humans remain speculative (as previously discussed in Section 10.4), and therefore, it is difficult to choose tests on the basis of a mechanistic rationale.

The popularity of standardised batteries is increasing (e.g. CANTAB, CDR); however, to date their application has been limited within the context of flavonoid interventions. These types of batteries offer good standardisation and norms, but it is important to consider whether such batteries are suitably sensitive to detect the subtle effects that might be anticipated following a flavonoid intervention. For example, a recent flavonoid-rich apple intervention in healthy adults had no effect on cognitive function as measured by the CDR (Bondonno et al., 2014). Perhaps the most sensible approach when selecting a cognitive test is to identify which tests have previously been found to be sensitive to flavonoid interventions in the population under consideration. For example, significant benefits have been observed with the California Verbal Learning Test in older adults with MCI following blueberry and grape juice interventions (Krikorian et al., 2010a,b, 2012). Therefore, it would be sensible to incorporate a test of verbal learning and memory into future flavonoid interventions in both older and younger adults, thus allowing a direct comparison across studies, provided that the cognitive testing procedures are similar.

## 10.5.2 METHOD OF FLAVONOID DELIVERY

Flavonoids are a group of phytochemicals which naturally occur in a wide range of foods and drinks such as berries, fruits, juices, vegetables and cocoa. These foods and drinks offer experimenters an easily available, palatable, natural source for delivering increased concentrations of flavonoids into the diet; thus, the effects of flavonoids on cognition in humans have rarely been examined in isolation or in their pure form. An obvious limitation of this approach is that the flavonoid-rich food being consumed may also contain other nutrients and ingredients which affect cognitive function. For example, cocoa contains caffeine and theobromine, both of which have well-established effects on cognitive performance; indeed, the effects of caffeine are likely to be greater than any flavonoid-induced effects. Berries, fruits and juices also contain very high quantities of vitamins and minerals, which have been associated with cognitive outcomes (see Chapter 8 for details of vitamins and minerals associated with cognitive outcomes). Furthermore, fruits and particularly juices typically have high levels of sugars (carbohydrate), as does chocolate, and variations in the ratio of fat and protein can also affect cognitive performance (Dye et al., 2000; Hoyland et al., 2008). It is therefore of critical importance to carefully consider the vehicle of flavonoid delivery in any intervention and to design a suitable placebo which is matched for calories, macronutrients, vitamins and minerals. The effects of psychological confounds such as palatability and satiety should not be overlooked, particularly with interventions lasting several weeks, and ideally, these characteristics should be confirmed with pilot work prior to the intervention. Matching for palatability can be tricky, as often the process of removing flavonoids can impair the taste of chocolate- and fruit-based drinks. Experimenters using cordial or squash as a control condition for juice-based interventions should carefully check for presence of flavonoids in the squash; these are often surprisingly high, particularly if the squash or cordial has real fruit extract. On the whole, these confounds have been successfully controlled in the majority of interventions; however, there are some notable omissions, for example, data from a blueberry juice intervention were compared with the control group from a previous grape juice intervention (Krikorian et al., 2010a); see Section 10.3.1 for more details. It is also essential to accurately measure the specific quantities and concentrations of flavonoids and their subclasses which are present *specifically* in the intervention vehicle. The publication of open access databases such as *Phenol-Explorer* (Neveu et al., 2010) is useful as a guide for indicating the general type and concentrations of flavonoids in different foods; however, experimenters should not rely on these as exact for a specific intervention. Ideally, the intervention product should be tested by the manufacturer or in-house high-performance liquid chromatography analysis. There are some instances in the literature where the specific concentrations of flavonoids in the intervention have not been reported in the manuscript (e.g. Crews et al., 2005; Krikorian et al., 2010a), which severely limits interpretation and comparisons between studies. Finally, the rate of absorption and metabolism of flavonoids will differ between individuals, populations and flavonoid subclasses; therefore, the gold standard approach is to confirm the intake of flavonoids by assessment of metabolites and biomarkers from urine and blood samples. This analysis is arguably more important during chronic interventions to ensure compliance of procedures and may also shed light on the mechanisms underlying cognitive effects. To date, few cognitive interventions have assessed metabolite concentrations of flavonoids; future studies should seek to address this limitation.

### 10.5.3 HABITUAL DIETARY ASSESSMENT

Given that flavonoids are present in high concentrations in a wide range of commonly consumed foods, it is essential that the effects of the intervention are not confounded by flavonoid consumption from the habitual diet. A number of flavonoid-based cognitive interventions have failed to consider the effect of habitual dietary flavonoid intake prior to or during the trial (e.g. Crews et al., 2005; Francis et al., 2006; Hendrickson & Mattes, 2008). This is particularly important for chronic interventions over several weeks. Arguably, participants should be advised to avoid foods containing high concentrations of flavonoids. One method is to give participants a list of specific foods and drinks to avoid. However, a limitation of this approach is that directly restricting intake of certain foods may result in an artificial reduction in habitual flavonoid consumption and circulation of the associated metabolites in the body. Subsequently, the intervention may only serve to return an individual's flavonoid consumption to baseline; thus, effects on cognitive function are less likely to be observed. Perhaps more concerning is the possibility that reducing habitual flavonoid intake over several weeks could impair cognitive performance (a form of withdrawal effect); therefore, the intervention may only serve to attenuate or prevent this impairment. This has been observed in pharmacological interventions whereby the effect of caffeine is moderated by levels of caffeine dependency or habitual caffeine intake; habitually high-caffeine consumers show cognitive impairments when forced to abstain from caffeine, and the consumption of caffeine only serves to reverse the impairment, whilst participants who rarely consume caffeine demonstrate improved reaction time and psychomotor skills following caffeine consumption relative to everyday baseline performance (James & Rogers, 2005). To address this, habitual diet should be measured before and during any flavonoid intervention.

This will allow experimenters to consider including baseline dietary characteristics as covariates in the analyses or compare outcomes between high and low habitual consumers. This approach will also provide welcome details regarding the dietary characteristics of the sample. An alternative systematic approach is to specifically recruit participants who consume low levels of flavonoids in their habitual diet (as indicated by food frequency questionnaires, food diaries or assessment of plasma flavonoid metabolites), but this limits generalisability. A recent review of the poly-phenol literature recommended that baseline and follow-up dietary measurements should coincide as closely as possible with the cognitive assessments in order to maximise the reliability and validity of conclusions (Lamport et al., 2012), which is particularly pertinent for longitudinal epidemiological studies (see Chapter 2 by Andreeva and Kesse-Guyot). In sum, the recommendation here is to ensure that a measure of habitual dietary flavonoid intake is incorporated into any intervention investigating the effects of flavonoids on cognitive function.

### 10.5.4 STUDY DESIGN

When designing a flavonoid intervention, it is important to carefully consider whether a parallel-group or crossover design is most appropriate. Following a crossover design allows control of individual differences in baseline cognitive per-formance, habitual nutritional intake and any other between-subjects variability. However, a major limitation which may particularly apply to studies of polyphenols is carry-over effects. The timescale over which chronic consumption of flavonoid-rich foods, drinks or supplements may benefit cognition is currently unknown, and it is entirely possible that cognitive benefits may persist several weeks follow-ing the termination of a trial. Having a clearer understanding of the mechanisms which underlie flavonoid-associated cognitive benefits will significantly enhance our understanding of this timescale, but at present this remains speculative (see Section 10.4). For example, if flavonoids can induce neurogenesis and enhance neu-ronal signalling within a time frame of 12 weeks, then participants might experi-ence enduring benefits from exposure to a flavonoid treatment in the first arm of a trial which do not wash out before the placebo or control arm commences. As our understanding of flavonoid-induced carry-over effects advances, the appropriate duration for the washout will become clearer. Presently, researchers should address this potential confound by including treatment order as a between-groups variable in the analysis of flavonoid treatment effects. Carry-over effects as described earlier would be indicated by significant treatment by order interactions and main effects of order.

A few flavonoid intervention studies enforce a comprehensive fasting period prior to cognitive testing. Doing so would reduce the acute effects of recent macronutrient and stimulant consumption (e.g. caffeine) which may mask any flavonoid effects. Hence at the very least, a 2 h fast should be applied, although researchers should note that the gold standard for clinical trials is an 8 h or overnight fast. It is of course a legitimate approach to incorporate a flavonoid intervention into a standardised meal (e.g. Hendrickson & Mattes, 2008) which perhaps more accurately reflects how such interventions might be consumed in everyday life, particularly juices.

However, researchers should be aware that subtle flavonoid effects may be masked by macronutrient effects exerted by the meal (for discussion of macronutrient effects, see Dye et al., 2000; Hoyland et al., 2008). Recent physical activity should also be carefully controlled or documented, particularly if the proposed mechanism by which the flavonoids are exerting their cognitive effects is via increased CBF (see Section 10.4), since exercise is associated with increased glucose and oxygen uptake in the brain, even following cessation of physical activity (Ide & Secher, 2000). Furthermore, exercise has been directly associated with improvements in cognitive function (Colcombe & Kramer, 2003).

There is now a suitable body of evidence with which to make sample size and power calculations prior to the commencement of a flavonoid intervention. Such calculations should be based on the population and the cognitive outcomes. Research dissemination is increasing via all forms of the media, and as a result, participants are becoming increasing knowledgeable and are often aware of the hypotheses that increased consumption of flavonoid-rich foods such as blueberries is associated with beneficial health outcomes such as improved cardiovascular health and enhanced cognitive function. It is therefore important that double-blind procedures are incorporated and adequately described. Similarly, the blinding of researchers actively collecting and analysing cognitive test data should not be overlooked as unconscious bias is difficult to identify and eliminate. Flavonoid intervention studies should always ask participants at debrief which condition they suspected contained the 'active' flavonoid (crossover design) or if they believed they had been assigned to the placebo or flavonoid condition (parallel-group design) (Table 10.1).

## 10.6 FUTURE DIRECTIONS

Based upon our current knowledge, this section outlines areas of interest and potential avenues of future research which should advance our understanding of the relationship between flavonoid consumption and cognitive function. As discussed earlier (see Section 10.4), several mechanisms have been proposed which potentially underlie the relationship between flavonoids and cognition. However, there is an absence of research in humans to support these mechanisms. As such, a key area which must be addressed is investigating these mechanisms in more detail. For example, developments in fMRI technology now allow for the assessment of CBF within the context of an acute intervention over the course of several hours. It would certainly be of interest to measure CBF simultaneously with cognitive testing to examine whether flavonoid-induced changes in blood flow and neuronal activation occur concomitantly with the mental effort required to complete a cognitively demanding task. Currently, data supporting a relationship between flavonoids and increased CBF are almost exclusively from interventions with cocoa flavanols. There is evidence that different flavonoid subclasses are metabolised within the body at different rates, and therefore the time points at which cognitive benefits are observed may vary between subclasses. For example, cocoa flavanols have been consistently shown to exert improvements in blood pressure, blood flow and vasodilation approximately 2 h after consumption, whereas the peak in

## TABLE 10.1
## Summary of Flavonoid Research Studies

| Authors | Participants | Design and Interventions | Key Findings |
|---|---|---|---|
| Bondonno et al. (2014) Apple | 30 adults (6 males), mean age 47 years (sd 13) | Acute crossover (i) Control (LF apple) (ii) HF apple (iii) Nitrate-rich spinach (iv) HF apple and spinach | No effects on cognitive function or mood with the CDR computerised cognitive assessment battery. Plasma nitrate and nitrite concentrations increased following intervention (iv) relative to control. |
| Camfield et al. (2012) Cocoa | 63 adults, mean age 52 years (sd 7), gender not stated | Chronic (30-day) parallel groups (i) Control (low-flavanol cocoa) (ii) 250 mg flavanol cocoa drink (iii) 500 mg flavanol cocoa drink | No effects on cognitive function. However, chronic consumption of the cocoa flavanols was associated with increased neural efficiency during a working memory task as measured by SSVEP. |
| Crews et al. (2005) Cranberry juice | 50 adults (21 males), mean age 69 (sd 6) | Chronic (6-week) parallel groups (i) Control (ii) HF cranberry juice 32 oz/day (United States) | No effects on cognitive function. |
| Desideri et al. (2012) Cocoa | 90 elderly adults with MCI (43 males), mean age 71 years (sd 5) | Chronic (8-week) parallel groups (i) Control 45 mg flavanol cocoa (ii) 520 mg flavanol cocoa (iii) 900 mg flavanol cocoa | Performance on the Trail Making Test was significantly better for the medium- and high-flavanol groups relative to the control. Verbal fluency was significantly better for the high-flavanol group relative to the control. |
| Field et al. (2011) Cocoa | 30 young adults (8 males) aged 18–25 years | Acute crossover (i) Control (white chocolate) (ii) 773 mg flavanol dark chocolate | Significantly better spatial working memory and choice reaction time was observed 2 h following consumption of the 773 mg flavanol chocolate relative to the control. |
| Francis et al. (2006) Cocoa | 16 young female adults aged 18–30 years | Acute (5-day) crossover (i) Control 13 mg/day flavanol cocoa drink (ii) 172 mg/day flavanol cocoa drink | No significant difference in attention switching performance between the drinks; however, increased CBF was observed following the high-flavanol drink. |

*(Continued)*

**TABLE 10.1 (*Continued*)**
**Summary of Flavonoid Research Studies**

| Authors | Participants | Design and Interventions | Key Findings |
|---|---|---|---|
| Hendrickson & Mattes (2008) Grape juice | 35 young adults (17 males), mean age 26 years (sd 8) | Acute crossover (i) Control drink (ii) Grape juice, 1.7 g polyphenols per 70 kg | No effects on cognitive function. |
| How et al. (2008) Blueberry *Abstract only* | 16 young adults, mean age 23 years (sd 3), and 16 older adults, mean age 68 years (sd 4) | Acute, crossover (i) Control drink (ii) Blueberry drink (235 mg flavonoids) | Both young and older adults showed improved attention 5 h post consumption of the flavonoid-rich blueberry drink relative to the control drink. |
| Kean et al. (2014) Orange juice | 37 older adults (13 males), mean age 67 years (sd 5) | Chronic (8-week) crossover (i) Control, 13 mg flavanones (ii) HF orange juice, 305 mg flavanones | Global cognitive function was significantly better following an 8-week consumption of flavanone-rich juice relative to an 8-week consumption of the low flavanone control. |
| Kennedy et al. (2000) Ginkgo | 20 young adults (2 males), mean age 20 years (19–24) | Acute crossover (i) Control (ii) 120 mg Ginkgo (iii) 240 mg Ginkgo (iv) 360 mg Gingko | Compared with control, Ginkgo was associated with a dose-dependent improvement of 'speed of attention' at 2.5 and 6 h post consumption. |
| Krikorian et al. (2010a) Grape juice | 12 adults with MCI (8 males), mean age 78 years (sd 5) | Chronic (12-week) parallel groups (i) Control (ii) Grape juice (18–27 ml/kg/day) | The grape juice was associated with significantly better verbal memory acquisition at 12 weeks. |
| Krikorian et al. (2010b) Blueberry juice | 9 adults with MCI (5 males), mean age 76 years (sd 5) | Chronic (12-week) parallel groups (i) Placebo (grape juice flavoured) (ii) Blueberry juice (1.8 g polyphenols/day) | The blueberry juice group showed significantly better verbal paired associate learning at 12 weeks compared to the control; however, baseline performance was not considered. |
| Krikorian et al. (2012) Grape juice | 21 adults with MCI (11 males), mean age 77 years (68–90) | Chronic (16-week) parallel groups (i) Control drink (ii) Grape juice (7.8 mL/kg/day) | The grape juice group showed significantly fewer word recognition interference errors and increased activation in cortical brain regions at follow-up. |

*(Continued)*

## TABLE 10.1 (*Continued*)
## Summary of Flavonoid Research Studies

| Authors | Participants | Design and Interventions | Key Findings |
|---|---|---|---|
| Mix & Crews (2000) Ginkgo | 48 adults (21 males) aged 55–86 years | Chronic (6-week) parallel groups (i) Control (ii) 180 mg/day Ginkgo | Significantly greater improvements in processing speed were observed for Ginkgo at follow-up relative to the control. |
| Mohamed et al. (2013) Ginkgo | 30 young healthy adults | Chronic (2-month) parallel groups (i) Control (ii) Catechin-rich leaf extract (50 mg/day) | Relative to the control group, the catechin group showed significantly improved short-term memory, processing speed and spatial visualisation at 2 months. |
| Pase et al. (2013) Polyphenol supplement | 72 adults (23 males), mean age 52 years (sd 8) | Acute and chronic (30-day) parallel groups (i) Control (ii) 250 mg polyphenols (iii) 500 mg polyphenols | No effects for cognitive function; however, after 30 days, the 500 mg dose was associated with significantly increased self-rated calmness and contentedness. |
| Pipingas et al. (2008) Polyphenol supplement | 42 males, mean age 58 (sd 4) | Chronic (5-week) parallel groups (i) Placebo (vitamin C) (ii) 960 mg Enzogenol/ day | Significantly faster spatial working memory and word recognition was observed following the polyphenol supplement. |
| Remington et al. (2010) Apple juice | 21 adults with Alzheimer's disease, mean age 82 years (sd 5) | Chronic (1 month) One glass of apple juice 24 oz/day (United States) (No control) | No change in scores on the Dementia Rating Scale 2 was observed between baseline and follow-up; however, mood scores improved significantly at follow-up. |
| Ryan et al. (2008) Polyphenol extract | 101 adults (46 males), mean age 69 years (sd 6) | Chronic (3-month) parallel groups (i) Control (ii) 150 mg flavonoids per day (Pycnogenol) | Significantly better spatial working memory was observed for the supplement group at 3-month follow-up. |
| Scholey et al. (2010) Cocoa | 30 adults (13 males), mean age 22 years (sd 1) | Acute crossover (i) Control drink (46 mg flavanol cocoa) (ii) 520 mg flavanol cocoa drink (iii) 994 mg cocoa drink | Significantly better working memory was observed following the 520 and 994 mg cocoa drinks relative to the 46 mg control. In addition, the 994 mg drink significantly improved attention. |

(*Continued*)

**TABLE 10.1 (*Continued*)**
**Summary of Flavonoid Research Studies**

| Authors | Participants | Design and Interventions | Key Findings |
|---|---|---|---|
| Watson et al. (2012) Berry extract *Abstract only* | 35 young adults | Acute crossover (i) Control (ii) Powdered berry extract (521 mg/60 kg) (iii) Juiced berry extract (528 mg/60 kg) | Both berry extract improved attention relative to the control. The powdered extract increased attention accuracy, whilst the juiced extract improved reaction times during an attention task. |
| Whyte & Williams (2012) Blueberry | 24 children aged 7–9 years (10 males) | Acute crossover (i) Control (ii) 126.5 mg flavonoid blueberry drink (iii) 253 mg flavonoid blueberry drink | Significantly improved immediate recall, delayed recall and attention were observed following the 253 mg drink relative to the control. Benefits for recall were also observed following the 126.5 mg drink relative to the control. |
| Whyte & Williams (2014) Blueberry | 14 children aged 8–9 years (11 males) | Acute crossover (i) Control (ii) Blueberry drink | The flavonoid-rich blueberry drink was associated with significantly improved delayed verbal recall; however, in contrast, greater proactive interference was observed following the blueberry drink. |

LF, low flavonoid; HF, high flavonoid; sd, standard deviation; MCI, mild cognitive impairment.

plasma metabolite concentration following flavanone-rich orange juice consumption occurs approximately 6 h post ingestion (Mullen et al., 2008). This raises the intriguing possibility that consuming a variety of flavonoids simultaneously may induce cumulative cognitive benefits over a prolonged time course, and to this end, the individual and synergistic effects of different flavonoid subclasses should be systematically examined.

The evidence reviewed in this chapter has concentrated on juice and cocoa interventions which are the most commonly studied flavonoids in humans to date (notwithstanding isoflavones which have not been included here due to the confounds which arise from oestrogen effects). This may be because juices and cocoa are easily available, palatable, naturally rich sources of flavonoids. It is also important that the effects of other sources are examined. For example, there is a distinct absence of interventions with flavonoid-rich vegetables, yet epidemiological data suggest strong links between vegetable consumption over the lifespan and beneficial cognitive outcomes (Lamport et al., 2014). Conversely, there needs to be greater consideration of juice-based flavonoids in epidemiological research (see Chapter 2). A recent review of fruits, vegetables, juices and cognitive function indicated that there are only two epidemiological studies which show cognitive benefits following chronic juice consumption (Dai et al., 2006; Nurk et al., 2010), whilst one study reported no relationship (Nooyens et al., 2011). Further examination of vegetable-based flavonoids may shed light on whether the cognitive benefits are specific to the flavonoids in certain food groups or whether flavonoids per se may enhance cognition when present in any food or drink. With this in mind, future interventions should examine the effects of pure flavonoid consumption possibly in capsulated form and consider the possibility of adding pure flavonoid compounds to a variety of different foods and drinks to artificially enhance the flavonoid concentration. Furthermore, this allows an investigation of the hypothesis that a dose–response relationship may exist between quantity of flavonoid consumption and cognitive benefits. This has been observed in epidemiological trials (e.g. Devore et al., 2012) although it is unclear whether the observed benefits plateau above a certain level of consumption or whether a threshold dose exists at which effects become discernible. This will depend on the proposed mechanisms by which flavonoids may affect cognitive function (see Section 10.4). Interestingly, a recent review of the polyphenol literature concluded that there is currently very little evidence for a relationship between dose, duration of intervention and cognitive outcomes predominantly due to the lack of systematic examination of this hypothesis (Lamport et al., 2012). Therefore, future intervention studies which follow a randomised, placebo-controlled, double-blind design should systematically investigate acute effects of a range of flavonoid doses on cognitive, physiological and metabolic outcomes.

It is evident that the majority of flavonoid interventions have been conducted in older adults (aged 60+ years). This is not surprising given that western nations are experiencing an increasingly ageing population and a concomitant increase in ageing-related neuropsychological disorders such as dementia and Alzheimer's disease. It is essential that future epidemiological and acute intervention studies continue to examine the benefits of flavonoid consumption for cognitive health in ageing, but we also need to examine whether flavonoid-based dietary interventions are effective for improving cognition in those who are healthy and young. This will ultimately provide a clearer picture of how specific flavonoids affect cognitive function at specific points over the lifespan ranging from the developing brain to the elderly brain. One approach that has not been considered is examining cognitive function in those who are malnourished. It would be of interest to examine whether flavonoid treatment could reverse any cognitive decrements associated with malnourishment and indeed whether an absence of flavonoids in the diet is associated with cognitive impairments. It would be challenging to identify whether cognitive decrements are due to LF intake or an absence of vitamins, minerals and other nutrients which are likely to be reduced in a malnourished population. Assessment of biomarkers and plasma metabolites in such interventions would be essential to provide a stronger case for a cause–effect relationship between flavonoids and cognitive function.

In summary, future intervention studies in this field should adopt the gold standard approach recognised and adopted by clinical trials: the randomised, double-blind, placebo-controlled design. Brain imaging technology should be utilised, and assessment of biomarkers and plasma flavonoid metabolites should be assessed concomitantly with cognitive function in order to further our understanding of the underlying mechanisms of different flavonoid subclasses. The individual and synergistic cognitive effects of specific flavonoid subclasses should be investigated given that they are digested and metabolised at different rates. There is clearly potential for designing foods and drinks which are enriched with flavonoids, but as of yet, it is unknown whether artificially enhancing the flavonoid content of a product will lead to cognitive benefits which are directly associated with the size of the flavonoid dose.

## TOP 5 SUMMARY POINTS FROM THIS CHAPTER

- There is good evidence that interventions with flavonoids and flavonoid-rich foods are associated with cognitive benefits.
- Eighteen of the 26 interventions (69%) reported in this chapter show significant cognitive benefits following flavonoid consumption.
- There is a large degree of methodological inconsistency within the field which limits comparisons between studies.
- Further work in humans is required to understand the acute and enduring mechanisms by which flavonoid consumption can lead to cognitive benefits.
- Future studies should aim to adopt a randomised, placebo-controlled, double-blind, crossover (or parallel-group) design and carefully document cognitive test procedures.

## WHAT'S UNDER DEBATE?

- What are the mechanisms that underlie the relationship between flavonoid consumption and cognitive function?
- Has research identified a dose–response relationship between flavonoid consumption and cognitive function?
- What methodological limitations are evident in the flavonoid research to date?
- Are flavonoids particularly beneficial for specific populations, for example, adults with MCI, or are cognitive improvements observed equally across the lifespan?
- What are the key points to consider when designing a flavonoid intervention study in humans?

## TOP 5 METHODOLOGICAL RECOMMENDATIONS

- Select appropriate, reliable cognitive tests which are known to be sensitive to the flavonoid intervention.
- Adopt a gold standard randomised, placebo-controlled, double-blind, cross-over (or parallel-group) design.
- Design an appropriate placebo which is matched for nutrients, macronutrients and psychological characteristics such as palatability and satiety.
- Assess habitual dietary intake of flavonoids in as much detail as possible at baseline and follow-up, and when adopting a crossover design, ensure that the washout period is of suitable duration.
- Assess the bioavailability of the flavonoids and their metabolites with urine and blood plasma samples.

# REFERENCES

Beking, K., & Vieira, A. (2011). An assessment of dietary flavonoid intake in the UK and Ireland. *International Journal of Food Sciences, 62*(1), 17–19.

Bondonno, C. P., Downey, L. A., Croft, K. D., Scholey, A., Stough, C., Yang, X., ... Hodgson, J. M. (2014). The acute effect of flavonoid-rich apples and nitrate-rich spinach on cognitive performance and mood in healthy men and women. *Food and Function, 5*, 849–858.

Camfield, D. A., Scholey, A., Pipingas, A., Silberstein, R., Kras, M., Nolidin, K., ... Stough, C. (2012). Steady state visually evoked potential (SSVEP) topography changes associated with cocoa flavanol consumption. *Physiology & Behaviour, 105*, 948–957.

Canter, P. H., & Ernst, E. (2007). *Ginkgo biloba* is not a smart drug: An updated systematic review of randomised clinical trials testing the nootropic effects of *G. biloba* extracts in healthy people. *Human Psychopharmacology: Clinical and Experimental, 22*(5), 265–278.

Colcombe, S., & Kramer, A. F. (2003). Fitness effects on the cognitive function of older adults: A meta-analytic study. *Psychological Science, 14*(2), 125–130.

Crews, W. D., Harrison, D. W., Griffin, M. L., Addison, K., Yount, A. M., Giovenco, M. A., & Hazell, J. (2005). A double-blinded, placebo-controlled, randomized trial of the neuropsychologic efficacy of cranberry juice in a sample of cognitively intact older adults: Pilot study findings. *The Journal of Alternative and Complementary Medicine, 11*(2), 305–309.

Crews, W. D., Harrison, D. W., & Wright, J. W. (2008). A double-blind, placebo-controlled, randomized trial of the effects of dark chocolate and cocoa on variables associated with neuropsychological functioning and cardiovascular health: Clinical findings from a sample of healthy, cognitively intact older adults. *American Journal of Clinical Nutrition, 87*, 872–880.

Dai, Q., Borenstein, A. R., Wu, Y., Jackson, J. C., & Larson, E. B. (2006). Fruit and vegetable juices and Alzheimer's disease: The Kame project. *Amercian Journal of Medicine, 119*(9), 751–759.

de Jager, C.A., Dye, L., de Bruin, E.A., Butler, L., Fletcher, J., Lamport, D.J., Latulippe, M.E., Spencer, J.P.E., & Wesnes, K. ( 2014). Criteria for validation and selection of cognitive tests for investigating the effects of foods and nutrients. *Nutrition Reviews, 72*, 162–179.

Desideri, G., Kwik-Uribe, C., Grassi, D., Necozione, S., Ghiadoni, L., Mastroiacovo, D., … Ferri, C. (2012). Benefits in cognitive function, blood pressure, and insulin resistance through cocoa flavanol consumption in elderly subjects with Mild Cognitive Impairment: The Cocoa, Cognition, and Aging (CoCoA) study. *Hypertension, 60*, 794–801.

Devore, E. E., Kang, J. H., Breteler, M. M. B., & Grodstein, F. (2012). Dietary intakes of berries and flavonoids in relation to cognitive decline. *Annals of Neurology, 72*(1), 135–143.

Dye, L., Lluch, A., & Blundell, J. E. (2000). Macronutrients and mental performance. *Nutrition, 16*(10), 1021–1034.

Field, D. T., Williams, C. M., & Butler, L. T. (2011). Consumption of cocoa flavanols results in acute improvement in visual and cognitive functions. *Physiology and Behaviour, 103*, 255–260.

Francis, S. T., Morris, P. G., & Macdonald, I. A. (2006). The effect of flavanol-rich cocoa on the fMRI response to a cognitive task in healthy young people. *Journal of Cardiovascular Pharmacology, 47*, S215–S220.

Halliwell, B. (2008). Are polyphenols antioxidants or pro-oxidants? What do we learn from cell culture and in vivo studies? *Archives of Biochemistry and Biophysics, 476*(2), 107–112.

Hendrickson, S. J., & Mattes, R. D. (2008). No acute effects of grape juice on appetite, implicit memory and mood. *Food and Nutrition Research, 52*, doi: 10.3402/fnr.v52i0.1891

How, P. S., Ellis, J. A., Spencer, J. P. E., & Williams, C. M. (2008). The impact of plant-derived flavonoids on mood, memory and motor skills in UK adults. *Appetite, 51*, 754.

Hoyland, A., Lawton, C. L., & Dye, L. (2008). Acute macronutrient manipulations on cognitive test performance in healthy young adults: A systematic research review. *Neuroscience and Biobehavioral Reviews, 31*(1), 72–85.

Ide, K., & Secher, N. H. (2000). Cerebral blood flow and metabolism during exercise. *Progress in Neurobiology, 61*(4), 397–414.

James, J. E., & Rogers, P. J. (2005). Effects of caffeine on performance and mood: Withdrawal reversal is the most plausible explanation. *Psychopharmacology, 182*, 1–8.

Kean, R. J., Lamport, D. J., Dodd, G. F., Freeman, J. E., Williams, C. M., Ellis, J. A., … Spencer, J. P. E. (2014). Chronic consumption of flavanone-rick orange juice is associated with cognitive benefits: An 8-week randomised double-blind placebo-controlled trial in healthy older adults. *American Journal of Clinical Nutrition*. doi:10.3945/ajcn.114.088518.

Kennedy, D. O., Scholey, A. B., & Wesnes, K. A. (2000). The dose-dependent cognitive effects of acute administration of *Ginkgo biloba* to healthy young volunteers. *Psychopharmachology, 151*, 416–423.

Krikorian, R., Boespflug, E. L., Fleck, D. E., Stein, A. L., Wightman, J. D., Shidler, M. D., & Sadat-Hossieny, S. (2012). Concord grape juice supplementation and neurocognitive function in human aging. *Journal of Agricultural and Food Chemistry, 60*(23), 5736–5742.

Krikorian, R., Nash, T. A., Shidler, M. D., Shukitt-Hale, B., & Joseph, J. A. (2010a). Concord grape juice supplementation improves memory function in older adults with mild cognitive impairment. *British Journal of Nutrition, 103*, 730–734.

Krikorian, R., Shidler, M. D., Nash, T. A., Kalt, W., Vinqvist-Tymchuk, M. R., Shukitt-Hale, B., & Joseph, J. A. (2010b). Blueberry supplementation improves memory in older adults. *Journal of Agricultural and Food Chemistry, 58*, 3996–4000.

Lamport, D. J., Dye, L., Wightman, J. D., & Lawton, C. L. (2012). The effects of flavonoid and other polyphenol consumption on cognitive performance: A systematic research review of human experimental and epidemiological studies. *Nutrition and Aging, 1*, 5–25.

Lamport, D. J., Saunders, C. Butler, L. T., & Spencer, J. P. E. (2014). Fruits, vegetables, 100% juices, and cognitive function: A critical review of the evidence. *Nutrition Reviews, 72*, 774–189.

Le Bars, P. L., Velasco, F. M., Ferguson, J. M., Dessain, E. C., Kieser, M., & Hoerr, R. (2002). Influence of the severity of cognitive impairment on the effect of the *Ginkgo biloba* extract EGb 761® in Alzheimer's disease. *Neuropsychobiology, 45*(1), 19–26.

Lee, Y.-B., Lee, H. J., & Sohn, H. S. (2005). Soy isoflavones and cognitive function. *The Journal of Nutritional Biochemistry, 16*(11), 641–649.

Letenneur, L., Proust-Lima, C., Le Gouge, A., Dartigues, J. F., & Barberger-Gateau, P. (2007). Flavonoid intake and cognitive decline over a 10 year period. *American Journal of Epidemiology, 165*(12), 1364–1371.

Luo, Y., Smith, J. V., Paramasivam, V., Burdick, A., Curry, K. J., Buford, J. P., ... Butko, P. (2002). Inhibition of amyloid-beta aggregation and capase-3 activation by the *Ginkgo biloba* extract EGb761. *Proceedings of the National Academy of Sciences of the USA, 99*(19), 12197–12202.

Macready, A. L., Kennedy, O. B., Ellis, J. A., Williams, C. M., Spencer, J. P. E., & Butler, L. T. (2009). Flavonoids and cognitive function: A review of human randomised controlled trial studies and recommendations for future studies. *Genes and Nutrition, 4*, 227–242.

Manach, C., Williamson, G., Morand, C., Scalbert, A., & Remesy, C. (2005). Bioavailability of polyphenols in humans. I. Review of 97 bioavailability studies. *American Journal of Clinical Nutrition, 81*, 230S–242S.

Mix, J. A., & Crews, W. D. (2000). An examination of the efficacy of *Ginkgo biloba* extract EGb 761 on the neuropsychological functioning of cognitively intact older adults. *The Journal of Alternative and Complementary Medicine: Research on Paradigm, Practice, and Policy, 6*(3), 219–229.

Mohamed, S., Lee, M. T., & Jaffri, J. M. (2013). Cognitive enhancement and neuroprotection by catechin-rich oil palm leaf extract supplement. *Journal of the Science of Food and Agriculture, 94*(4), 819–827.

Mullen, W., Archeveque, M.-A., Edwards, C. A., Matsumoto, H., & Crozier, A. (2008). Bioavailability and metabolism of orange juice flavanones in humans: Impact of a full-fat yoghurt. *Journal of Agricultural and Food Chemistry, 56*(23), 11157–11164.

Nagahama, Y., Nabatame, H., Okina, T., Yamauchi, H., Narita, M., Fujimoto, N., ... Matsuda, M. (2003). Cerebral correlates of the progression rate of the cognitive decline in probable Alzheimer's disease. *European Neurology, 50*(1), 1–9.

Neveu, V., Perez-Jimenez, J., Vos, F., Crespy, V., du Chaffaut, L., Mennen, L., ... Scalbert, A. (2010). Phenol-explorer: An online comprehensive database on polyphenol contents in foods. Database, doi: 10.1093/database/bap024

Nooyens, A. C. J., Bueno-de-Mesquita, H. B., van Boxtel, M. P. J., van Gelder, B. M., Verhagen, H., & Verschuren, M. (2011). Fruit and vegetable intake and cognitive decline in middle-aged men and women: The Doetinchem cohort study. *British Journal of Nutrition, 106*(5), 752–761.

Nurk, E., Refsum, H., Drevon, C. A., Tell, G. S, Nygaard, H. A., Engedal, K., & Smith, D. (2010). Cognitive performance among the elderly in relation to the intake of plant foods: The Hordaland health study. *British Journal of Nutrition, 104*(8), 1190–1201.

Ohab, J. J., Fleming, S., Blesch, A., & Carmichael, S. T. (2006). A neurovascular niche for neurogenesis after stroke. *The Journal of Neuroscience, 26*(50), 13007–13016.

Pase, M. P., Scholey, A. B., Pipingas, A., Kras, M., Nolidin, K., Gibbs, A., ... Stough, C. K. (2013). Cocoa polyphenols enhance positive mood states but not cognitive performance: A randomised, placebo-controlled trial. *Journal of Psychopharmacology, 27*(5), 451–458.

Pipingas, A., Silberstein, R. B., Vitetta, L., Van Rooy, C., Harris, E. V., Young, J. M., ... Nastasi, J. (2008). Improved cognitive performance after dietary supplementation with a pinus radiate bark extract formulation. *Phytotherapy Research, 22*, 1168–1174.

Remington, R., Chan, A., Lepore, A., Kotlya, E., & Shea, T. B. (2010). Apple juice improved behavioural but not cognitive symptoms in moderate-to-late stage Alzheimer's disease in an open-label pilot study. *American Journal of Alzheimer's Disease and Other Dementias, 25*(4), 367–371.

Rendeiro, C., Foley, A., Lau, V. C., Ring, R., Rodriguez-Mateos, A., Vauzour, D., ... Spencer, J. P. E. (2014). A role for hippocampal PSA-NCAM and NMDA-NR2B receptor function in flavonoid-induced spatial memory improvements in young rats. *Neuropharmacology, 79*, 335–44.

Rendeiro, C., Vauzour, D., Rattray, M., Waffo-Teguo, P., Merillonm, J. M., Butler, L. T., ... Spencer, J. P. E. (2013). Dietary levels of pure flavonoids improve spatial memory performance and increase hippocampal brain derived neurotrophic factor. *PLoS One, 8*(5), e63535

Ryan, J., Croft, K., Mori, T., Wesnes, K., Spong, J., Downey, L., ... Stough, C. (2008). An examination of the effects of the antioxidant Pycnogenol on cognitive performance, serum lipid profile, endocrinological and oxidate stress biomarkers in an elderly population. *Journal of Psychopharmacology, 22*(5), 553–562.

Saunders, C. (2010). Cocoa flavonols and their effects on cognitive function and risk factors for Alzheimer's disease. PhD thesis, University of Reading, Reading, MA.

Scholey, A., & Owen, L. (2013). Effects of chocolate on cognitive function and mood: A systematic review. *Nutrition Reviews, 71*(10), 665–681.

Scholey, A. B., French, S. J., Morris, J. P., Kennedy, D. O., Milne, A. L., & Haskell, C. F. (2010). Consumption of cocoa flavanols results in acute improvements in mood and cognitive performance during sustained mental effort. *Journal of Psychopharmacology, 24*(10), 1505–1514.

Schroeter, H., Heiss, C., Balzer, J., Kleinbongard, P., Keen, C. L., Hollenberg, N. K., ... Kelm, M. (2006). (-)-Epicatechin mediates beneficial effects of flavanol-rich cocoa on vascular function in humans. *Proceedings of the National Academy of Sciences of the USA, 106*, 1024–1029.

Shukitt-Hale, B., Lau, F.C., Carey, A.N., Galli, R.L., Spangler, E.L., Ingram, D.K., & Joseph, J.A. (2008). Blueberry polyphenols attenuate kainic acid-induced decrements in cognition and alter inflammatory gene expression in rat hippocampus. *Nutritional Neuroscience, 11*, 172–182.

Sorond, F. A., Lipsitz, L. A., Hollenberg, N. K., & Fisher, N. D. L. (2008). Cerebral blood flow response to flavanol-rich cocoa in healthy elderly humans. *Neuropsychiatric Disease and Treatment, 4*(2), 433–440.

Spencer, J. P. E. (2009). Flavonoids and brain health: Multiple effects underpinned by common mechanisms. *Genes and Nutrition, 4*, 243–250.

Spencer, J. P. E. (2010). Beyond antioxidants: The cellular and molecular interactions of flavonoids and how these underpin their actions on the brain. *Proceedings of the Nutrition Society, 69*, 244–260.

Taubert, D., Roesen, R., Lehmann, C., Jung, N., & Schomig, E. (2007). Effects of low habitual cocoa intake on blood pressure and bioactive nitric oxide: A randomised controlled trial. *Journal of the American Medical Association, 287*, 2212–2213.

Toda, N., Ayajiki, K., & Okamura, T. (2009). Cerebral blood flow regulation by nitric oxide: Recent advances. *Pharmacological Reviews, 61*, 62–97.

Vauzour, D., Rodriguez-Mateos, A., Corona, G., Oruna-Concha, M. J., & Spencer, J. P. E. (2010). Polyphenols and human health: Prevention of disease and mechanisms of action. *Nutrients, 2*(11), 1106–1131.

Watson, A. W., Kennedy, D. O., Haskell, C. F., & Scheepens, A. (2012). A double blind placebo controlled study measuring the effect of two berry fruit extracts on mood, cognition and monamine oxidase B inhibition in healthy young adults. *Appetite, 59*(2), 636.

Whyte, A. R., & Williams, C. M. (2012). The cognitive effects of acute blueberry anthocyanin interventions on 7–9 year old children. *Appetite, 59*, 637.

Whyte, A. R., & Williams, C. M. (2014). A pilot study investigating the effects of a single dose of flavonoid-rich blueberry drink on memory in 8–10 year old children. *Nutrition, 31*(3), 531–534. doi: 10.1016/j.nut.2014.09.013

Williams, C.M., El Mohsen, M.A., Vazour, D., Rendeiro, C., Butler, L.T., Ellis, J.A., Whiteman, M., & Spencer, J.P.E. (2008). Blueberry-induced changes in spatial working memory correlate with changes in hippocampal CREB phosphorylation and brain-derived neurotrophic factor (BDNF) levels. *Free Radical Biology and Medicine, 45*, 295–305.

# Section IV

## Technology and Brain Function

# 11 Using Technology to Improve Cognitive Function

## Fact or Fiction?

*Wei-Peng Teo*

## CONTENTS

## SUMMARY

In the last two decades, the advent of noninvasive brain stimulation (NBS) techniques has allowed us to systematically study the functionality of various brain regions in great detail. NBS methods such as transcranial magnetic stimulation (TMS) and transcranial direct current stimulation (tDCS) not only can function as a tool to establish the interconnectivity of different brain networks (i.e. cognitive, motor, executive and inter-hemispheric) but can also be used as an interventional non-pharmacological means of treating various mental health and neurological disorders. The mechanism of action of NBS is centred on modulating neurophysiological processes that underpin brain plasticity, which is vital for the brain to adapt to the external environment (i.e. learning), injury or disease. The effects of TMS and tDCS are thought to primarily act upon the release of excitatory and inhibitory neurotransmitters at the synaptic junction and the polarity of the neuronal membrane that ultimately impacts upon the strength of communication between neurons. Particularly intriguing is that the neuro-modulatory effects of TMS and tDCS may outlast the period of stimulation. Thus NBS techniques have the potential as adjunctive or stand-alone treatments for various mental health and neurological conditions. This chapter provides an overview of the history and evidence regarding the use of NBS to measure brain function and will explore the interventional effects of NBS on cognition in healthy and clinical populations. Lastly, this chapter will discuss the strengths and limitations of current NBS systems and the potential for combining micronutrients (using the example of caffeine) and NBS to improve cognitive function.

## 11.1   WHAT IS NBS?

There is often a pervading misconception surrounding the term *brain stimulation*. In the past, particularly from the 1950s to 1970s, brain stimulation was synonymous with the treatment of mental illnesses such as severe depression, psychotic illnesses and bipolar disorders that were resistant to drug therapy. In particular, electroconvulsive therapy (ECT), for many people, conjures up images of the 1975 movie 'One Flew Over the Cuckoo's Nest', with Jack Nicholson thrashing about, forced against his will to endure painful, violent seizures. Today, however, modern-day ECT is a far cry from the old methods that earned its sinister reputation. Despite the stigma attached to ECT, better understanding of electrophysiology and electromagnetism in the mid-1980s saw the emergence of a separate branch of brain stimulation techniques known as NBS. As the name implies, NBS is a form of painless and noninvasive stimulation technique that is performed with the participant fully awake and seated comfortably in a chair. Fundamentally, the mechanisms underlying NBS differs from ECT. Whilst ECT consists of inducing convulsive activity, NBS induces physiological changes to brain function by influencing the release of excitatory and inhibitory neurotransmitter at the synaptic junction that alters the strength of communication between neurons. NBS, unlike ECT, causes no memory disturbances or loss of consciousness; neither does it require sedation or muscle relaxants. There are two common forms of NBS, albeit other variants have since been developed based on these two forms: (1) TMS and (2) tDCS. The purpose of this chapter is therefore to provide readers with an introduction and overview to the world of NBS and how it can be used to study cognition and brain health in both healthy and clinical populations. This chapter will be divided into three main areas of focus:

1. Provide a brief historical background of the evolution of NBS and the mechanisms of action associated with TMS and tDCS.
2. Highlight the uses of NBS as a method for probing cognitive and executive functions of the brain, and review its use as a rehabilitative tool in cognitive-impaired populations.
3. Discuss the strengths, limitations and future direction of NBS techniques for clinical application.

Advancements in neurophysiological techniques and electromagnetic technology over the last two decades have allowed scientists to systematically investigate the different functions of the central nervous system (CNS – consisting of the brain and spinal cord). Various techniques have been developed that generate low-intensity electric currents within the CNS to influence neuronal activity, cognition and behaviour (Wagner et al., 2007b). TMS has become a standard stimulation technique for the noninvasive exploration of cognitive function, whereby neurons are stimulated using the principles of electromagnetic induction to activate or inhibit specific regions of the brain (Ziemann, 2010). When TMS currents are applied with the appropriate pulse frequency, duration and intensity, a neuro-modulatory effect is induced by which neural function and behaviour are altered during (online) and after (offline) the stimulation period (Hallett, 2007; Thickbroom, 2007). Due to this multifunctional role that TMS can offer (i.e. as a diagnostic and intervention tool), it has become the equipment of choice for many neuroscientists who wish to study the mechanisms of cognitive and executive functions in the brain.

Similar to TMS, the use of tDCS in recent years has received great attention (Nitsche et al., 2008; Tanaka & Watanabe, 2009). Historically, the use of direct currents (DCs) to treat various ailments such as psychiatric disorders and pain has been widely documented (refer to Section 11.2); however, the development of ECT and psychotropic medications in the mid-1900s hindered the development of tDCS. However, seminal studies at the turn of the century demonstrated that weak, direct electric currents could be delivered effectively and safely to either increase or inhibit brain activity depending on the stimulation polarity used (anodal/positive tDCS, increases brain excitability; cathodal/negative tDCS, inhibits brain excitability) (Nitsche & Paulus, 2000; Priori et al., 1998).

Due to this inherent ability to modulate brain function, several studies have shown that tDCS induces specific changes in psychological, physiological and motor activity by targeting different brain areas (Bikson et al., 2009; Miranda et al., 2006; Wagner et al., 2007a). This has sparked an increase in clinical studies using tDCS particularly for, but not limited to, neuropsychiatric disorders such as severe mood disorders (Fregni et al., 2006; Nitsche, 2002), chronic and acute pain (Knotkova & Cruciani, 2010; O'Connell et al., 2013), stroke rehabilitation (Schlaug & Renga, 2008; Schlaug et al., 2008) and addiction (Fecteau et al., 2007; Fraser & Rosen, 2012). Moreover, tDCS has appealing characteristics over TMS such as, for most people, it is well tolerated, not associated with adverse effects, relatively cheap, portable and easy to set up.

## 11.2   BRIEF HISTORICAL BACKGROUND OF BRAIN STIMULATION

The first reference of the use of electricity to alter brain function can be found in literature from almost 2000 years ago (Ceccarelli, 1962). Between AD 43 and 48, Scribonius Largus, a Roman physician, observed that placing a torpedo fish (a species of electric ray) on the scalp of patients with headaches elicited a state of transient stupor that provided pain relief. He soon realised that the benefits to the patient were due to the numbness and narcotic effect induced by the electric ray. Similarly, other reports of pain relief using the torpedo fish were documented by Gaius Plinius Secundus (AD 23–79), also known as Pliny the Elder, and the Greek physician Claudius Galen (AD 131–401) (Kellaway, 1946). Reference made by Ibn Sidah (AD 1007–1066), a Muslim physician, further suggested that a live electric catfish on the frontal bone of the skull might treat patients with epilepsy (Kellaway, 1946).

Building on the work of Scribonius Largus and his contemporaries, it was the systematic study of the torpedo fish with modern scientific methods (Walsh, 1773) and the work of Italian physician Luigi Galvani (Bresadola, 1998; de Micheli, 1991) and physicist Alessandro Volta (Pancaldi, 2003) that led to a greater understanding of electro-neurophysiology. Galvani's nephew, Giovanni Aldini, was one of the first to report the successful treatment of patients suffering from melancholia (a mood disorder of nonspecific depression) by applying DC over the head. He also assessed the effects of DC applied to himself and reported an unpleasant sensation followed by insomnia for several days (Aldini, 1804). Although these early observations used extremely variable procedures and only qualitative clinical description, a consistent finding was the opposite effect induced by reversing stimulating polarities (further discussed in the subsequent section).

## 11.3   MECHANISM OF ACTION UNDERLYING TMS AND tDCS

### 11.3.1   TMS

The earliest attempts to study CNS function and its involvement in motor performance were performed using open surgery on animals (Adrian & Moruzzi, 1939; Patton & Amassian, 1954). These studies involved removing the skull so that electrodes could be placed directly over the exposed brain region(s) to be stimulated. A major drawback to this approach was that it is highly invasive and produced profound perturbations to the brain. Merton and Morton (1980) were the first to successfully use transcranial electrical stimulation (TES) to stimulate the primary motor cortex (part of the brain that controls movement) without removing the scalp. The procedure involved placing two electrodes over the scalp and using a high-voltage current bypassing the skull to induce weak electrical currents in the superficial layers of the brain. Although successful, the procedure proved to be very uncomfortable to the subject due to the localised pain and contraction of the scalp muscles caused by the electric currents. It was not until 5 years later that Barker and colleagues

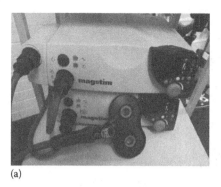
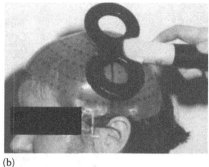

(a)                                                    (b)

**FIGURE 11.1**   An example of (a) setup of two transcranial magnetic stimulators positioned on top of each other to deliver paired-pulsed TMS and (b) stimulation of the primary motor cortex using a figure-of-eight coil.

(1985) used Faraday's principle of magnetic induction to safely and painlessly deliver electrical stimulations across the scalp and skull (refer to Figure 11.1).

According to Faraday's principle of electromagnetic induction, a changing magnetic field will induce an electrical current in a nearby circuit (Halliday et al., 2002). In TMS, a high-current pulse is produced in a magnetic coil of wires that is placed tangentially across the scalp. The magnetic fields produced by the coil generate fluxes that run perpendicular to the field. The rapidly changing magnetic fields induce a secondary loop of electrical current, which travels parallel to the plane of the coil. This brief electric current evoke pulses in the brain, which can trigger action potentials in cortical neurons, particularly those found within superficial areas of the cerebral cortex.

## 11.3.2   tDCS

tDCS differs from TES or TMS such that it does not induce neuronal firing, but rather modulate spontaneous neuronal network activity (Nitsche et al., 2008; Priori et al., 2009). At the neuronal level, the primary mechanism of action for tDCS is a polarity-dependent change (polarisation) in resting membrane potential. Specifically, positive anodal tDCS increases neuronal excitability, whereas negative cathodal tDCS suppresses neuronal excitability. It is this primary polarisation mechanism that underlies the acute effects of low-intensity DC stimulation on neuronal excitability in humans (see Figure 11.2).

However, tDCS also elicits after-effects that can last for up to 1 h following a session of stimulation (Nitsche et al., 2003b; Nitsche & Paulus, 2001). Thus, mechanisms of action cannot be solely attributed to changes in resting membrane potential. In fact, studies have showed that tDCS also influences the microenvironment at the synaptic junction (connection between neurons and other tissues) by modulating NMDA receptor (a glutamate receptor) activity or altering GABAergic activities (Liebetanz et al., 2002; Nitsche et al., 2003a; Stagg et al., 2009). Both glutamate and GABA have been suggested as the predominant neurotransmitters that are responsible for controlling overall plasticity of the brain (Myhrer, 2003).

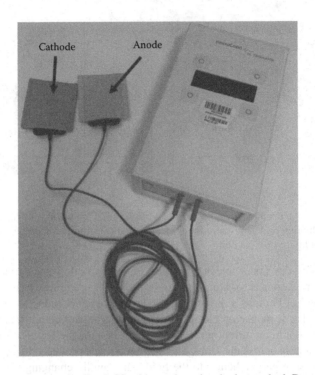

**FIGURE 11.2** An example of a tDCS with anode and cathode attached. Depending on the intended stimulation outcome, cathodal stimulation of the intended site of stimulation inhibits neuronal activity, whilst anodal stimulation is used to increase neuronal excitability. The anode and cathode may be placed on different areas of the scalp to target specific superficial regions of the brain.

## 11.4 USING NBS TO STUDY BRAIN FUNCTION

To date, there has been a plethora of TMS and tDCS studies ranging from investigating relationships between different brain regions (i.e. inter- vs. intra-hemispheric interactions) to assessing brain function associated with various neurological and mental health conditions. In this section, functional differences between NBS and neuroimaging techniques (see Camfield and Scholey, Chapter 12, for details of neuroimaging techniques) and the interpretation of TMS measures (i.e. what do these measures tell us?) for application to brain health will be discussed.

### 11.4.1 MEASURES FROM NBS: WHAT DO THEY REPRESENT?

As described previously in Section 11.1, TMS and tDCS differ in terms of the underlying mechanism of action and its application. Functionally, TMS systems can operate as either a diagnostic or an interventional tool, whilst tDCS is primarily used for interventional purposes. However, it is not uncommon to find TMS being used in conjunction with tDCS to measure any neurophysiological changes associated with tDCS interventions. This section will focus on the use of TMS as a diagnostic tool to measure changes in brain function, and the common measures used to assess CNS functionality will be discussed. As a diagnostic tool, TMS can provide information about the status of the CNS by measuring the level of excitation and/or inhibition of neurons using various TMS paradigms. The four most common TMS measures are (1) motor threshold, (2) central motor conduction time, (3) intra-cortical inhibition/facilitation and (4) cortical silent period, of which a combination of these measures can provide an overview of the relative integrity and functional status of the CNS. The four common outcome measures of TMS are described as follows:

1. *Resting motor threshold*: Resting motor threshold is defined as the least amount of single-pulse TMS intensity that is required to elicit a small visible physical response or an electromyographic (EMG) recording of 0.05–0.1 mV in a targeted muscle that forms the basic measure of TMS. It is thought to reflect the membrane excitability of neurons within the brain as well as the excitability of the spinal tract and motor neurons innervating the target muscle (Ziemann, 2004). The EMG response is a single-pulse TMS known as a motor-evoked potential (MEP) and is usually recorded by stimulating the primary motor cortex and measuring the EMG activity of the corresponding muscle. For example, stimulating the hand representation on the primary motor cortex will result in a physical activation of the muscles controlling the hand (refer to Figure 11.3). An increase in the size of MEP at resting motor threshold, or a reduction in the TMS stimulus intensity required to elicit motor threshold, indicates an overall increase in

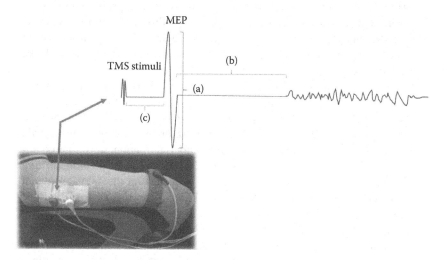

**FIGURE 11.3**   An illustration of an MEP recording collected via EMG electrodes from the wrist extensor muscle. The MEP recording shows the (a) MEP amplitude, (b) cortical silent period and (c) central motor conduction time. Changes in the size/amplitude of MEP indicate a change in excitability of the CNS, whilst change in the duration/length of cortical silent period is indicative of inhibitory changes in the brain particularly that of $GABA_B$. Central motor conduction time remains generally unaffected in most pathologies, unless the structural integrity of the CNS is affected.

the excitability of the CNS. In most, if not all, TMS studies, stimulation of the primary motor cortex to measure resting motor threshold is used as a surrogate measure for brain excitability as the outputs (i.e. EMG responses) are easily recorded compared to any other areas of the brain. For example, in patients with structural damage/lesions to the CNS (i.e. stroke, brain and spinal cord injury), it is common to observe higher motor thresholds (*less brain excitability*) relative to healthy age-matched controls (Bashir et al., 2012; Foltys et al., 2003; Pennisi et al., 2002). However, lower motor thresholds (*greater brain excitability*) are also synonymous with neurological conditions such as, but not limited to, Alzheimer's (AD) and Parkinson's disease (PD) where the production of inhibitory neurotransmitters may be impaired (Berardelli et al., 1996; Di Lazzaro et al., 2004; Hoeppner et al., 2012; Ueki et al., 2006).

2. *Central motor conduction time*: Central motor conduction time refers to the time between activating a TMS stimulus and the recording of an EMG response in the muscle (refer to Figure 11.3). The central motor conduction time provides an indication of the speed in which an action potential travels along the cortical motor pathway before activating the intended muscle. Prolongation of central motor conduction time often occurs due to the slowing of conduction that is associated with demyelinating diseases (i.e. multiple sclerosis), amyotrophic lateral sclerosis, structural lesions to the brain such as stroke, and neurodegenerative disorders that result in structural damage of the neurons (Kidd et al., 1998; Shimizu et al., 2001). As central motor conduction time is almost always prolonged in these neurological conditions, clinicians often use this measure in diagnostic assessments. It is also used as a prognostic marker for some neurological conditions, such as myelopathy and multiple sclerosis (Kidd et al., 1998; Nakamae et al., 2010).

3. *Short intra-cortical inhibition and facilitation*: Short intra-cortical inhibition and facilitation are obtained with paired-pulse TMS (*two successive TMS pulses separated by a rapid inter-pulse interval*) and are a reflection of interneuron influences in the brain (Di Lazzaro et al., 2006; Kujirai et al., 1993). To elicit short intra-cortical inhibition/facilitation, an initial conditioning stimulus is given (*strong enough to activate neurons of the brain*), but small enough so that no descending influence on the spinal cord can be detected in which no MEP is produced (*sub-threshold*). A second test stimulus, at a supra-threshold level, is delivered at a short interval. The outcome is that the intra-cortical influences initiated by the conditioning (*first*) stimulus affects the amplitude of the MEP produced by the test stimulus. At very short intervals, less than 5 ms, there is inhibition of the test stimulus MEP, and at intervals between 8 and 30 ms, there is facilitation (refer to Figure 11.4). The elicitation of SICI is attributed to a GABAergic effect, specifically the inhibitory neurotransmitter – $GABA_A$ – by which the short inter-pulse interval (<5 ms) of paired-pulse TMS is thought to facilitate the release of $GABA_A$ at the synaptic junction (DiLazzaro et al., 2000; Kujirai et al., 1993).

(a)                          (b)                          (c)

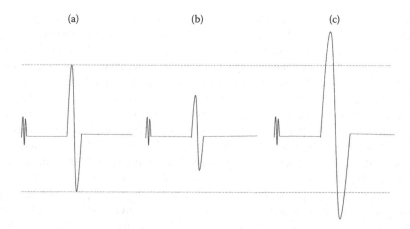

**FIGURE 11.4** An illustration of an MEP recording following (a) single-pulse TMS and (b and c) paired-pulse TMS. Short-interval intra-cortical inhibition is produced by applying a preceding sub-threshold TMS stimulus followed by a supra-threshold stimulus separated by 1–8 ms inter-pulse interval. Similarly, intra-cortical facilitation is produced by applying a preceding sub-threshold TMS stimulus followed by a supra-threshold stimulus separated by 8–30 ms inter-pulse interval.

4. *Cortical silent period*: A cortical silent period refers to a period of no EMG activity following TMS during a tonic muscle contraction (refer to Figure 11.3). The cortical silent period is believed to be mediated by the neurotransmitter $GABA_B$ and represents different aspects of cortical inhibition. Patients with amyotrophic lateral sclerosis and PD and AD often have shortened duration of silent periods due to a lack in intra-cortical inhibition that can be reversed by anti-glutamatergic, cholinergic or dopaminergic medication (Khedr et al., 2011; Siciliano et al., 1999; Van Der Werf et al., 2007).

## 11.4.2 Combining NBS with Neuroimaging Techniques

Whilst the use of NBS techniques has greatly enhanced our understanding of how the brain works, it still does not provide a complete picture of the causal relationships between activation of different brain regions and its associated behavioural outcomes. To fully comprehend the relationship between neurophysiological changes and how it affects behavioural measures (i.e. cognitive and motor), NBS techniques can be paired with existing neuroimaging techniques. For example, functional magnetic resonance imaging (fMRI), electroencephalography (EEG), near-infrared spectroscopy (NIRS) and positron-emission tomography (PET) can be combined with NBS to illustrate cause-and-effect relationships and determine how other interconnected networks of the brain are involved in a specific outcome. For example, a simple finger-tapping task by the left hand is controlled largely by the right contralateral motor cortex. The involvement of the right primary motor cortex is verified because when TMS is applied to the right-hand representation of the motor cortex, it disrupts the tapping movement performed by the left hand. However, there are other associated motor areas of the brain, such as those involved in movement speed, amplitude and rhythm of the finger-tapping task that are just as likely to be activated during the finger-tapping action that cannot be targeted using TMS. Consequently, a combination of NBS and neuroimaging techniques is necessary to provide a global picture of the different motor networks working in sync to produce a smooth and uninterrupted finger-tapping action. The benefits of using neuroimaging techniques are that they provide for greater spatial resolution (i.e. investigating larger areas of the brain) whilst TMS provides better focal, temporal resolution (i.e. understanding the function of specific neurons at a specific time point). Both forms of investigative techniques are therefore highly complementary and are useful in characterising functional changes in the brain that are associated with disease or injury.

For example, a synchronised TMS and functional imaging measurement can answer several methodological questions concerning neurophysiological effects and their dependence on the different TMS stimulation parameters. One of the earliest attempts to correlate TMS changes with neuroimaging measures was performed by Bohning et al. (1999). In this study, changes in blood–oxygen level–dependent (BOLD) signal was measured with fMRI, in local and remote brain areas, associated with varying intensities of TMS. Specifically, the left primary motor cortex of seven healthy subjects was stimulated with a figure-of-eight coil at two different intensities (110% motor threshold vs. 80% of the motor threshold) whilst simultaneously acquiring fMRI images. The higher intensity TMS led to a greater activation of BOLD signals in the primary motor cortex in comparison to lower intensity TMS. In addition, higher intensity TMS showed a greater level of activation at the local stimulation sites. To confirm the direction of the findings, Bohning and colleagues (2000) compared TMS-induced finger movements to voluntary finger movements of a similar movement pattern and found similar concomitant increase in BOLD signals as the speed of the finger movement increased. These data suggest that activation of cortical brain areas via TMS is similar to natural volitional brain activation and support the use of TMS to investigate normal and abnormal cortical processes. In a separate study, Baudewig et al. (2001) combined repetitive TMS (rTMS) and fMRI to investigate the direct effects of rTMS over both motor cortices. Specifically, they investigated the differences between voluntary and rTMS-induced finger movements and systematically compared the effects of sub-threshold and supra-threshold rTMS. They observed BOLD signal changes in the primary motor cortex only either when the subjects voluntarily performed a real finger movement or when a finger movement was induced by supra-threshold rTMS over the contralateral primary motor cortex. Neither sub-threshold rTMS over the primary motor cortex nor supra-threshold rTMS over the lateral premotor cortex resulted in respective BOLD signal changes in the primary motor cortex.

In another example, by combining TMS with PET, Paus et al. (1997) revealed a dose-dependent (number of TMS pulses) effect of TMS stimulation, that is, an increase of cerebral blood flow followed by high-frequency stimulation over the visual cortex at the stimulation site and, paradoxically, a dose-dependent decrease in regional cerebral blood flow after high-frequency TMS over the motor cortex (Paus et al., 1998). These results by Paus and colleagues suggest not only that TMS has different neurophysiological effects that depend on the stimulation parameters but that these different effects (e.g. excitatory vs. inhibitory) might differ between different regions of the brain. Baudewig and Paus and colleagues performed one of the first studies to illustrate the use of neuroimaging such as fMRI and PET and NBS techniques to answer fundamental questions about how the brain works and the interconnected relationship between different brain regions.

## 11.5 NBS AS A REHABILITATIVE TO IMPROVE BRAIN FUNCTION

The use of NBS interventions as a form of treatment clinical populations has gained increasing popularity over the last two decades. Initially driven by psychiatric applications and modelled on the effectiveness of ECT, there is increasing interest in how neuro-modulation by NBS might be extended to impairments in mental and cognitive health and neurological disorders. Whilst there is strong evidence for brain plasticity and the underlying mechanisms of mental health and neurological disorders (Cheetham & Finnerty, 2007; Peled, 2005), the relationship between using NBS to alter brain plasticity to elicit the desired functional outcome is less clear and somewhat theoretical. One of the biggest conundrums in NBS literature is determining the optimal stimulation approach for different neurological or cognitive impairments as most studies investigating the interventional effects of NBS in clinical have no standardised treatment methodology (i.e. they use different stimulation paradigms and parameters). The following section provides an overview of the key findings and the theoretical framework underpinning the potential use of interventional TMS and tDCS in mental illness and neurological disorders.

### 11.5.1 ALZHEIMER'S DISEASE

To date, there have only been a few reports that have directly investigated the effects of NBS on cognitive functions in dementia and cognitively impaired patients (Bentwich et al., 2011; Boggio et al., 2009; Cotelli et al., 2011, 2006; Ferrucci et al., 2008; Rabey et al., 2013). One of the first studies conducted by Cotelli et al. (2006) investigated the effects of high-frequency rTMS on 15 mild to moderate AD patients all currently receiving medication (20 Hz real and sham rTMS over the left or right dorsolateral prefrontal cortex [DLPFC]). A picture-naming task, using pictures of actions or objects, was used as a measure of cognitive function. The results showed a significant improvement for action naming after both the left and right DLPFC stimulation as compared to sham stimulation. In a subsequent study using the same rTMS paradigm, Cotelli et al. (2008) investigated the effects of rTMS on 24 AD patients with varying degrees of disease severity. Consistent with the previous study, rTMS of both left and right DLPFC resulted in an improvement in action naming in the mild AD group, but more importantly, the results showed an improvement in both action and object naming after rTMS in patients with moderate to severe AD. However, as rTMS was applied in a single session as an acute intervention in both studies, any chronic effects could not be ascertained.

To investigate the cumulative effects of repeated consecutive sessions and possible chronic effects, Cotelli et al. (2011) investigated the effects of a high-frequency rTMS paradigm for 4 weeks on ten patients with moderate AD. Patients were allocated to one of two groups in which they received either 4 weeks of active rTMS of the left DLPFC or

2 weeks of sham rTMS followed by 2 weeks of active rTMS over the same area. A series of cognitive measures including picture-/object-naming task, sentence comprehension and mini-mental state examination were taken at baseline and at 2 (mid-intervention), 4 (immediately post-intervention) and 12 weeks (8 weeks post-intervention) after the onset of the rTMS treatment. The results showed a significant improvement in auditory sentence comprehension and picture/object naming in the group receiving real rTMS as early as 2 weeks into the intervention, and the improvements lasted up to 8 weeks post-intervention. The authors concluded that 2 weeks of active rTMS was sufficient to promote specific language improvements that may last up to 8 weeks post-treatment.

Following the studies by Cotelli and colleagues, there is also emerging evidence supporting the combination of cognitive training with NBS for improving working memory and sentence comprehension. A study by Bentwich et al. (2011) investigated the effects of combined cognitive training with rTMS sessions in eight patients with probable AD (determined by the mini-mental state examination and AD assessment scale) for which each patient received daily cognitive training interspersed with high-frequency rTMS over several regions of the brain (Broca's area, Wernicke's area, left/right DLPFC and left/right somatosensory association cortex) for 6 weeks. The cognitive training included a series of computer tasks that focused on visuo-spatial pattern recognition, sentence comprehension and word recall. Following the intervention, there was a maintenance phase that included two sessions per week, for an additional 3 months. Results from the study showed significant improvements in cognitive scores up to four and a half months post-intervention as assessed by the AD assessment scale, which included word recall, sentence comprehension and visuospatial recognition tasks.

By contrast, there are only two tDCS studies investigating the effects of this technique on AD patients (Boggio et al., 2009; Ferrucci et al., 2008). Ferrucci et al. (2008) compared the effects of tDCS over the temporo-parietal junction in ten patients with probable AD, which showed a significant improvement on a verbal recognition memory task after a single session of tDCS. Building on the work of Ferrucci and colleagues, Boggio et al. (2009) investigated the effects of tDCS on a recognition memory test. Ten AD patients received tDCS in three different sessions – active tDCS over the left DLPFC and left temporal cortex and sham tDCS. Neuropsychological assessment included three cognitive domains (selective attention, working memory and visual recognition memory), which were all were administered during tDCS. Boggio and colleagues found an improvement of 18% and 13% on the visual recognition memory task during temporal and prefrontal cortex stimulation, respectively. Overall, the current literature provides emerging evidence for the clinical application of NBS in AD particularly with interventional TMS protocols. However, the long-term effects of NBS are still inconclusive and will require more large-scale randomised control trials that are needed to confirm the chronic effects of NBS.

### 11.5.2 DEPRESSION

The use of interventional TMS as an acute treatment for depression has probably received the greatest attention. To date, more than 20 individual randomised, placebo-controlled clinical trials, including more than a thousand patients who had major depressive episodes, have been conducted investigating the effects of NBS as an antidepressant (Lam et al., 2008). Whilst there are disparate findings, trials with sample sizes of more than 20 participants, which include a treatment time frame of at least 2 weeks, have reliably demonstrated improved symptoms of depression over sham TMS interventions (Couturier, 2005; Gaynes et al., 2014; Holtzheimer et al., 2001; Martin et al., 2003). A meta-analysis conducted in 2006 investigated 33 individual trials with 877 clinically diagnosed depressive patients and found active rTMS to be more effective than sham with an average reduction of 33.6% in depression scores after active rTMS compared with 17.4% after sham rTMS using clinical depression measures such as the Beck Depression Inventory and the Hamilton Depression Rating Scale (Herrmann & Ebmeier, 2006). Despite the positive outcome of this meta-analysis, there are limited data on the optimal stimulation parameters such as the frequency, duration and intensity of TMS. There is some evidence to suggest that a higher intensity or longer duration of TMS may lead to improved and longer lasting therapeutic effects (Fitzgerald et al., 2003; Rossini et al., 2005); however, this has yet to be systematically validated. Despite the accumulating body of emerging evidence that supports the use of NBS in mental illness such as depression, there are still no large multisite trials of TMS that demonstrate the potential efficacy of TMS treatments as an antidepressant compared to pharmaceutical interventions.

Recently, one TMS equipment manufacturer – Neuronetics – conducted such a double-blind multisite study that included 301 medication-free patients with major depression randomly assigned to either active or sham rTMS five times a week for 4–6 weeks (O'Reardon et al., 2007). Results from the study showed that active rTMS has significantly improved scores on the Montgomery–Asberg Depression Rating Scale and Hamilton Depression Rating Scale compared to sham TMS at weeks 4 and 6. Active rTMS was also found to be very well tolerated with a low dropout rate for adverse events (4.5%) that were generally mild and limited to transient scalp discomfort or pain. An open-label extension of the Neuronetics randomised control trial further showed a 46% response rate in depressed patients, which varied as a function of the level of treatment resistance to conventional antidepressants, with more treatment-resistant patients having poorer response (Avery et al., 2008). Given these potential benefits of rTMS on depressive patients, there is now a greater emphasis to determine the optimal stimulation parameters such as stimulation location, frequency and intensity to ensure the best clinical outcome (Blumberger et al., 2012; Chen et al., 2014; Fitzgerald et al., 2012).

### 11.5.3 NEUROLOGICAL DISORDERS

The application of NBS to treat chronic neurological disorders is a challenge as the progression of these diseases occurs over the longer term and the trajectory may change constantly. Furthermore, NBS is difficult to administer chronically, and because interventional forms of NBS have only been introduced in the last decades, the long-term effects (positive and/or negative) are still unknown. PD is a progressive movement disorder related to loss of dopaminergic neurons in the substantia nigra and depletion of dopamine in the basal ganglia. Although the origins of PD stem from deep brain structures, secondary abnormalities manifest in the superficial layer of the brain, including changes in cortical inhibition and shifts in the cortical motor representation of hand muscles, which can occur in both early and late stages of the disease (Kagerer et al., 2003; Thickbroom et al., 2006). Shifts in cortical motor representation correlate with the severity of clinical symptoms (UPDRS) and suggest an ongoing process of cortical reorganisation with functional consequences (Thickbroom et al., 2006). Dopamine has been implicated in the modulation of brain plasticity (Calabresi et al., 2007), and the loss of dopaminergic neurons in PD may have secondary effects on functional reorganisation of the brain or limit the natural ability of the brain to compensate for disease-related processes. It is likely that brain plasticity may be functional in the earlier stages of PD, as the brain adapts to the initial loss of dopaminergic neurons, but becomes dysfunctional later in the stages as a result of the gradual depletion in endogenous dopamine production. This suggests that the therapeutic effects of NBS may be increased when applied in conjunction with levodopa therapy, when plasticity (due to increased dopamine levels in the brain) may be more functional (Fierro et al., 2008; Rodrigues et al., 2008). However, it is unclear as to whether NBS can induce a lasting clinically beneficial effect in PD. A number of NBS interventions have been trialled in PD patients and have shown some modest if not transient improvement in motor function. For example, a meta-analysis of randomised controlled trials in PD indicates that active NBS can be beneficial in improving brain plasticity and motor function over and above sham NBS paradigms (Fregni et al., 2005b).

Apart from PD, dystonia is another neurological condition that may likely to benefit from NBS. Dystonia results from unwanted contraction of muscles that may be focal, generalised or task specific and is thought to arise from alterations in basal ganglion regulatory loops involving premotor cortical areas and motor cortex (Hallett, 2011; Vitek et al., 2011). Some studies have shown that plasticity is upregulated in dystonia and probably dysfunctional, evidenced by greater changes in brain excitability with NBS interventions that is less spatially restricted and longer lasting (Quartarone et al., 2008). TMS cortical mapping studies reveal changes in the cortical representation of muscles that are primarily involved in the dystonic posture as well as muscles that are not dystonic (Byrnes et al., 1998; Thickbroom et al., 2003). Alleviation of symptoms following injection of botulinum toxin into affected muscles is associated with normalisation of TMS maps, suggesting that reorganisation is an ongoing and dynamic process perhaps maintained by abnormal afferent inputs to cortical regions (Byrnes et al., 1998; Thickbroom et al., 2003). How NBS could be applied therapeutically in dystonia is uncertain, although alleviation of symptoms has been reported with an excitability-reducing NBS protocol delivered over an fMRI-identified region of hyperactivity within DLPFC (Murase et al., 2005; Siebner et al., 1999).

### 11.5.4 BRAIN INJURIES AND STROKE

The stroke or traumatic brain injury model offers most promise for the application of NBS if the intervention can facilitate a longer lasting recovery in the absence of further brain damage. The contribution of brain plasticity in recovery from stroke and traumatic brain injury may be evidenced by a normalisation of cortical map representation of the limbs, as ascertained by TMS, and brain activation patterns observed with functional imaging techniques (Butefisch et al., 2006; Byrnes et al., 2001). In the case of TMS, a correlation has been reported between grip strength in the affected hand and the extent of cortical map shifts, suggesting this form of brain plasticity may be beneficial to function (Thickbroom et al., 2004). Although there has been some modest functional improvement reported after NBS interventions, however, the longer term clinical benefits remain unproven (Hummel & Cohen, 2006). It is likely that NBS will need to be administered in combination with other therapies for more lasting effects; however, the relative timing and the nature of the intervention and the therapy remain to be determined.

Accordingly, two advances have been proposed for the use of NBS in stroke rehabilitation: (1) application of NBS to facilitate the affected hemisphere to enhance plasticity therefore promoting functional recovery and (2) application of inhibitory NBS on the unaffected hemisphere to reduce inter-hemispheric competition from the affected side. These advances are based on the theory of inter-hemispheric imbalance (i.e. unaffected hemisphere takes over certain function of the affected hemisphere) following stroke. tDCS applied to the affected motor cortex has been studied in patients with chronic stroke in sham-controlled double-blind crossover experimental designs (Fregni et al., 2005a; Hummel et al., 2005; Hummel & Cohen, 2005). In the first double-blind sham-controlled study in 6 patients, each with a single ischemic stroke, the authors documented transient improvements in performance of the Jebsen–Taylor hand-function test with one single session of stimulation but not with sham (Hummel et al., 2005). This improvement was evident in all patients studied, representing approximately a 10% reduction in the time required to perform the Jebsen–Taylor hand-function test, and persisted for more than 30 min after the end of the stimulation period. Another study by Kim et al. (2006) showed that high-frequency rTMS to the affected primary motor cortex resulted in a significantly larger increase in MEP amplitudes than sham rTMS; this increase was associated with an enhanced accuracy during performance of a finger motor sequence task. Similarly, in a study performed in subacute instead of chronic stroke patients, with multiple sessions of rTMS applied to the affected primary motor cortex, Khedr et al. (2005) used rTMS combined with customary rehabilitative treatment for 10 days within the first 2 weeks after stroke. They reported improvements in fine motor function hand function with active rTMS relative to sham lasting for at least 10 days after the end of the treatment period.

Based on the idea that inter-hemispheric interactions can influence motor performance (Swinnen, 2002), it should be possible, in theory, to improve motor function in the paretic hand by decreasing excitability in the unaffected primary motor cortex possibly through modulation of inter-hemispheric imbalance (Murase et al., 2004). Studies in normal, healthy volunteers show that decreasing excitability in one motor cortex result in increased excitability in the opposite motor cortex (Plewnia et al., 2003; Schambra et al., 2003) and even in performance improvements in motor function of the ipsilateral hand (Kobayashi et al., 2003). In patients with stroke, it was shown that inhibitory tDCS applied to the unaffected primary motor cortex may improve performance in the paretic hand, possibly by suppressing the imbalance in inter-hemispheric inhibition proposed to interfere with stroke recovery in some patients (Fregni et al., 2005a). Decreasing activity in the unaffected primary motor cortex with low-frequency rTMS was found to decrease inter-hemispheric inhibition from the unaffected to affected hemisphere of chronic stroke patients (Takeuchi et al., 2005) with the decrease in inter-hemispheric inhibition elicited by rTMS correlated with functional improvements in a finger pinch acceleration task. Another study, using low-frequency rTMS to the unaffected motor cortex, found behavioural improvements in the paretic hand in simple reaction time and on the Purdue Pegboard test (Mansur et al., 2005).

## 11.6   CAN NUTRITION AND NBS BE COMPLIMENTARY?

Evidence from epidemiological studies (see Chapter 2 by Andreeva and Kesse-Guyot for more details) has consistently demonstrated beneficial effects of dietary compounds for healthy brain function that may attenuate cognitive decline associated with aging and disease (Mishra & Palanivelu, 2008; Yehuda et al., 2005). Findings from animal-model studies have provided insight into the potential mechanism that micronutrients act upon across various neurophysiological processes to confer neuro-protective effects on brain function. It therefore begs the question as to whether nutrition and NBS can be complimentary to maximise neurophysiological and functional performance benefits.

To date, little is known about the interactions between nutrition and NBS or indeed if these interventions could act synergistically. Evidence from pharmacological studies suggests that drugs used to modulate neuronal communication can potentiate or inhibit changes in brain plasticity induced by NBS (Gerdelat-Mas et al., 2005; Reis et al., 2006; Robol et al., 2004). However, these changes are often abolished once the effects of the drug wear off. It is therefore logical to postulate that dietary components may be able to influence NBS-related changes in brain plasticity if they can cross the blood–brain barrier (as has been demonstrated for caffeine and turmeric). However, the ability for any dietary component to exert a lasting effect on brain plasticity changes elicited by NBS will be dependent on the availability (*how much*) of the micronutrient after it crosses the blood–brain barrier and its half-life (*how long it stays in the body*) following consumption. Other important considerations are the homeostatic mechanisms that regulate brain plasticity, which come into play should any external perturbations to the CNS exceed a pre-set physiological threshold

(Abraham & Bear, 1996). Evidence from interventional NBS studies has shown that increasing the intensity and duration of NBS does not necessarily equate to an amplification of changes in brain plasticity (Kidgell et al., 2013; Murray et al., 2011), which suggests some form of regulatory homeostatic effect towards any forms of external influences. It could be that homeostatic regulatory processes may buffer or prevent any neurophysiological changes associated with nutrition and NBS interventions if the brain deems that the changes exceed the normal physiological threshold.

Although there is limited evidence to suggest any form of interaction between nutrition and NBS, certain micronutrients such as caffeine have often been considered to be potential confounders in NBS-related research. From a mechanistic standpoint, caffeine is a powerful source of neuro-stimulant that readily crosses the blood–brain barrier, and it exerts a stimulatory effect by blocking adenosine receptor function that produces a sedative-like effect in the brain. At the spinal level, a study by Walton et al. (2003) found that neuronal excitability is increased as measured by an increase in amplitude of H-reflexes following caffeine consumption. In a separate study, Cerqueira et al. (2006) investigated the effects of a single 200 mg dose of caffeine consumption on brain excitability and found that measures of the cortical silent period were significantly reduced compared to a sham-controlled caffeine group. They concluded that a single dose of caffeine is strong enough to elicit changes in brain excitability and should be a consideration in any TMS research. Another study investigated the effects of Lucozade (a common energy drink with high concentrations of glucose and caffeine) and found significant increase in brain excitability measure by TMS compared with a sham energy drink that endured at 90 min post-consumption (Specterman et al., 2005). Taken together, these two studies suggest a significant effect of certain macro- and micronutrients, especially those that can cross the blood–brain barrier easily, to modulate brain excitability. By contrast, a study by Ortha et al. (2005) found no significant effects of caffeine on measures of brain excitability such as resting motor threshold, cortical inhibition and facilitation.

What are the prospects of combining nutrition and NBS to treat neuro-cognitive disorders? Most certainly, both nutrition and NBS interventions individually (as discussed throughout the previous chapters) have demonstrated strong potential to attenuate age-/disease-related declines in cognition; however, the effects of combined nutrition and NBS intervention have yet to be systematically explored. There is also the question of how much and, more importantly, how long does it take for a certain micronutrient to have a significant lasting effect on NBS-induced plasticity for any functional and behavioural changes to be observed (see Camfield and Scholey, Chapter 12, for more discussion of techniques for assessing functional and behavioural changes). In summary, not only the combination of nutrition and NBS represents an exciting potential for treating neuro-cognitive and neurological disorders, but these methods are also a cheap and effective alternative to traditional forms of pharmacological treatments for preventing functional declines in the aging and diseased human brain.

## 11.7 FUTURE DIRECTION FOR NBS

The application of NBS has provided a unique way of exploring the brain and has advanced the understanding of neuronal networks that govern emotion, movement and perception. There remains, however, several technical and ethical challenges that need to be addressed in future studies. The first challenge relates to the focal point, intensity and direction of effects associated with NBS techniques such as rTMS and tDCS. As with most current NBS methods, stimulation focal point is a highly debatable issue due to the relatively large surface area of stimulation electrodes/coils use, particularly with tDCS. Although fMRI and PET imaging provide us with evidence of increased cortical activation (*as indexed by increase cerebral blood flow*) at the site of stimulation, the resulting area of cortical activation from NBS may be larger than the intended target of stimulation. In such cases, it is unclear if any effects of NBS are due to the direct stimulation of the intended brain area or whether the effects are caused by indirect stimulation of the adjacent areas. Further to that, noninvasive cortical stimulation involves inducing electromagnetic currents through the skin and bone of the skull. This method of current induction through various layers of human tissue that consists largely of water is likely to result in current refraction (*distortion of current flow*), resulting in a lower stimulation intensity (*increased resistance*) and directionality (*increased multidirectional current spread*). To date, most evidences for stimulation intensity and direction of NBS techniques are derived from computational modelling that does not take into account the size and shape of the individual's head and also the thickness of each individual layer of tissue (Bijsterbosch et al., 2012; Laakso & Hirata, 2012).

Another highly debatable area in the NBS literature relates to the use of NBS in children and adolescents. Several studies so far have undertaken the use of TMS to explore how cognitive, emotional, behavioural and motor functions develop with age. However, due to the plasticity-inducing nature of NBS techniques, some critics have argued their concerns about interfering with important functional development associated with brain plasticity in children. At this point, no studies have yet to explore the use of interventional forms of NBS in an adolescent population due to a lack of established safety guidelines (Frye et al., 2008). Aside from an adolescent population, there are also some concerns about the application of NBS techniques in a healthy adult population for the purpose of inducing behavioural changes to moral judgement (Fumagalli et al., 2010), decision-making (Boggio et al., 2010) and deception (Luber et al., 2009). Although most behavioural-inducing experiments are conducted across a single session with short-lasting effects, the ethical concern is whether longer term stimulation would lead to unwanted behavioural changes that may persist. Future studies will therefore need to establish safety limits and guidelines to optimise the use of NBS not only in clinical settings as a treatment tool for neuro-cognitive and neurological disorders but also in experimental settings involving children and behavioural modification.

**TOP 4 SUMMARY POINTS FROM THE CHAPTER**

- TMS and tDCS are noninvasive methods of brain stimulation that can be used to investigate the structural integrity and function of the CNS.
- Repetitive use of TMS and tDCS can elicit long-term changes in brain plasticity that can help to improve cognitive and motor functions in individuals suffering from neuro-cognitive and neurological disorders.
- Despite having the ability to influence brain plasticity, it is unclear if combining nutritional interventions and NBS may yield greater results compared to either intervention alone.
- Future studies will need to elucidate potential interactions between nutrition and NBS protocols in healthy and clinical populations.

**WHAT'S UNDER DEBATE?**

- Although most studies favour the use of NBS as a potential tool for treating neuro-cognitive disorders, these studies often have small sample sizes and only show acute changes following NBS. This therefore limits the interpretation of the efficacy of NBS as a tool for treating neuro-cognitive and mental health disorders.
- There is still no consensus on the most optimal NBS protocol to be used with treating various conditions. More importantly, it is still unclear as to how long-term NBS may affect the overall health and function of the brain. It remains to be seen if long-term stimulation may positively or adversely affect brain function, particularly in clinical populations.
- Current methods of NBS can only target cortical (superficial) areas that are responsible for executive motor and cognitive functions, as the penetration depth of TMS and tDCS is approximately about 2–3 cm. This brings into question the relevance and efficacy of NBS in treating neurological disorders that affect deeper, subcortical brain structures (i.e. PD, subcortical strokes and traumatic brain injury).

## REFERENCES

Abraham, W. C., & Bear, M. F. (1996). Metaplasticity: The plasticity of synaptic plasticity. *Trends in Neuroscience, 19*(4), 126–130.

Adrian, E. D., & Moruzzi, G. (1939). Impluses in the pyramidal tract. *Journal of Physiology, 97*(2), 153–199.

Aldini, G. (1804). *Essai théorique et expérimental sur le galvanisme, avec une série d'expériences faites devant des commissaires de l'Institut national de France, et en divers amphithéâtres anatomiques de Londres.* Paris, France: Fournier Fils.

Avery, D. H., Isenberg, K. E., Sampson, S. M., Janicak, P. G., Lisanby, S. H., Maixner, D. F., ... George, M. S. (2008). Transcranial magnetic stimulation in the acute treatment of major depressive disorder: Clinical response in an open-label extension trial. *Journal of Clinical Psychiatry, 69*(3), 441–451.

Barker, A. T., Jalinous, R., & Freeston, I. L. (1985). Non-invasive magnetic stimulation of human motor cortex. *Lancet, 1*(8437), 1106–1107.

Bashir, S., Vernet, M., Yoo, W. K., Mizrahi, I., Theoret, H., & Pascual-Leone, A. (2012). Changes in cortical plasticity after mild traumatic brain injury. *Restorative Neurology and Neuroscience, 30*(4), 277–282.

Baudewig, J., Siebner, H. R., Bestmann, S., Tergau, F., Tings, T., Paulus, W., & Frahm, J. (2001). Functional MRI of cortical activations induced by transcranial magnetic stimulation (TMS). *Neuroreport, 12*(16), 3543–3548.

Bentwich, J., Dobronevsky, E., Aichenbaum, S., Shorer, R., Peretz, R., Khaigrekht, M., ... Rabey, J. M. (2011). Beneficial effect of repetitive transcranial magnetic stimulation combined with cognitive training for the treatment of Alzheimer's disease: A proof of concept study. *Journal of Neural Transmission, 118*(3), 463–471.

Berardelli, A., Rona, S., Inghilleri, M., & Manfredi, M. (1996). Cortical inhibition in Parkinson's disease. A study with paired magnetic stimulation. *Brain, 119*(Pt 1), 71–77.

Bijsterbosch, J. D., Barker, A. T., Lee, K. H., & Woodruff, P. W. (2012). Where does transcranial magnetic stimulation (TMS) stimulate? Modelling of induced field maps for some common cortical and cerebellar targets. *Medical & Biological Engineering & Computing, 50*(7), 671–681.

Bikson, M., Datta, A., & Elwassif, M. (2009). Establishing safety limits for transcranial direct current stimulation. *Clinical Neurophysiology, 120*(6), 1033–1034.

Blumberger, D. M., Mulsant, B. H., Fitzgerald, P. B., Rajji, T. K., Ravindran, A. V., Young, L. T., ... Daskalakis, Z. J. (2012). A randomized double-blind sham-controlled comparison of unilateral and bilateral repetitive transcranial magnetic stimulation for treatment-resistant major depression. *The World Journal of Biological Psychiatry, 13*(6), 423–435.

Boggio, P. S., Campanha, C., Valasek, C. A., Fecteau, S., Pascual-Leone, A., & Fregni, F. (2010). Modulation of decision-making in a gambling task in older adults with transcranial direct current stimulation. *European Journal of Neuroscience, 31*(3), 593–597.

Boggio, P. S., Khoury, L. P., Martins, D. C., Martins, O. E., de Macedo, E. C., & Fregni, F. (2009). Temporal cortex direct current stimulation enhances performance on a visual recognition memory task in Alzheimer disease. *Journal of Neurology, Neurosurgery & Psychiatry, 80*(4), 444–447.

Bohning, D. E., Shastri, A., McConnell, K. A., Nahas, Z., Lorberbaum, J. P., Roberts, D. R., ... George, M. S. (1999). A combined TMS/fMRI study of intensity-dependent TMS over motor cortex. *Biological Psychiatry, 45*(4), 385–394.

Bohning, D. E., Shastri, A., McGavin, K. A., McConnell, K. A., Nahas, Z., Lorberbaum, J. P., ... George, M. S. (2000). Motor cortex brain activity induced by 1-Hz transcranial magnetic stimulation is similar in location and level to that for volitional movement. *Investigative Radiology, 35*(11), 676–683.

Bresadola, M. (1998). Medicine and science in the life of Luigi Galvani (1737–1798). *Brain Research Bulletin, 46*(5), 367–380.

Butefisch, C. M., Kleiser, R., & Seitz, R. J. (2006). Post-lesional cerebral reorganisation: Evidence from functional neuroimaging and transcranial magnetic stimulation. *Journal of Physiology Paris, 99*(4–6), 437–454.

Byrnes, M. L., Thickbroom, G. W., Phillips, B. A., & Mastaglia, F. L. (2001). Long-term changes in motor cortical organisation after recovery from subcortical stroke. *Brain Research, 889*(1–2), 278–287.

Byrnes, M. L., Thickbroom, G. W., Wilson, S. A., Sacco, P., Shipman, J. M., Stell, R., & Mastaglia, F. L. (1998). The corticomotor representation of upper limb muscles in writer's cramp and changes following botulinum toxin injection. *Brain, 121*(Pt 5), 977–988.

Calabresi, P., Picconi, B., Tozzi, A., & Di Filippo, M. (2007). Dopamine-mediated regulation of corticostriatal synaptic plasticity. *Trends in Neurosciences, 30*(5), 211–219.

Ceccarelli, U. (1962). The 1st pharmacopoeia: The "De compositionibus medicamentorum" of Scribonio Largo. *Minerva Medica, 53,* 2398–2402.

Cerqueira, V., de Mendonça, A., Minez, A., Dias, A. R., & de Carvalho, M. (2006). Does caffeine modify corticomotor excitability? *Clinical Neurophysiology, 36*(4), 219–226.

Cheetham, C., & Finnerty, G. (2007). Plasticity and its role in neurological diseases of the adult nervous system. *Advances in Clinical Neuroscience & Rehabilitation, 7*(3), 8–9.

Chen, J. J., Liu, Z., Zhu, D., Li, Q., Zhang, H., Huang, H., ... Xie, P. (2014). Bilateral vs. unilateral repetitive transcranial magnetic stimulation in treating major depression: A meta-analysis of randomized controlled trials. *Psychiatry Research, 219*(1), 51–57.

Cotelli, M., Calabria, M., Manenti, R., Rosini, S., Zanetti, O., Cappa, S. F., & Miniussi, C. (2011). Improved language performance in Alzheimer disease following brain stimulation. *Journal of Neurology, Neurosurgery & Psychiatry, 82*(7), 794–797.

Cotelli, M., Manenti, R., Cappa, S. F., Geroldi, C., Zanetti, O., Rossini, P. M., & Miniussi, C. (2006). Effect of transcranial magnetic stimulation on action naming in patients with Alzheimer disease. *Archives of Neurology, 63*(11), 1602–1604.

Cotelli, M., Manenti, R., Cappa, S. F., Zanetti, O., & Miniussi, C. (2008). Transcranial magnetic stimulation improves naming in Alzheimer disease patients at different stages of cognitive decline. *European Journal of Neurology, 15*(12), 1286–1292.

Couturier, J. L. (2005). Efficacy of rapid-rate repetitive transcranial magnetic stimulation in the treatment of depression: A systematic review and meta-analysis. *Journal of Psychiatry & Neuroscience, 30*(2), 83–90.

de Micheli, A. (1991). From Galvani's De viribus electricitatis... to modern electrovectorcardiography. *Archivos del Instituto de Cardiologia de Mexico, 61*(1), 7–13.

Di Lazzaro, V., Oliviero, A., Meglio, M., Cioni, B., Tamburrini, G., Tonali, P., & Rothwell, J. C. (2000). Direct demonstration of the effect of lorazepam on the excitability of the human motor cortex. *Clinical Neurophysiology, 111*(5), 794–799.

Di Lazzaro, V., Oliviero, A., Pilato, F., Saturno, E., Dileone, M., Marra, C., ... Tonali, P. A. (2004). Motor cortex hyperexcitability to transcranial magnetic stimulation in Alzheimer's disease. *Journal of Neurology, Neurosurgery & Psychiatry, 75*(4), 555–559.

Di Lazzaro, V., Pilato, F., Oliviero, A., Dileone, M., Saturno, E., Mazzone, P., ... Rothwell, J. C. (2006). Origin of facilitation of motor-evoked potentials after paired magnetic stimulation: Direct recording of epidural activity in conscious humans. *Journal of Neurophysiology, 96*(4), 1765–1771.

Fecteau, S., Pascual-Leone, A., Zald, D. H., Liguori, P., Theoret, H., Boggio, P. S., & Fregni, F. (2007). Activation of prefrontal cortex by transcranial direct current stimulation reduces appetite for risk during ambiguous decision making. *Journal of Neuroscience, 27*(23), 6212–6218.

Ferrucci, R., Mameli, F., Guidi, I., Mrakic-Sposta, S., Vergari, M., Marceglia, S., ... Priori, A. (2008). Transcranial direct current stimulation improves recognition memory in Alzheimer disease. *Neurology, 71*(7), 493–498.

Fierro, B., Brighina, F., D'Amelio, M., Daniele, O., Lupo, I., Ragonese, P., ... Savettieri, G. (2008). Motor intracortical inhibition in PD: LDOPA modulation of high-frequency rTMS effects. *Experimental Brain Research, 184,* 521–528.

Fitzgerald, P. B., Brown, T. L., Marston, N. A., Daskalakis, Z. J., De Castella, A., & Kulkarni, J. (2003). Transcranial magnetic stimulation in the treatment of depression: A double-blind, placebo-controlled trial. *Archives of General Psychiatry, 60*(10), 1002–1008.

Fitzgerald, P. B., Hoy, K. E., Herring, S. E., McQueen, S., Peachey, A. V., Segrave, R. A., ... Daskalakis, Z. J. (2012). A double blind randomized trial of unilateral left and bilateral prefrontal cortex transcranial magnetic stimulation in treatment resistant major depression. *Journal of Affective Disorders, 139*(2), 193–198.

Foltys, H., Krings, T., Meister, I. G., Sparing, R., Boroojerdi, B., Thron, A., & Topper, R. (2003). Motor representation in patients rapidly recovering after stroke: A functional magnetic resonance imaging and transcranial magnetic stimulation study. *Clinical Neurophysiology, 114*(12), 2404–2415.

Fraser, P. E., & Rosen, A. C. (2012). Transcranial direct current stimulation and behavioral models of smoking addiction. *Frontiers in Psychiatry, 3*, 79.

Fregni, F., Boggio, P. S., Mansur, C. G., Wagner, T., Ferreira, M. J., Lima, M. C., ... Pascual-Leone, A. (2005a). Transcranial direct current stimulation of the unaffected hemisphere in stroke patients. *Neuroreport, 16*(14), 1551–1555.

Fregni, F., Boggio, P. S., Nitsche, M. A., Marcolin, M. A., Rigonatti, S. P., & Pascual-Leone, A. (2006). Treatment of major depression with transcranial direct current stimulation. *Bipolar Disorders, 8*(2), 203–204.

Fregni, F., Simon, D. K., Wu, A., & Pascual-Leone, A. (2005b). Non-invasive brain stimulation for Parkinson's disease: A systematic review and meta-analysis of the literature. *Journal of Neurology, Neurosurgery & Psychiatry, 76*(12), 1614–1623.

Frye, R. E., Rotenberg, A., Ousley, M., & Pascual-Leone, A. (2008). Transcranial magnetic stimulation in child neurology: Current and future directions. *Journal of Child Neurology, 23*(1), 79–96.

Fumagalli, M., Vergari, M., Pasqualetti, P., Marceglia, S., Mameli, F., Ferrucci, R., ... Priori, A. (2010). Brain switches utilitarian behavior: Does gender make the difference? *PLoS One, 5*(1), e8865.

Gaynes, B. N., Lloyd, S. W., Lux, L., Gartlehner, G., Hansen, R. A., Brode, S., ... Lohr, K. N. (2014). Repetitive transcranial magnetic stimulation for treatment-resistant depression: A systematic review and meta-analysis. *Journal of Clinical Psychiatry, 75*(5), 477–489; quiz 489.

Gerdelat-Mas, A., Loubinoux, I., Tombari, D., Rascol, O., Chollet, F., & Simonetta-Moreau, M. (2005). Chronic administration of selective serotonin reuptake inhibitor (SSRI) paroxetine modulates human motor cortex excitability in healthy subjects. *Neuroimage, 27*(2), 314–322.

Hallett, M. (2007). Transcranial magnetic stimulation: A primer. *Neuron, 55*(2), 187–199.

Hallett, M. (2011). Neurophysiology of dystonia: The role of inhibition. *Neurobiology of Disease, 42*(2), 177–184.

Halliday, D., Resnick, R., & Walker, J. (2002). *Fundamentals of physics* (6th ed.). Philadelphia, PA: Wiley.

Herrmann, L. L., & Ebmeier, K. P. (2006). Factors modifying the efficacy of transcranial magnetic stimulation in the treatment of depression: A review. *Journal of Clinical Psychiatry, 67*(12), 1870–1876.

Hoeppner, J., Wegrzyn, M., Thome, J., Bauer, A., Oltmann, I., Buchmann, J., & Teipel, S. (2012). Intra- and inter-cortical motor excitability in Alzheimer's disease. *Journal of Neural Transmission, 119*(5), 605–612.

Holtzheimer, P. E., 3rd, Russo, J., & Avery, D. H. (2001). A meta-analysis of repetitive transcranial magnetic stimulation in the treatment of depression. *Psychopharmacology Bulletin, 35*(4), 149–169.

Hummel, F. C., Celnik, P., Giraux, P., Floel, A., Wu, W. H., Gerloff, C., & Cohen, L. G. (2005). Effects of non-invasive cortical stimulation on skilled motor function in chronic stroke. *Brain, 128*(Pt 3), 490–499.

Hummel, F. C., & Cohen, L. G. (2005). Improvement of motor function with noninvasive cortical stimulation in a patient with chronic stroke. *Neurorehabilitation and Neural Repair, 19*(1), 14–19.

Hummel, F. C., & Cohen, L. G. (2006). Non-invasive brain stimulation: A new strategy to improve neurorehabilitation after stroke? *The Lancet Neurology, 5*(8), 708–712.

Kagerer, F. A., Summers, J. J., Byblow, W. D., & Taylor, B. (2003). Altered corticomotor representation in patients with Parkinson's disease. *Movement Disorders, 18*(8), 919–927.

Kellaway, P. (1946). The part played by electric fish in the early history of bioelectricity and electrotherapy. *Bulletin of the History of Medicine, 20*(2), 112–137.

Khedr, E. M., Ahmed, M. A., Darwish, E. S., & Ali, A. M. (2011). The relationship between motor cortex excitability and severity of Alzheimer's disease: A transcranial magnetic stimulation study. *Clinical Neurophysiology, 41*(3), 107–113.

Khedr, E. M., Ahmed, M. A., Fathy, N., & Rothwell, J. C. (2005). Therapeutic trial of repetitive transcranial magnetic stimulation after acute ischemic stroke. *Neurology, 65*(3), 466–468.

Kidd, D., Thompson, P. D., Day, B. L., Rothwell, J. C., Kendall, B. E., Thompson, A. J., … McDonald, W. I. (1998). Central motor conduction time in progressive multiple sclerosis. Correlations with MRI and disease activity. *Brain, 121*(Pt 6), 1109–1116.

Kidgell, D. J., Daly, R. M., Young, K., Lum, J., Tooley, G., Jaberzadeh, S., … Pearce, A. J. (2013). Different current intensities of anodal transcranial direct current stimulation do not differentially modulate motor cortex plasticity. *Neural Plasticity, 1*–9. doi: http://dx.doi.org/10.1155/2013/603502.

Kim, Y. H., You, S. H., Ko, M. H., Park, J. W., Lee, K. H., Jang, S. H., … Hallett, M. (2006). Repetitive transcranial magnetic stimulation-induced corticomotor excitability and associated motor skill acquisition in chronic stroke. *Stroke, 37*(6), 1471–1476.

Knotkova, H., & Cruciani, R. A. (2010). Non-invasive transcranial direct current stimulation for the study and treatment of neuropathic pain. *Methods in Molecular Biology, 617*, 505–515.

Kobayashi, M., Hutchinson, S., Schlaug, G., & Pascual-Leone, A. (2003). Ipsilateral motor cortex activation on functional magnetic resonance imaging during unilateral hand movements is related to interhemispheric interactions. *Neuroimage, 20*(4), 2259 –2270.

Kujirai, T., Caramia, M. D., Rothwell, J. C., Day, B. L., Thompson, P. D., Ferbert, A., … Marsden, C. D. (1993). Corticocortical inhibition in human motor cortex. *The Journal of Physiology, 471*, 501–519.

Laakso, I., & Hirata, A. (2012). Fast multigrid-based computation of the induced electric field for transcranial magnetic stimulation. *Physics in Medicine and Biology, 57*(23), 7753–7765.

Lam, R. W., Chan, P., Wilkins-Ho, M., & Yatham, L. N. (2008). Repetitive transcranial magnetic stimulation for treatment-resistant depression: A systematic review and metaanalysis. *Canadian Journal of Psychiatry, 53*(9), 621–631.

Liebetanz, D., Nitsche, M. A., Tergau, F., & Paulus, W. (2002). Pharmacological approach to the mechanisms of transcranial DC-stimulation-induced after-effects of human motor cortex excitability. *Brain, 125*(Pt 10), 2238–2247.

Luber, B., Fisher, C., Appelbaum, P. S., Ploesser, M., & Lisanby, S. H. (2009). Non-invasive brain stimulation in the detection of deception: Scientific challenges and ethical consequences. *Behavioral Science & the Law, 27*(2), 191–208.

Mansur, C. G., Fregni, F., Boggio, P. S., Riberto, M., Gallucci-Neto, J., Santos, C. M., … Pascual-Leone, A. (2005). A sham stimulation-controlled trial of rTMS of the unaffected hemisphere in stroke patients. *Neurology, 64*(10), 1802–1804.

Martin, J. L., Barbanoj, M. J., Schlaepfer, T. E., Thompson, E., Perez, V., & Kulisevsky, J. (2003). Repetitive transcranial magnetic stimulation for the treatment of depression. Systematic review and meta-analysis. *The British Journal of Psychiatry, 182*, 480–491.

Merton, P. A., & Morton, H. B. (1980). Stimulation of the cerebral cortex in the intact human subject. *Nature, 285*(5762), 227.

Miranda, P. C., Lomarev, M., & Hallett, M. (2006). Modeling the current distribution during transcranial direct current stimulation. *Clinical Neurophysiology, 117*(7), 1623–1629.

Mishra, S., & Palanivelu, K. (2008). The effect of curcumin (turmeric) on Alzheimer's disease: An overview. *Annals of Indian Academy of Neurology, 11*(1), 13–19.

Murase, N., Duque, J., Mazzocchio, R., & Cohen, L. G. (2004). Influence of interhemispheric interactions on motor function in chronic stroke. *Annals of Neurology, 55*(3), 400–409.

Murase, N., Rothwell, J. C., Kaji, R., Urushihara, R., Nakamura, K., Murayama, N., ... Shibasaki, H. (2005). Subthreshold low-frequency repetitive transcranial magnetic stimulation over the premotor cortex modulates writer's cramp. *Brain, 128*(Pt 1), 104–115.

Murray, L. M., Nosaka, K., & Thickbroom, G. W. (2011). Interventional repetitive I-wave transcranial magnetic stimulation (TMS): The dimension of stimulation duration. *Brain Stimulation, 4*(4), 261–265.

Myhrer, T. (2003). Neurotransmitter systems involved in learning and memory in the rat: A meta-analysis based on studies of four behavioral tasks. *Brain Research Reviews, 41*(2–3), 268–287.

Nakamae, T., Tanaka, N., Nakanishi, K., Fujimoto, Y., Sasaki, H., Kamei, N., ... Ochi, M. (2010). Quantitative assessment of myelopathy patients using motor evoked potentials produced by transcranial magnetic stimulation. *European Spine Journal, 19*(5), 685–690.

Nitsche, M. A. (2002). Transcranial direct current stimulation: A new treatment for depression? *Bipolar Disorders, 4*(Suppl. 1), 98–99.

Nitsche, M. A., Cohen, L. G., Wassermann, E. M., Priori, A., Lang, N., Antal, A., ... Pascual-Leone, A. (2008). Transcranial direct current stimulation: State of the art 2008. *Brain Stimulation, 1*(3), 206–223.

Nitsche, M. A., Fricke, K., Henschke, U., Schlitterlau, A., Liebetanz, D., Lang, N., ... Paulus, W. (2003). Pharmacological modulation of cortical excitability shifts induced by transcranial direct current stimulation in humans. *Journal of Physiology, 553*(Pt 1), 293–301.

Nitsche, M. A., Liebetanz, D., Antal, A., Lang, N., Tergau, F., & Paulus, W. (2003). Modulation of cortical excitability by weak direct current stimulation – Technical, safety and functional aspects. *Supplements to Clinical Neurophysiology, 56*, 255–276.

Nitsche, M. A., & Paulus, W. (2000). Excitability changes induced in the human motor cortex by weak transcranial direct current stimulation. *Journal of Physiology, 527*(Pt 3), 633–639.

Nitsche, M. A., & Paulus, W. (2001). Sustained excitability elevations induced by transcranial DC motor cortex stimulation in humans. *Neurology, 57*(10), 1899–1901.

O'Connell, N. E., Cossar, J., Marston, L., Wand, B. M., Bunce, D., De Souza, L. H., ... Moseley, G. L. (2013). Transcranial direct current stimulation of the motor cortex in the treatment of chronic nonspecific low back pain: A randomized, double-blind exploratory study. *Clinical Journal of Pain, 29*(1), 26–34.

O'Reardon, J. P., Solvason, H. B., Janicak, P. G., Sampson, S., Isenberg, K. E., Nahas, Z., ... Sackeim, H. A. (2007). Efficacy and safety of transcranial magnetic stimulation in the acute treatment of major depression: A multisite randomized controlled trial. *Biological Psychiatry, 62*(11), 1208–1216.

Ortha, M., Amann, B., Ratnarajc, N., Patsalosc, P. N., & Rothwell, J. C. (2005). Caffeine has no effect on measures of cortical excitability. *Clinical Neurophysiology, 116*(2), 308–314.

Pancaldi, G. (2003). *Volta: Science and culture in the age of enlightenment*. Princeton, NJ: Princeton University Press.

Patton, H. D., & Amassian, V. E. (1954). Single and multiple-unit analysis of cortical stage of pyramidal tract activation. *Journal of Neurophysiology, 17*(4), 345–363.

Paus, T., Jech, R., Thompson, C. J., Comeau, R., Peters, T., & Evans, A. C. (1997). Transcranial magnetic stimulation during positron emission tomography: A new method for studying connectivity of the human cerebral cortex. *The Journal of Neuroscience, 17*(9), 3178–3184.

Paus, T., Jech, R., Thompson, C. J., Comeau, R., Peters, T., & Evans, A. C. (1998). Dose-dependent reduction of cerebral blood flow during rapid-rate transcranial magnetic stimulation of the human sensorimotor cortex. *Journal of Neurophysiology, 79*(2), 1102–1107.

Peled, A. (2005). Plasticity imbalance in mental disorders the neuroscience of psychiatry: Implications for diagnosis and research. *Medical Hypotheses, 65*(5), 947–952.

Pennisi, G., Alagona, G., Rapisarda, G., Nicoletti, F., Costanzo, E., Ferri, R., ... Bella, R. (2002). Transcranial magnetic stimulation after pure motor stroke. *Clinical Neurophysiology, 113*(10), 1536–1543.

Plewnia, C., Lotze, M., & Gerloff, C. (2003). Disinhibition of the contralateral motor cortex by low-frequency rTMS. *Neuroreport, 14*(4), 609–612.

Priori, A., Berardelli, A., Rona, S., Accornero, N., & Manfredi, M. (1998). Polarization of the human motor cortex through the scalp. *Neuroreport, 9*(10), 2257–2260.

Priori, A., Hallett, M., & Rothwell, J. C. (2009). Repetitive transcranial magnetic stimulation or transcranial direct current stimulation? *Brain Stimulation, 2*(4), 241–245.

Quartarone, A., Rizzo, V., & Morgante, F. (2008). Clinical features of dystonia: A pathophysiological revisitation. *Current Opinion in Neurology, 21*(4), 484–490.

Rabey, J. M., Dobronevsky, E., Aichenbaum, S., Gonen, O., Marton, R. G., & Khaigrekht, M. (2013). Repetitive transcranial magnetic stimulation combined with cognitive training is a safe and effective modality for the treatment of Alzheimer's disease: A randomized, double-blind study. *Journal of Neural Transmission, 120*(5), 813–819.

Reis, J., John, D., Heimeroth, A., Mueller, H. H., Oertel, W. H., Arndt, T., & Rosenow, F. (2006). Modulation of human motor cortex excitability by single doses of amantadine. *Neuropsychopharmacology, 31*(12), 2758–2766.

Robol, E., Fiaschi, A., & Manganotti, P. (2004). Effects of citalopram on the excitability of the human motor cortex: A paired magnetic stimulation study. *Journal of Neurological Sciences, 221*(1–2), 41–46.

Rodrigues, J. P., Walters, S. E., Stell, R., Thickbroom, G. W., & Mastaglia, F. L. (2008). Repetitive paired-pulse transcranial magnetic stimulation at I-wave intervals (iTMS) increases cortical excitability andimproves movement initiation in Parkinson's disease. *Clinical Neurophysiology, 119*, e25. doi: 10.1016/j.clinph.2007.10.055.

Rossini, D., Lucca, A., Zanardi, R., Magri, L., & Smeraldi, E. (2005). Transcranial magnetic stimulation in treatment-resistant depressed patients: A double-blind, placebo-controlled trial. *Psychiatry Research, 137*(1–2), 1–10.

Schambra, H. M., Sawaki, L., & Cohen, L. G. (2003). Modulation of excitability of human motor cortex (M1) by 1 Hz transcranial magnetic stimulation of the contralateral M1. *Clinical Neurophysiology, 114*(1), 130–133.

Schlaug, G., & Renga, V. (2008). Transcranial direct current stimulation: A noninvasive tool to facilitate stroke recovery. *Expert Reviews of Medical Devices, 5*(6), 759–768.

Schlaug, G., Renga, V., & Nair, D. (2008). Transcranial direct current stimulation in stroke recovery. *Archives of Neurology, 65*(12), 1571–1576.

Shimizu, H., Shiga, Y., Fujihara, K., Obhnuma, A., & Itoyama, Y. (2001). Clinical and physiological significance of abnormally prolonged central motor conduction time in HAMrTSP. *Journal of Neurological Sciences, 185*, 39–42.

Siciliano, G., Manca, M. L., Sagliocco, L., Pastorini, E., Pellegrinetti, A., Sartucci, F., ... Murri, L. (1999). Cortical silent period in patients with amyotrophic lateral sclerosis. *Journal of the Neurological Sciences, 169*(1–2), 93–97.

Siebner, H. R., Tormos, J. M., Ceballos-Baumann, A. O., Auer, C., Catala, M. D., Conrad, B., & Pascual-Leone, A. (1999). Low-frequency repetitive transcranial magnetic stimulation of the motor cortex in writer's cramp. *Neurology, 52*(3), 529–537.

Specterman, M., Bhuiya, A., Kuppuswamy, A., Strutton, P. H., Catley, M., & Davey, N. J. (2005). The effect of an energy drink containing glucose and caffeine on human corticospinal excitability. *Physiology & Behavior, 83*(5), 723–728.

Stagg, C. J., Best, J. G., Stephenson, M. C., O'Shea, J., Wylezinska, M., Kincses, Z. T., ... Johansen-Berg, H. (2009). Polarity-sensitive modulation of cortical neurotransmitters by transcranial stimulation. *Journal of Neuroscience, 29*(16), 5202–5206.

Swinnen, S. P. (2002). Intermanual coordination: From behavioural principles to neural-network interactions. *Nature Reviews Neuroscience, 3*(5), 348–359.

Takeuchi, N., Chuma, T., Matsuo, Y., Watanabe, I., & Ikoma, K. (2005). Repetitive transcranial magnetic stimulation of contralesional primary motor cortex improves hand function after stroke. *Stroke, 36*(12), 2681–2686.

Tanaka, S., & Watanabe, K. (2009). Transcranial direct current stimulation – A new tool for human cognitive neuroscience. *Brain and Nerve, 61*(1), 53–64.

Thickbroom, G. W. (2007). Transcranial magnetic stimulation and synaptic plasticity: Experimental framework and human models. *Experimental Brain Research, 180*(4), 583–593.

Thickbroom, G. W., Byrnes, M. L., Archer, S. A., & Mastaglia, F. L. (2004). Motor outcome after subcortical stroke correlates with the degree of cortical reorganization. *Clinical Neurophysiology, 115*(9), 2144–2150.

Thickbroom, G. W., Byrnes, M. L., Stell, R., & Mastaglia, F. L. (2003). Reversible reorganisation of the motor cortical representation of the hand in cervical dystonia. *Movement Disorders, 18*(4), 395–402.

Thickbroom, G. W., Byrnes, M. L., Walters, S., Stell, R., & Mastaglia, F. L. (2006). Motor cortex reorganisation in Parkinson's disease. *Journal of Clinical Neuroscience, 13*(6), 639–642.

Ueki, Y., Mima, T., Kotb, M. A., Sawada, H., Saiki, H., Ikeda, A., ... Fukuyama, H. (2006). Altered plasticity of the human motor cortex in Parkinson's disease. *Annals of Neurology, 59*(1), 60–71.

Van Der Werf, Y. D., Berendse, H. W., van Someren, E. J., Stoffers, D., Stam, C. J., & Wolters, ECh. (2007). Observations on the cortical silent period in Parkinson's disease. *Journal of Neural Transmission, (Suppl. 72)*, 155–158.

Vitek, J. L., Delong, M. R., Starr, P. A., Hariz, M. I., & Metman, L. V. (2011). Intraoperative neurophysiology in DBS for dystonia. *Movement Disorders, 26*(Suppl. 1), S31–S36.

Wagner, T., Fregni, F., Fecteau, S., Grodzinsky, A., Zahn, M., & Pascual-Leone, A. (2007a). Transcranial direct current stimulation: A computer-based human model study. *Neuroimage, 35*(3), 1113–1124.

Wagner, T., Valero-Cabre, A., & Pascual-Leone, A. (2007b). Noninvasive human brain stimulation. *Annual Review of Biomedical Engineering, 9*, 527–565.

Walsh, J. (1773). On the electric property of torpedo: In a letter to B. Franklin. *Philosophical Transcactions for the Royal Society, 63*, 478–489.

Walton, C., Kalmar, J., & Cafarelli, E. (2003). Caffeine increases spinal excitability in humans. *Muscle Nerve, 28*(3), 359–364.

Yehuda, S., Rabinovitz, S., & Mostofsky, D. I. (2005). Essential fatty acids and the brain: From infancy to aging. *Neurobiology of Aging, 26*(Suppl. 1), 98–102.

Ziemann, U. (2004). TMS and drugs. *Clinical Neurophysiology, 115*(8), 1717–1729.

Ziemann, U. (2010). TMS in cognitive neuroscience: Virtual lesion and beyond. *Cortex, 46*(1), 124–127.

# 12 Use of Neuroimaging Techniques in the Assessment of Nutraceuticals for Cognitive Enhancement

*Methodological and Interpretative Issues*

*David Alan Camfield and Andrew Scholey*

## CONTENTS

## SUMMARY

The following review provides a comparison of neuroimaging techniques (electrophysiology [EEG], steady-state topography [SST], near-infrared spectroscopy [NIRS], functional magnetic resonance imaging [fMRI] and positron-emission tomography [PET]) which have been used to study nutraceutical interventions for cognition in healthy adults. Recent research in the area is summarised for the following substances: glucose, green tea extracts, caffeine, theanine, chlorogenic acid, *Panax ginseng*, nicotine, *Ginkgo biloba*, multivitamins, fish oils, soybean peptide, resveratrol, creatine, guaraná and cocoa flavanols. A brief outline of the individual neuroimaging techniques, together with methodological and interpretative issues associated with each of these technologies, is presented. A review of acute and chronic neurocognitive intervention studies featuring nutraceutical substances over the past 20 years is also presented for each of these neuroimaging modalities. Following this, a general discussion of common pitfalls associated with neuroimaging and psychopharmacology is also included, including the importance of directional hypothesis testing, the careful selection of difficulty level when specifying a cognitive *activation* task and how to correct for multiple comparisons whilst maintaining an acceptable level of statistical power. Recommendations for future research using neuroimaging in conjunction with nutraceutical interventions are outlined.

## 12.1   INTRODUCTION

The recording of changes in neural activity associated with human psychopharmacology requires very precise and accurate measurement, as well as a nuanced interpretation which takes into account a number of important factors. The most fundamental questions that need to be answered before embarking on a neurocognitive intervention study are as follows: (1) Why is neuroimaging data required? (2) Would another physiological measurement be more appropriate? And (3) if neuroimaging is necessary, then which technique would be best suited to your study hypotheses? Valid answers to question (1) may include the following: a desire to better understand the underlying mechanism(s) of action of a substance in the brain or the desire to measure subtle changes in sensory or cognitive functioning that cannot be captured using standard behavioural measures of reaction time and accuracy. Invalid answers are numerous but are generally subsumed under the guise of wanting to provide some *objective* measure of *brain activation* that infers some ill-defined benefit to the substance under study. In regard to the second question, it is worth keeping in mind that there are a multitude of physiological measures other than neuroimaging techniques which may better answer underlying mechanistic questions. These include, but are not limited to, autonomic measures such as skin conductance response and startle reflexes, cardiovascular measurements such as heart-rate variability or Doppler blood flow effects and finally haematological and saliva assays. The answer to the third question requires a much more in-depth analysis and is the subject of this chapter.

In the following chapter, the functional neuroimaging techniques of EEG, power spectral analysis, event-related potentials (ERPs) and SST will be discussed, together with NIRS, fMRI and PET. A review of selected studies in healthy non-clinical adult samples, specifically concerned with acute and/or chronic cognitive effects of nutraceutical substances, will also be presented separately for each of these neuroimaging modalities. A review of structural imaging techniques such as voxel-based morphometry, as well as magnetic resonance spectroscopy, is beyond the scope of this chapter. Similarly, there are too few studies in the nutraceutical literature to permit an examination of magnetoencephalography (MEG) and single-photon computerised emission tomography. The interested reader is referred to the excellent review by Sizonenko et al. (2013) for coverage of these other techniques in the more general context of nutritional neuroscience.

## 12.2 ELECTROPHYSIOLOGY

Due to the relatively low cost associated with EEG recording and analysis in comparison to other neuroimaging technologies, EEG has been used extensively in nutraceutical intervention studies, in particular those involving acute administration. The two paradigms used predominantly in EEG research over the past 50 years have been ERPs and power spectral analysis. However, in recent years, the more advanced technique of steady-state probe topography (SST) has also begun to gain prominence in studies of the human psychopharmacology associated with nutraceuticals.

### 12.2.1 POWER SPECTRAL ANALYSIS

Power spectral analysis of continuous EEG in the traditional frequency bands of delta (<4 Hz), theta (4–7 Hz), alpha (8–15 Hz), beta (15–30 Hz) and gamma (30+ Hz) are typically measured during a resting state, either with the eyes open or closed. The latter, eyes closed EEG, is the preferred method in the majority of studies, due to the fact that the degree of external stimulation is standardised and the results are more easily interpretable across participants. The lower frequency bands are associated with more synchronised and higher amplitude power, whereas the higher frequency bands with oscillations in more regional brain regions and are of lower amplitude. In addition to analysis of the EEG spectral power at rest, changes in EEG power can also be observed whilst completing a cognitive task. The technique of event-related synchronisation/desynchronisation (Pfurtscheller, 1992) is a more precise method for these types of analyses, which compares the percentage decrease or increase in spectral power in relation to a pre-stimulus baseline period. More recently, time–frequency analysis of the EEG, using either short fast-Fourier transforms or wavelets, has also been used in order to measure changes in oscillatory activity with millisecond temporal resolution (see Herrmann et al., 2014). However, this approach is yet to be applied in nutraceutical intervention studies.

The alpha rhythm is the dominant frequency of the EEG spectrum which reflects activity in thalamocortical feedback loops as well as inhibitory control (Klimesch et al., 2007). Alpha activity is maximal over posterior recording sites during resting, eyes closed. Typically, alpha activity is found to decrease, or desynchronise, during cognitive processing, whilst higher frequency activity (e.g. in the beta band) will begin to increase. This is due to the activation of neural networks that start to oscillate at different frequencies and with different phases (Klimesch, 1999). An exception to this pattern of alpha desynchronisation during cognition is observed in tasks which require the online maintenance of material in short-term memory. Here, upper alpha power has been found to increase, or synchronise, in order to inhibit task-irrelevant information (Klimesch et al., 1999). Theta activity has also been found to be modulated by cognitive demands, with theta power found to increase, and synchronise, in tasks which require the encoding of new episodic memories. Klimesch et al. (1999) propose that theta is specifically linked to activity in cortico-hippocampal feedback loops and the encoding of new information. EEG activity in the gamma range (>30) is more difficult to record and analyse due to the fact that muscle EMG activity, as well as 50 Hz electrical interference, can often confound the results. One approach to overcoming this problem is to focus analysis on central, rather than temporal, recording sites and to restrict the analysis of gamma band activity to the 35–45 Hz frequency range (Barry et al., 2010). An interesting finding in relation to gamma power is that it forms strong correlations with metabolic activity (Oakes et al., 2004).

In relation to nutraceutical intervention studies involving cognitive effects in healthy adults, there have been around 12 EEG power spectral studies conducted over the past 20 years (see Table 12.1). In studies involving acute caffeine administration, the most consistent finding has been that of reduced alpha power during a resting state (Barry et al., 2011; Kenemans & Lorist, 1995) as well as during the completion of an n-back task (Gevins et al., 2002), although other findings have included reduced delta power (Keane & James, 2008) as well as increased theta and beta power (Keane & James, 2008; Keane et al., 2007). For studies involving acute administration of green tea extracts/epigallocatechin gallate (EGCG), increases in frontal alpha, beta and theta power were observed during a resting state (Scholey et al., 2012), whilst reduced delta power together with increased frontal delta/theta was observed during a reading task (Dimpfel et al., 2007). In relation to the tea constituent L-theanine administered in isolation, a reduction in alpha power was observed during a visuospatial attention task (Gomez-Ramirez et al., 2009). For *Panax ginseng*, reduced alpha power was observed during a resting state (Kennedy et al., 2003), whilst reduced delta power (Dimpfel et al., 2006) as well as reduced frontal theta and beta power was also observed when ginseng was administered in combination with *Ginkgo biloba* during a resting state (Kennedy et al., 2003). Decreased delta power was also observed following combined supplementation with *Panax ginseng* and *Ginkgo biloba* during a reading task (Dimpfel et al., 2006). When *Ginkgo biloba* was administered in isolation, a dose-dependent increase in alpha power was observed from 1–7 h post-dose (Itil et al., 1996). Finally, one study by Fontani et al. (2005) investigated the effects of chronic (35-day) supplementation with 4 g/day of fish oil high in ω-3 fatty acids (FAs) and revealed greater theta and alpha power following fish oil supplementation in comparison to placebo.

**TABLE 12.1**

**Nutraceutical Neurocognitive Intervention Studies in Healthy Adults**

| Study | Nutraceutical Treatment | Sample/Design | Cognitive Task(s) | Summary of Findings |
|---|---|---|---|---|
| *EEG frequency analysis* | | | | |
| Scholey et al. (2012) | EGCG (300 mg acute) | N = 31 (46–95 years) Acute crossover | Resting eyes open | Frontal alpha, beta and theta power increased with EGCG in comparison to placebo |
| Barry et al. (2011) | Caffeine (250 mg acute) | N = 22 (17–36 years) Acute crossover | Resting eyes open and closed | Global alpha power reduced with caffeine in comparison to placebo |
| Gomez-Ramirez et al. (2009) | Theanine (250 mg acute) | N = 35 (M = 23.5 years) Acute crossover | Visuo-spatial attention | Reduction in tonic alpha power with theanine, but no sig. change in cue-related phasic alpha |
| Keane& James (2008) | Caffeine (5.25 mg/day) | N = 15 (17–19 years) 4-week crossover | Resting eyes open/closed, SART | Decreased delta power and increased beta power with caffeine in comparison to placebo |
| Keane et al. (2007) | Caffeine (5.25 mg/day) | N = 22 (17–44 years) 4-week crossover | Resting eyes open/closed, SART | Increased theta power in response to caffeine acutely and after acute caffeine withdrawal |
| Dimpfel et al. (2007) | Green tea, theanine | N = 12 (40–65 years) Acute crossover | Resting, reading | Reduced delta, increased frontal delta/theta during reading for green tea vs. placebo |
| Dimpfel et al. (2006) | *Panax ginseng* (0.232 g), *Ginkgo biloba* (2 g) | N = 10 (35–55 years) Acute crossover | Resting eyes open, closed and story reading | Decreased delta power in resting eyes open/closed and increased delta power during reading for active drink compared to placebo |
| Fontani et al. (2005) | Omega-3 PUFA (4 g/day chronic) | N = 33 (22–51 years) 35 day, parallel group | Resting eyes closed | Greater theta and alpha power following ω – 3s vs. placebo |
| Kennedy et al. (2003) | *Panax ginseng* (0.200 g), *Ginkgo biloba* (0.360 g) | N = 15 (19–39 years) Acute crossover | Resting eyes closed | Reduced frontal theta and beta power with resting eyes closed (both ginseng and ginkgo) and reduced alpha power (ginseng only) |
| Gevins et al. (2002) | Caffeine (200 mg acute) | N = 16 (21–32 years) Acute crossover | *n*-back working memory, resting eyes open/closed | Decreased posterior alpha power in both low- and high-load *n*-back conditions vs. placebo |

*(Continued)*

**TABLE 12.1 (*Continued*)**

**Nutraceutical Neurocognitive Intervention Studies in Healthy Adults**

| Study | Nutraceutical Treatment | Sample/Design | Cognitive Task(s) | Summary of Findings |
|---|---|---|---|---|
| Itil et al. (1996) | *Ginkgo biloba* (40–240 mg acute) | N = 12 (18–65) Dose escalation | Resting eyes closed, SRT | Dose-dependent increase in alpha power from 1 to 7 hrs post-dose |
| Kenemans & Lorist (1995) *ERP analysis* | Caffeine (3 mg/kg acute) | N = 16 (19–29 years) Acute crossover | Resting eyes open | Decreased alpha power with caffeine vs. placebo |
| Scholey et al. (2014) | Glucose (25 g acute) | N = 12 (65 years+) Acute crossover | Word recognition | Left parietal (LP) old–new component enhanced for glucose in comparison to placebo |
| Brown & Riby (2013) | Glucose (25 g acute) | N = 35 (18–35 years) Acute parallel groups | Episodic memory | LP old–new component enhanced for glucose in comparison to placebo |
| Cropley et al. (2012) | Coffee enriched with CGA | N = 39 Acute crossover | RVIP – P300/ CNV MMN | No sig ERP effects |
| Riby et al. (2008) | Glucose (25 g acute) | N = 15 (M = 28.7 years) Acute crossover | Visual oddball | Reduction in P3b amplitude with glucose in comparison to placebo |
| Dimpfel et al. (2007) | Green tea, theanine | N = 12 (40–65 years) Acute crossover | Visual oddball | Decreased P3 latency for green tea vs. placebo |
| Tieges et al. (2007) | Caffeine (3 mg/kg acute) | N = 18 (18–31 years) Acute crossover | Task-switch paradigm | Enhanced ERP negativity in response to caffeine, during interval preceding task shifting |
| Barry et al. (2007) | Caffeine (250 mg acute) | N = 24 (17–46) Acute parallel groups | Auditory Go/ NoGo | Increased P1, P2 and P3b amplitude to Go stimuli with caffeine, in comparison to placebo |
| Baldeweg et al. (2006) | Nicotine (2 × 2 mg gum) | N = 24 (20–35 years) Acute parallel groups | Auditory sensory memory | Mismatch negativity (MMN) amplitude was augmented for nicotine vs. placebo |
| Fontani et al. (2005) | Omega-3 PUFA/ (4 g/day chronic) | N = 33 (22–51 years) 35 day, parallel group | SRT, CRT, Go/ NoGo, SA | P3 amplitude increased for Go and NoGo trials for Omega 3 vs. placebo |

*(Continued)*

## TABLE 12.1 *(Continued)*
## Nutraceutical Neurocognitive Intervention Studies in Healthy Adults

| Study | Nutraceutical Treatment | Sample/Design | Cognitive Task(s) | Summary of Findings |
|---|---|---|---|---|
| Tieges et al. (2004) | Caffeine (3.5 mg/kg acute) | N = 15 (18–26 years) Acute crossover | Task switching | Enhanced error-related negativity (ERN) amplitude for both caffeine doses vs. placebo |
| Kennedy et al. (2003) | *Panax ginseng* (0.200 g), *Ginkgo biloba* (0.360 g) | N = 15 (19–39 years) Acute crossover | Auditory oddball, CNV, | Reduced P3 latency with ginseng vs. placebo |

*ERP: Steady-state visual evoked potentials*

| | | | | |
|---|---|---|---|---|
| Camfield et al. (2013) | *Hypericum perforatum* (500 mg/day), NRT | N = 20 (18–60 years) 10-week, parallel group. | Spatial working memory (SWM) | Increased SSVEP amplitude in posterior-parietal regions for HP and NRT, as well as decreased fronto-central SSVEP latency with HP |
| Camfield et al. (2012) | *Cocoa flavanols* (250,500 mg/ day chronic) | N = 63 (40–65 years) 30-day, parallel group | SWM | Decreased posterior SSVEP amplitude at retest during SWM hold period and decreased posterior SSVEP phase lag at retest during SWM encoding/retrieval, for CF vs. placebo |
| Macpherson et al. (2012) | Multivitamins (1 tablet/day chronic) | N = 41 (64–79 years) 16 week, parallel group | SWM | Increased SSVEP phase lag in right temporal and left frontal regions at retest during SWM retrieval period, for MV vs. placebo |
| Stough et al. (2011) | *Ginkgo biloba* (80 mg/day chronic) | N = 19 (50–61 years) Chronic 14-day crossover | Object working memory (OWM) | Increased SSVEP amplitude at occipital and frontal sites, increased SSVEP latency at left temporal and left frontal sites during OWM hold period, for ginkgo vs. placebo |
| Thompson et al. (2000) | Nicotine (0.8 mg acute) | N = 13 (M = 25 years) Acute crossover | Visual vigilance | Increased SSVEP amplitude in central and occipital sites and reduced SSVEP latency in bilateral frontal and right parietal regions for nicotine vs. placebo |

*(Continued)*

**TABLE 12.1 (Continued)**
**Nutraceutical Neurocognitive Intervention Studies in Healthy Adults**

| Study | Nutraceutical Treatment | Sample/Design | Cognitive Task(s) | Summary of Findings |
|---|---|---|---|---|
| *NIRS* | | | | |
| Wightman et al. (2012) | EGCG (135,270 mg acute) | N = 27 (18–30 years) Acute crossover | Serial subtract, oddball, RVIP, stroop, SRT | Reduced oxygenated and total haemoglobin in frontal cortex during cognitive tasks for EGCG vs. placebo |
| Jackson et al. (2012a) | Fish oil (1 g DHA-rich, 1 g EPA-rich chronic) | N = 22 (M = 21.96 years) 12-week parallel group | Stroop, peg and ball, 3-back WM and WCST | Increased oxy-Hb and total Hb in frontal cortex during cognitive tasks for DHA-rich fish oil vs. placebo |
| Jackson et al. (2012b) | Fish oil (1 g DHA-rich, 2 g DHA-rich chronic) | N = 65 (18–29 years) 12-week parallel group | Numeric WM, 3-back, SRT, CRT, RVIP, serial subtract, stroop, corsi blk. | Increased oxy-Hb and total Hb in PFC during cognitive tasks for both doses of DHA-rich fish oil vs. placebo |
| Yimit et al. (2012) | Soybean peptide (8 g acute) | N = 10 (20–25 years) Acute crossover | Resting state | Increased theta, alpha-2 and beta-L amplitudes in premotor cortex, primary motor cortex, DLPFC and frontal polar region for soybean peptide vs. placebo |
| Kennedy & Haskell (2011) | Caffeine (75 mg acute) | N = 20 (19–28 years) Acute crossover | Serial subtract, RVIP | Reduced total Hb in frontal cortex during cognitive tasks for caffeine vs. placebo but only for non-habitual consumers |
| Kennedy et al. (2010) | Resveratrol (250,500 mg acute) | N = 22 (18–25 years) Acute crossover | Serial subtract, RVIP | Increased total Hb and deoxy-Hb in frontal cortex during cognitive tasks for resveratrol vs. placebo |
| Watanabe et al. (2002) | Creatine (8/g day chronic) | N = 24 (M = 24.3 years) 5 day, parallel groups | Serial numeric calculation | Reduced oxy-Hb in frontal cortex during cognitive tasks for creatine vs. placebo |
| Gagnon et al. (2012) | Glucose (50 g acute) | N = 20 (M = 69.4 years) Acute crossover | Single and dual task (colour and letter discrimination) | Glucose was associated with increased activation in lateral and ventral sites as participants moved from single to dual discrimination tasks |

*(Continued)*

## TABLE 12.1 (*Continued*)
## Nutraceutical Neurocognitive Intervention Studies in Healthy Adults

| Study | Nutraceutical Treatment | Sample/Design | Cognitive Task(s) | Summary of Findings |
|---|---|---|---|---|
| *fMRI* | | | | |
| Schmidt et al. (2014) | EGCG (13.75, 27.5 g GTE acute) | N = 12 (M = 24.1 years) Acute crossover | n-back working memory | Increased connectivity between right superior parietal lobe and middle frontal gyrus for EGCG vs. placebo |
| Scholey et al. (2013) | Multivitamins/ Guaraná (G) (MV,MV+G acute) | N = 20 (21–39 years) Acute crossover | Inspection time, RVIP | Increased activation in R precentral gyrus and L/R cerebellum for MV vs. placebo, increased activation in R precentral gyrus, L middle frontal gyrus, frontal medial gyri and L/R superior parietal lobes for MV+G vs. placebo |
| Park et al. (2014) | Caffeine (200 mg acute) | N = 14 (M = 30.3 years) Acute within subj | Visuomotor task | Increased BOLD activation in the L cerebellum, putamen, insula, thalamus and R primary motor cortex for caffeine |
| Haller et al. (2013) | Caffeine (200 mg acute) | N = 24 (62–80 years) Acute crossover | n-back working memory | −22.7% reduction in whole-brain perfusion with caffeine. Increased activation in L/R striatum, R middle and inferior frontal gyrus, L/R insula, L superior and inferior parietal lobule and L/R cerebellum, with caffeine vs. placebo |
| Klaassen et al. (2013) | Caffeine (100 mg acute) | N = 20 (40–61 years) Acute crossover | Sternberg working memory | Increased activation in L/R DLPFC during WM encoding and decreased activation in L thalamus during WM maintenance with caffeine vs. placebo |
| Tal et al. (2013) | Caffeine (200 mg acute) | N = 10 (21–33 years) Acute crossover | Resting eyes closed, eyes open | Widespread reductions in resting-state fMRI and beta MEG connectivity, with caffeine vs. placebo |

*(Continued)*

**TABLE 12.1 (*Continued*)**
**Nutraceutical Neurocognitive Intervention Studies in Healthy Adults**

| Study | Nutraceutical Treatment | Sample/Design | Cognitive Task(s) | Summary of Findings |
|---|---|---|---|---|
| Wong et al. (2012) | Caffeine (200 mg acute) | N = 10 (24–33 years) Acute crossover | Resting eyes closed, eyes open | Anticorrelation between default-mode (DMN) and task-positive (TPN) networks during resting eyes closed, with caffeine vs. placebo |
| Diukova et al. (2012) | Caffeine (250 mg acute) | N = 14 (20–32 years) Acute crossover | Visual task, visuomotor task, auditory oddball | Decreased BOLD activation in visual and primary motor cortex during visual and visuomotor tasks. Increased BOLD activation during auditory oddball and decreased EEG P3 latency, with caffeine vs. placebo |
| Borgwardt et al. (2012) | EGCG (250, 500 mL drink, 0.05% GT extract) | N = 12 (21–28 years) Acute crossover | n-back working memory | Increased activation in the DLPFC for the green tea extract vs. placebo |
| Griffeth et al. (2011) | Caffeine (200 mg acute) | N = 10 (not reported) Acute within subj | Visual checkerboard (8 Hz) | CBF reduced by 27%, whilst $CRMO_2$ increased by 22%. Evoked $CRMO_2$ in response to visual stimulus increased by 61%. Net result of similar pre- and post-caffeine BOLD response |
| Parent et al. (2011) | Glucose (50 g) | N = 14 (M = 24.1 years) Acute crossover | Emotional and neutral memory encoding | Increased activation in, and increased connectivity between, brain loci associated with memory encoding (including hippocampus) |
| Serra-Grabulosa et al. (2010) | Glucose/caffeine (75 mg glu, 75 mg caff, combination) | N = 40 (18–25 years) Acute parallel groups | Numeric CPT | Combined caffeine and glucose resulted in decreased BOLD activation in L/R parietal and left PFC, yet similar behavioural performance |

*(Continued)*

## TABLE 12.1 (*Continued*)
## Nutraceutical Neurocognitive Intervention Studies in Healthy Adults

| Study | Nutraceutical Treatment | Sample/Design | Cognitive Task(s) | Summary of Findings |
|---|---|---|---|---|
| Liau et al. (2008) | Caffeine (200 mg acute) | N = 10 (M = 33 years) Acute within subj | Resting state, visual checkerboard (8 Hz) | Decreased CBF activation, but not the BOLD activation with caffeine. |
| Perthen et al. (2008) | Caffeine (200 mg acute) | N = 10 (M = 33 years) Acute within subj | Resting state, visual checkerboard (8 Hz) | CBF decreased by 34.5% whilst $CMRO_2$ did not change significantly, with caffeine. Contribution of CBF to BOLD signal was calibrated pre-dose using mild hypercapnia ($CO_2$ inhalation) |
| Koppelstaetter et al. (2008) | Caffeine (100 mg acute) | N = 16 (25–47 years) Acute crossover | n-back working memory | Increased BOLD activation in L/R medial frontopolar cortex and R ACC, with caffeine vs. placebo |
| Bendlin et al. (2007) | Caffeine (222 mg acute) | N = 21 (18–40 years) Acute parallel groups | Word stem completion | Reduction in baseline CBF, but no effect on baseline BOLD or response to WSC task with caffeine vs. placebo |
| Francis et al. (2006) | Cocoa flavanols (13, 172 mg chronic) | N = 16 (18–30 years) 5-day crossover | Task switching | Increased BOLD activation during switch condition in DLPFC, parietal cortex and ACC for high vs. low flavanol drinks. Pilot study (N = 4) revealed increased CBF associated with acute (450 mg) dose of flavanols |
| Stone et al. (2005) | Glucose (50 g) | N = 8 DSM IV schizophrenia (18–59) Acute within subj | Verbal encoding | Increased BOLD in left hippocampus with trend in DLPFC |

(*Continued*)

**TABLE 12.1 (*Continued*)**

**Nutraceutical Neurocognitive Intervention Studies in Healthy Adults**

| Study | Nutraceutical Treatment | Sample/Design | Cognitive Task(s) | Summary of Findings |
|---|---|---|---|---|
| Portas et al. (1998) | Caffeine (5 mg/kg acute) | N = 8 (25–38 years) Acute within subj | Visual checkerboard, blank screen, attentional task, passive viewing | Activation of ventrolateral thalamus during the attentional task was highest during a state of low arousal (following sleep deprivation) compared with normal and high arousal (following caffeine) |
| *PET* | | | | |
| Park et al. (2014) | Caffeine (200 mg acute) | N = 14 (M = 30.3 years) Acute within subj | Visuomotor task | Reduced metabolic activity in the putamen, caudate, nucleus, insula, pallidum and posterior medial cortex with caffeine |
| Nugent et al. (2011) | Fish oil (680 mg DHA/323 mg EPA chronic) | N = 11 (18–30 and 70+ years) 3-week open-label | Resting state | No effect of fish oil on cerebral glucose metabolism in young or healthy elderly |
| Small et al. (2006) | Healthy diet (chronic) | N = 17 (35–69 years) 14-day parallel group | Resting state | 5% decrease in cerebral glucose metabolism in the DLPFC for healthy diet group vs. usual lifestyle routine |

EGCG, epigallocatechin gallate; SART, sustained attention to response task; SRT, simple reaction time; RVIP, rapid visual information processing; Hb, haemoglobin; oxy-Hb, oxygenated haemoglobin; deoxy-Hb, deoxygenated haemoglobin; PUFA, polyunsaturated fatty acids; CNV, contingent negative variation; MMN, mismatch negativity; ERN, error-related negativity; SSVEP, steady-state visually evoked potential; SWM, spatial working memory; CF, cocoa flavanols; MV, multivitamin; OWM, object working memory; DLPFC, dorsolateral prefrontal cortex; BOLD, blood oxygen level dependent signal; WM, working memory; GTE, green tea extract; NRT, nicotine replacement therapy; G, guarana; CRMO2, cerebral metabolic rate of oxygen; CBF, cerebral blood flow; MEG, magnetoencephalography; fMRI, functional magnetic resonance imaging.

## 12.2.2 EVENT-RELATED POTENTIALS

ERP analysis lends itself well to the study of changes in brain activity associated with sensory and/or cognitive processing. However, in order to obtain an adequate signal-to-noise ratio associated with the ERP components, stimulus–response sequences must often be presented multiple times to each participant over the course of the experiment and averaged for analysis. Similarly, an adequate number of participants must be studied in order to ensure that statistical power is sufficient to uncover between or within-group differences. Another important issue associated with ERP analysis is the use of an appropriate technique to remove ocular artefact. This is achieved by recording the electro-occulogram (EOG) associated with eye movements and blinks in addition to the ongoing EEG, using two electrodes placed near the outer canthus of the left and right eyes, as well as two electrodes placed equi-distantly above and below either the right or the left eye (Croft & Barry, 2000c). Whilst there are a wide range of different techniques that may be used to remove eye movement and blink artefact during subsequent analysis, the high-quality regression-based revised aligned-artefact average (RAAA) technique, developed by Croft & Barry (2000b), which utilises an EOG calibration task at the beginning of the recording to estimate vertical, horizontal and radial eye movement coefficients, is recommended. More recently, techniques that rely on spatial independent components analysis (Li et al., 2006) or principal components analysis (PCA) of the raw EEG (Wallstrom et al., 2004) to estimate ocular artefact components and remove these components have also become popular. However, in comparison to the large number of validation studies that have been conducted using the regression-based techniques (Croft & Barry, 2000a; Croft et al., 2005; Pham et al., 2011) further empirical evidence is required in order to properly establish the effectiveness of the newer ICA and PCA techniques.

Whilst there are several different ERP components which have been found to be associated with various types of cognitive processing, the most well-researched components are the (1) P300, a positive component appearing around 300 ms post-stimulus which is related to the allocation of attentional resources and is typically elicited using an auditory or visual oddball paradigm (Donchin & Coles, 1988); (2) the N200, which is a negative component appearing around 200 ms post-stimulus and is often related to inhibitory processing in a Go/NoGo task; (3) contingent negative variation (CNV), which is a slow negative-going potential which is related to the anticipation of a stimulus; (4) error-related negativity (ERN), which is a negative deflection peaking around 100ms following an erroneous response in a Go/NoGo task; and (5) the left parietal (LP) old-new effect, which is associated with correct recognition of a previously memorised stimulus in comparison to a new stimulus. In relation to early sensory processing, the mismatch negativity (MMN) is also a commonly used paradigm, which is a frontal measure of pre-attentive auditory change detection (Näätänen et al., 2007). Traditionally, ERP components are identified by *peak picking* within specified post-stimulus time windows. However, more recently, there has been a shift toward the use of temporal principal components analysis (tPCA) in order to empirically derive the components which explain the greatest amount of variance in the data (Dien, 2012). This more objective approach to EEG analysis is being adopted by a growing number of prominent EEG researchers (see Barry & De Blasio, 2013; Barry et al., 2014).

As with power spectral analysis, there have also been a large number of studies utilising ERP paradigms in research involving nutraceuticals. However, whilst EEG power analysis has been applied primarily during a resting state, ERP analysis is the preferred method when conducting a precisely timed cognitive task.

In ERP studies involving acute caffeine administration, enhanced negativities have been observed in the interval preceding task switching (Tieges et al., 2007), as well as increased P1, P2 and P3b amplitudes in response to Go stimuli in an auditory Go/NoGo paradigm (Barry et al., 2007); see Figure 12.1. Enhanced ERN (see Figure12.1) has also been observed for caffeine versus placebo (Tieges et al., 2004).

More recently, the effect of acute glucose administration on cognition has also been investigated, with enhancement of the LP ERP component during a recognition memory task emerging as a consistent finding (Brown & Riby, 2013; Riby et al., 2008; Scholey et al., 2014). In an earlier study by Riby et al. (2008), evidence was also provided to suggest that the P3b amplitude is reduced with glucose in comparison to placebo when completing a visual oddball task. A study by Cropley et al. (2012) reported no effects on either P300, CNV or MMN in response to administration of decaffeinated coffee enriched with chlorogenic acids. In relation to green tea enriched with L-theanine, Dimpfel et al. (2007) reported that P3 latency was reduced in a visual oddball task. Baldeweg et al. (2006) found that MMN was augmented for nicotine gum in compared to placebo, whilst Kennedy et al. (2003) reported reduced P3 latency with *Panax ginseng* versus placebo in an auditory oddball task. Finally, for the chronic fish oil study by Fontani et al. (2005), P3 amplitude was found to be increased for both Go and NoGo trials in an oddball task following fish oil supplementation over 35 days.

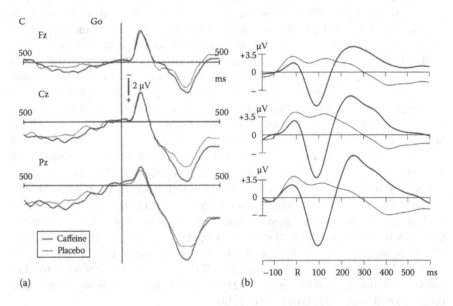

**FIGURE 12.1** (a) Effect of caffeine on P1, P2 and P3b amplitudes in response to Go stimuli in an auditory Go/NoGo paradigm. (From Barry, R.J. et al., *Clin. Neurophysiol.*, 118(12), 2692, 2007. doi: 10.1016/j.clinph.2007.08.023.) (b) Effect of caffeine on ERN amplitudes. (From Tieges, Z. et al., *Cognit. Brain Res.*, 21(1), 87, 2004. doi: 10.1016/j.cogbrainres.2004.06.001.)

## 12.2.3   STEADY-STATE PROBE TOPOGRAPHY

SST is an advanced electrophysiological technique that involves measuring the brain's response to visual stimuli at a set frequency. The resultant steady-state visually evoked potential (SSVEP) response to the stimulation frequency occurs primarily at the same frequency as the stimulation frequency, although spectral peaks at harmonic frequencies are also observed. In the SST method pioneered by Silberstein et al. (1995), a diffuse visual flicker is administered to the subject's peripheral vision at a frequency of 13 Hz via custom-built goggles which are fitted with half-silvered mirrors. Fourier analysis is subsequently used to extract information regarding the amplitude and phase of the SSVEP response at 13 Hz. This particular stimulation frequency typically sits just above the individual alpha peak, and, in studies which have compared a wide range of different stimulation frequencies, has been found to be optimal for the generation of maximal SSVEP amplitude (Bayram et al., 2011). The amplitude of the SSVEP response at this frequency has been theorised by Silberstein et al. (1995) to provide an index of activity in regional cortico-cortico and thalamocortical loops in the 8–18 Hz range.

The SST technique is ideally suited to the analysis of changes in oscillatory cortical activity during the concurrent completion of a cognitive task. In practical terms, the SST has some advantages over other EEG methodologies. For example, it is relatively robust to artefacts arising from task-irrelevant sensory or motor factors. In contrast to the traditional analysis technique of ERPs, changes to the 13 Hz SSVEP amplitude can be monitored at multiple time points during neural processing throughout the completion of a task, with a maximum temporal resolution of around 76 ms (1/13 s). In addition to analysis of changes to SSVEP amplitude, changes in the phase of the SSVEP can also be analysed. The latter measures ongoing differences in the lag time between the administration of the 13 Hz flicker and the resultant SSVEP response. Reductions in 13 Hz SSVEP amplitude during cognitive processing are typically interpreted in a similar fashion to alpha desynchronisation (ERD), whilst decreases in SSVEP phase lag are interpreted as evidence of increased synaptic excitation and/or decreases in synaptic inhibitory processes. Typically, both the amplitude and phase of the SSVEP response are normalised for each participant prior to conducting group averaging. This is often conducted using the average amplitude and phase values obtained during a low-demand reference task at the beginning of the study. The choice of baseline task, together with whether the normalisation process is repeated for each subsequent study visit, in the case of a chronic intervention study, is of particular importance when analysing SSVEP data associated with a nutraceutical intervention. For a more detailed discussion of the SST/SSVEP analysis method, please refer to Silberstein (1995).

Whilst application of the SSVEP technique to the study of psychopharmacology is still in its infancy, there have been a handful of intriguing studies to emerge from the literature in the past decade which suggest that this technique may be particularly informative for detecting subtle changes in cognitive function associated with nutraceutical intervention. In an early study by Thompson et al. (2000), acute nicotine administration was found to increase SSVEP amplitude in central and occipital brain regions, as well as reduce SSVEP latency in bilateral frontal and right parietal regions when compared to placebo. In a study investigating the chronic neurocognitive effects of *Ginkgo biloba*, Stough et al. (2011) found that 14-day supplementation brought about increases to occipital and frontal SSVEP amplitude as well as increases to SSVEP latency at left temporal and left frontal sites, during an object working memory task which required participants to hold one or two irregular polygons in working memory. In another chronic intervention study where multivitamins were administered for 16 weeks, MacPherson et al. (2012) reported decreased SSVEP latency in right temporal and left frontal regions during the retrieval period of a spatial working memory (SWM) task. More recently, Camfield et al. (2012) demonstrated that 30-day supplementation with cocoa flavanols resulted in decreased posterior SSVEP amplitude during the hold period of an SWM task, as well as increased posterior SSVEP latency during the encoding and retrieval periods of the task, when compared to placebo treatment (see Figure 12.2). In another study, Camfield et al. (2013) compared changes in the SSVEP during a SWM task at the beginning and the end of a 10-week treatment programme involving *Hypericum perforatum* (HP) and/or nicotine replacement therapy (NRT) for smokers attempting to quit cigarettes. Stronger SSVEP amplitudes in posterior-parietal regions were found with HP as well as NRT, and decreased fronto-central SSVEP latency was also evident following HP administration. Whilst behavioural data revealed a significant main effect of a reduction in the number of smokers over the course of the study, no significant differences in efficacy were found between treatments (Stough et al., 2013).

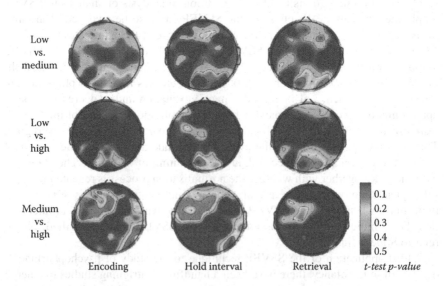

**FIGURE 12.2** Topographic mapping of significant SSVEP amplitude differences between low, medium and high cocoa flavanol treatment groups. (From Camfield, D.A. et al., *Physiol. Behav.*, 105(4), 948, 2012. doi: 10.1016/j.physbeh.2011.11.013.)

## 12.3 NEAR-INFRARED SPECTROSCOPY

NIRS is an imaging technique which measures the degree of absorption of light in the near-infrared frequency range when directed at cortical tissue directly underlying the intact skull. Due to the difference in absorption properties associated with oxygenated haemoglobin (oxy-Hb) and deoxygenated haemoglobin (deoxy-Hb), a measure of cerebral blood flow (CBF) in the cortex can be determined. The NIRS signal has been found to correspond closely with the blood oxygenation level-dependent (BOLD) signal obtained using fMRI (Steinbrink et al., 2006). In the context of nutraceutical intervention studies, NIRS is used primarily as a measure of changes in haemodynamic response and cerebral oxygenation following treatment. In light of the fact that the costs associated with NIRS are significantly less than MRI, this technology provides an affordable means of recording information on CBF that may complement electrophysiological data. The most commonly used, and least expensive, version of NIRS is the *continuous-wave* (CW) system which emits light at a constant amplitude and measures amplitude decay (Strangman et al., 2002). The other two available NIRS alternatives are time domain systems which emit short bursts of photons and frequency domain systems which emit amplitude-modulated light (Jackson & Kennedy, 2013). A methodological issue that is of concern in relation to many existing NIRS systems is that absolute values for oxy-Hb and deoxy-Hb are unable to be measured, and hence only relative change can be measured in response to an intervention. However, more recent quantitative CW NIRS systems have overcome this limitation. Another methodological issue that needs to be overcome is that the majority of NIRS studies to date have only investigated CBF changes in the prefrontal region, due to difficulties in placing optodes where there is thick hair cover. For a more detailed discussion of the use of NIRS in nutritional neuroscience, please refer to the excellent review by Jackson et al. (2013).

Six studies were identified in the literature which used CW NIRS to investigate changes to haemodynamic responses associated with nutraceutical interventions in healthy adults, although all of these used only two optodes focussed on the prefrontal cortex (PFC). Watanabe et al. (2002) found 5-day supplementation with creatine to result in reduced oxy-Hb in frontal cortex during a cognitively demanding numeric calculation task. In a study investigating the acute effects of resveratrol, Kennedy et al. (2010) reported increases to deoxy-Hb in frontal cortex during serial subtraction and rapid visual information processing (RVIP) tasks, when compared to placebo. In another study by Kennedy & Haskell (2011), investigating acute caffeine administration, reduced total Hb was reported in frontal cortex during serial subtraction and RVIP completion. Interestingly, this reduction in total Hb was found to only be significant for non-habitual caffeine consumers. The chronic effects of fish oil rich in docosahexaenoic acid (DHA) on haemodynamic response were investigated by Jackson and colleagues in two studies (Jackson et al., 2012a,b). In the first of these, 12-week supplementation with 1 g fish oil/day was compared for fish oil rich in DHA versus eicosapentaenoic acid (EPA) in 21 healthy young adults. After the end of the intervention period, increased oxy-Hb and total Hb were found for frontal cortex during the completion of a cognitive battery, but only for the fish oil rich in DHA. In the second study, using a larger sample of 65 young adults, DHA-rich fish oil was administered at doses of 1 and 2 g/day for 12 weeks, with oxy-Hb and total Hb in PFC again found to be significantly increased during the completion of a cognitive battery when compared to placebo. Wightman et al. (2012) investigated the acute effect of EGCG at two different doses (135 and 270 mg) using NIRS and reported that oxy-Hb and total Hb were both reduced in the frontal cortex during completion of the same cognitive battery used in the fish oil studies, when compared to placebo. It is interesting to note that five out of the six nutritional CW NIRS intervention studies where from the same laboratory (Jackson & Kennedy, 2013; Jackson et al., 2012a; Kennedy & Haskell, 2011; Kennedy et al., 2010; Wightman et al., 2012) and used similar cognitive test batteries (e.g. RVIP, serial subtraction, stroop) as well as the same prefrontal optode placements. Consistent reductions in prefrontal CBF, as evidenced by reduced oxy-Hb and total Hb, were observed for acute administrations of both EGCG (Wightman et al., 2012) and caffeine (Kennedy & Haskell, 2011) during sustained cognitive activity. Consistent prefrontal increases in CBF, as evidenced by increased oxy-Hb and total Hb, were also observed during cognitive batteries across both of the chronic fish oil intervention studies (Jackson et al., 2012a,b). Similarly, increased CBF, as evidenced by increased total Hb and deoxy-Hb, was also observed during cognitive tasks following acute administration of resveratrol, a finding attributable to the vasorelaxatory properties of this treatment (Kennedy et al., 2010).

In addition to the six studies which utilised CW NIRS, a study by Yimit et al. (2012) investigated the acute effects of soybean peptide using a multichannel frequency wave NIRS. Yimit et al. (2012) reported increases in theta, alpha-2 and beta-L frequency amplitudes across a number of brain regions including premotor cortex, primary motor cortex, dorsolateral PFC (DLPFC) and the frontal polar region following administration of soybean peptide versus placebo. Functional NIRS using two arrays of four sources and eight detectors has also been used to measure oxygenation changes following glucose administration in an older (>60 years) cohort. Gagnon et al. (2012) reported that, compared with placebo, glucose was associated with a greater increase in activation as participants moved from single to dual (colour/letter discrimination) tasks. This effect was most apparent in more lateral and ventral sites.

## 12.4   FUNCTIONAL MAGNETIC RESONANCE IMAGING

fMRI, as an indirect measure of brain activity, measures magnetic changes associated with fluctuations in the BOLD signal, rather than neural activity itself (Ritter & Villringer, 2006). For this reason, the temporal resolution of this technique is limited by the haemodynamic response function and is typically of the order of several seconds (Kim et al., 1997). The implication of this limited temporal resolution is that transient changes in brain activity which occur at higher frequencies cannot be captured. Due to being an indirect measure of neural activation, interpretations of BOLD changes associated with nutraceutical interventions need to be interpreted with some caution. Whilst many studies will equate an increase in BOLD as evidence of increased *brain activation*, this is not strictly the case. This is because the BOLD signal is influenced by both changes to CBF and by the cerebral metabolic rate of oxygen ($CMRO_2$). In a general sense, neural activity has a much greater effect on CBF than it does on $CMRO_2$. However, in the case of pharmaceutical or nutraceutical agents that alter either of these parameters, interpretation becomes more difficult. Caffeine (see Table 12.1) is one such substance which provides a particularly illuminating example. Across a number of studies, caffeine (which has known vasoconstrictor properties) has been found to *decrease* CBF whilst simultaneously *increasing* $CMRO_2$. In a quantitative fMRI study which measured blood flow in conjunction with the BOLD response following caffeine administration, Griffeth et al. (2011) reported that the net result of a 27% baseline reduction in blood flow, a 22% increase in oxygen metabolism and a 61% increase in the evoked metabolism response to visual stimulation was that pre- and post-BOLD responses remained largely unchanged.

By far, the majority of fMRI studies to investigate acute nutraceutical interventions for cognition in healthy adults have focussed on caffeine. Four studies, in addition to the one mentioned earlier by Griffeth et al. (2011), examined changes in the BOLD response following acute caffeine administration during a resting state or with simple visual stimulation using an 8 Hz checkerboard presentation. Liau et al. (2008) reported a decrease in CBF, but not the BOLD activation with caffeine, whilst Perthen et al. (2008) reported a 35% reduction in CBF, but no change to $CMRO_2$ when using mild hypercapnia ($CO_2$ inhalation) to calibrate the baseline BOLD signal. Wong et al. (2012) reported a negative correlation (commonly termed anticorrelation in the fMRI literature) between regions of the default-mode network (DMN) and the task-positive network (TPN) during resting eyes closed following acute caffeine administration, when compared to placebo. Similarly, Tal et al. (2013) reported widespread reduction in resting-state connectivity with eyes closed following acute caffeine administration.

Another four studies were identified which investigated the effects of acute caffeine administration on BOLD activation during the completion of working memory tasks. Using the n-back task, Koppelstaetter et al. (2008) reported increased BOLD activation bilaterally in medial frontopolar cortex and right anterior cingulate cortex (ACC) following acute caffeine administration. Haller et al. (2013) also used the n-back as a working memory activation task following acute caffeine administration and provided evidence of a 22.7% reduction in whole-brain perfusion together with increased BOLD activation in a large number of brain regions including the bilateral striatum, right middle and inferior frontal gyrus, bilateral insula, left superior and inferior parietal lobules as well as bilateral cerebellum. Klaassen et al. (2013) used the Sternberg WM task and reported increased BOLD activation bilaterally in the DLPFC during the WM encoding period, together with decreased activation in the left thalamus during WM maintenance following acute caffeine administration.

Using other tasks, Portas et al. (1998) provided evidence of increased BOLD activation in the ventrolateral thalamus during an attentional task that was highest during a state of low arousal, following sleep deprivation, in comparison to a state of high arousal with acute caffeine. Bendlin et al. (2007) reported a reduction in baseline CBF, but no effect on baseline BOLD or response to a word stem completion task, following acute caffeine administration. Diukova et al. (2012) reported decreased BOLD activation in visual and primary motor cortex during visual and visuomotor tasks, as well as increased BOLD activation during an auditory oddball task with acute caffeine administration. Similarly, Park et al. (2014) also reported increased BOLD activation in the (right) primary motor cortex following acute caffeine administration with a visuomotor task, although increased activation was also reported for the left cerebellum, putamen, insula and thalamus.

Only a handful of studies have been conducted to investigate the neurocognitive effects of other nutraceutical substances using fMRI, with only four identified in the literature. In relation to chronic cocoa flavanol administration for 5 days, Francis et al. (2006) reported increased BOLD activation during task switching in DLPFC, parietal cortex and ACC for high versus low flavanol drinks. For combined glucose and caffeine administered acutely, Serra-Grabulosa et al. (2010) reported a decrease in BOLD activation bilaterally in the parietal region, as well as left PFC. These

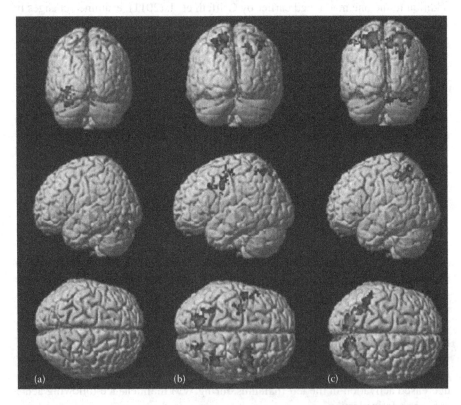

**FIGURE 12.3**  Posterior (top panel) and left lateral surface (middle) and dorsal (bottom) views of brain surfaces showing activation during the RVIP task for multivitamins drink > placebo (a), multivitamins+guaraná drink > placebo (b) and multivitamins+guaraná drink > multivitamins drink (c). (Diagram from Scholey, A. et al., *Nutrients*, 5(9), 3589, 2013. doi: 10.3390/nu5093589.)

results are not unlike those for glucose alone, albeit in a small sample of individuals with schizophrenia. Stone et al. (2005) reported that, during verbal encoding, glucose administration was associated with a trend for greater activation in the DLPFC with significantly greater activation in the parahippocampal area in this population. In healthy individuals, compared with placebo, glucose administration prior to memory tasks was associated with increased activation in areas associated with encoding (including both left and right hippocampi), which differed with respect to whether neutral or emotional material was being encoded (Parent et al., 2011). Further analysis of functional connectivity revealed that glucose was associated with increased connectivity between the hippocampus and a broad network of areas associated with declarative memory encoding (e.g. bilateral inferior and middle frontal cortices).

More recently, Scholey et al. (2013) investigated the acute neurocognitive effects of multivitamins with or without guaraná using inspection time and RVIP tasks. Increased BOLD activation was observed in right precentral gyrus and bilateral cerebellum for multivitamins versus placebo, whilst increased activation in the right precentral gyrus, left middle frontal gyrus, frontal medial gyri and bilateral superior parietal lobes was observed following the combined treatment of multivitamins with guaraná (see Figure 12.3). For green tea extract (EGCG), Borgwardt et al. (2012) reported increased DLPFC activation when green tea was administered acutely, compared to placebo, during the *n*-back WM task. In another study investigating the acute effect of green tea extract, Schmidt et al. (2014) provided evidence of increased connectivity between right superior parietal lobe and middle frontal gyrus for EGCG versus placebo.

## 12.5   POSITRON-EMISSION TOMOGRAPHY

PET is a technique that enables the direct observation of cerebral metabolism associated with specific substances. By injecting a radioactive tracer chemical into the body, the uptake of the radiotracer into the brain may be observed through the use of sensors placed around the participant's head which detect the emitted radiation. The most common radiotracer to be used in PET scans is [$^{18}$F]fluoro-2-deoxy-D-glucose (FDG), which can be used to observe regional cerebral glucose metabolism in the brain. To date, PET has not been used to a great extent in psychopharmacological studies, in the context of nutraceuticals. The two main reasons for its lack of use are its relative expense and the fact that it involves the use of radioisotopes.

For this reason, only three studies investigating the neurocognitive effects of nutraceutical interventions using FDG-PET were identified in the literature. Small et al. (2006) investigated the neurocognitive effect of a 14-day healthy diet containing high levels of fresh fruit and vegetables as well as omega-3 FAs. A 5% decrease in cerebral glucose metabolism was observed in the DLPFC at the end of the intervention for the healthy diet group in comparison to the participants who followed their usual lifestyle routine. Nugent et al. (2011) investigated the chronic effects of fish oil containing high levels of DHA and EPA in a 3-week open-label FDG-PET study. However, in this study, no effect of fish oil on cerebral glucose metabolism was found for either young or healthy elderly participants. Finally, Park et al. (2014), in a study of the acute effects of caffeine, reported that cerebral metabolic activity was reduced in the putamen, caudate nucleus, insula, pallidum and posterior medial cortex following caffeine administration.

## 12.6  GENERAL INTERPRETATIVE ISSUES

### 12.6.1  IMPORTANCE OF MAKING HYPOTHESES DIRECTIONAL

Of particular importance to the further advancement of scientific understanding of nutraceutical mechanisms of action in the brain is the proper specification of hypotheses. In this regard, hypotheses should be explicit as to the expected direction of change in brain activation following treatment administration. Whilst it may be acceptable for early *proof-of-concept* studies to simply explore general changes in brain activation associated with treatment, subsequent studies would be better served to specify whether increased or decreased activation is expected and in which brain regions. The problem with a directionless hypothesis is that a significant, and unexpected, decrease in brain activation can equally be used as evidence in support of improved brain function via increased neural efficiency (i.e. less activation being required to maintain a given level of cognitive performance [Neubauer & Fink, 2009]) as it can to refute cognitive benefits. Whilst Neubauer and colleagues (Grabner et al., 2004; Neubauer & Fink, 2009; Neubauer et al., 2002, 2005) have provided strong evidence in support of decreased brain activation being associated with more effective completion of cognitive tasks, this relationship is generally found to be specific to frontal brain regions and interacts with the difficulty of the task involved. If a prediction of decreased brain activation following treatment administration is made, on the basis of both available knowledge of the pharmacological action of the treatment and the nature/difficulty of the cognitive activation task used, then this needs to be explicitly stated at the outset of the experiment.

### 12.6.2  DIFFICULTY LEVEL OF THE COGNITIVE ACTIVATION TASK

A related issue that directly influences the likelihood of obtaining increased versus decreased brain activation during cognitive processing is the selection of an activation task which is appropriately difficult for the sample being studied. As reported by Neubauer and Fink (2009), in more intelligent individuals, relatively less brain activation is elicited by tasks of easy to medium difficulty and less brain activation is also observed when the task is very well practiced. In cases where the task demands become relatively more difficult, then high IQ individuals will display a greater degree of brain activation, whilst individuals with lower IQ will effectively give up on the task and display a lower level of activation (refer to Figure 12.4a).

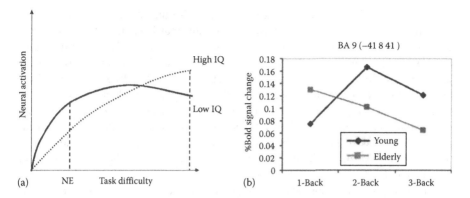

**FIGURE 12.4** (a) Neural efficiency (NE) as a function of task difficulty. (Adapted from Neubauer, A.C. and Fink, A., *Neurosci. Biobehav. Rev.*, 33(7), 1004, 2009. doi: 10.1016/j. neubiorev.2009.04.001.) (b) BOLD signal change in PFC for young versus elderly participants. (Adapted from Mattay, V.S. et al., *Neurosci. Lett.*, 392(1–2), 32, 2006. doi: 10.1016/j. neulet.2005.09.025.) BA 9: Brodmann's area 9, contributing to both dorsolateral and medial prefrontal cortex.

Similar findings have also been reported by Rypma et al. (2005, 2007) as well as Mattay et al. (2006) in normal ageing, whereby decreases in neural efficiency have been found in cognitive tasks which typically display processing speed deficits in older age. In analysis of fMRI activation patterns for young versus old adults whilst completing the *n*-back working memory task at varying levels of task difficulty, Mattay et al. (2006) reports that the relationship between behavioural performance and activation in the PFC follows an inverted U shape for younger participants, whilst activation steadily decreases with increasing task difficulty for older participants. Essentially, when older participants performed as well as younger participants on the 1-back WM task, they displayed greater PFC activation, yet when they were unable to perform as well as the younger participants (from 2-back onward), they started to display decreased PFC activity due to their inability to meet the task demands (refer to Figure 12.4b).

One of the important implications of these findings for neurocognitive intervention studies is that an activation task needs to be selected that is of a similar difficulty level across all participants. This issue may be of particular relevance when a sample is used which includes either a wide range of premorbid intelligence levels and/or age groups. In a typical example where the effect of an intervention is tested on young (e.g. 18–30 years) as well as older (65+ years) adults in the same study, then the use of an identical cognitive task in both groups may yield patterns of brain activation that are in different directions. If the task is found to be only moderately difficult for the younger group, then it may be expected that if the nutraceutical intervention is of cognitive benefit, then decreased activation will be observed in task-relevant brain regions following treatment. In contrast, if the task is found to be very difficult in the older age group at baseline, then regardless of whether the intervention is of benefit or not, the task may still be too difficult for significant changes in brain activation to be observed.

In order to avoid confounding task difficulty with the effect of the intervention in neuroimaging studies, it is therefore important that behavioural pilot data are collected beforehand in order to establish the difficulty level of the specific cognitive task for the sample in which it is intended to be used. As a rough guide, if the difficulty level of the task is set at a level that ensures that ceiling and floor effects are avoided on a behavioural level (e.g. 70%–80% accuracy), then this will ensure that changes in the neural activation outcome measures are also not range limited. If different age groups/IQ levels of participants are used, then it is worth considering setting task difficulty separately for each of the groups. One should also be aware, of course, that such an approach has ramifications for the interpretation of cognitive data.

Another potential approach to activation task selection, which is yet to be widely adopted in cognitive neuroscience, is to individually adjust task difficulty on a trial-by-trial basis as determined by ongoing task accuracy. An example of this approach is the Adjusting-Paced Serial Addition Test (Adjusting-PSAT) (Royan et al., 2004; Tombaugh et al., 2006) measure of processing speed, whereby inter-stimulus interval (ISI) is made contingent on accuracy of responding (increasing or decreasing on the basis of response). In contrast to conventional computerised cognitive tests, the main outcome measure for the Adjusting-PSAT is the threshold whereby the individual is no longer able to process information. It is foreseeable that a similar approach could also be used for neuroimaging studies in psychopharmacology, whereby ISI is individually adjusted until a stable level of performance accuracy is established, for example, 70% for 10 min. In this way, if the same level of performance accuracy is demonstrated, both pre- and post-dose, the findings are more clearly interpreted in terms of neural efficiency if decreased activation is observed. Alternatively, if time permits, then the task could also be administered at individually adjusted levels of 60%, 70% and 80% accuracy and the relationship between behavioural performance and neural activation pre- and post-dose could be investigated.

### 12.6.3 Importance of Accounting for Pharmacokinetics

Another important issue that is relevant not just for neuroimaging studies but also for cognitive testing involving psychopharmacological interventions in general is the importance of taking into account the pharmacokinetics (PK) associated with the given treatment, particularly in the context of acute intervention studies. Taking PK data into account is relatively straightforward for substances such as caffeine or glucose which have a single dominant active constituent, but this may be more difficult in the study of phytotherapies which contain multiple active constituents. However, even in the case of herbal medicine studies, it is advantageous to identify at least one or two main active constituents in the extract which have known human pharmacokinetic data (i.e. time to peak plasma level and elimination half-life), so that the timing of the neuroimaging assessments can be optimised to capture central changes.

### 12.6.4 STATISTICAL ANALYSIS OF NEUROIMAGING DATA, CORRECTING FOR MULTIPLE COMPARISONS

There are typically a very large number of outcome variables obtained when using neuroimaging techniques. This is due to the fact that data are often available for multiple brain regions and time points. As an illustrative example, in an acute crossover trial which records EEG whilst conducting a working memory task, there may be P300 amplitude data available for each of 64 EEG electrodes both pre- and post-dose across placebo and active treatment. The difficulty with mass univariate statistical analysis of treatment effects associated with changes across several spatial and temporal samples is that whilst leaving the data uncorrected will greatly inflate the chance of a type 1 error, applying a strict Bonferroni correction (i.e. 0.05/64) is also inappropriate, as this will over-correct the $p$-value and reduce statistical power to a level at which the possibility of detecting any real treatment effect is no longer possible.

There are a number of solutions to this dilemma. The most basic solution is to collapse the spatial data into a smaller selection of regions (e.g. left frontal, right frontal, LP and right parietal in the case of multichannel EEG data) and also to collapse the data across time by restricting analysis to peak amplitude or means across a specified time period. This type of data would then be suitable for analysis using common parametric statistical approaches such as repeated measures analysis of variance. Other methods of data reduction include identifying the sensor/electrode in which the effect is maximal and restricting analysis only to this channel or using a region-of-interest (ROI) or *cluster-based* technique. The ROI approach is popular in the fMRI literature (Poldrack, 2007) but can also be applied to electrophysiological data (Groppe et al., 2011). This approach typically involves reducing the whole-brain voxel-wise data into a new activation map consisting only of voxels/sensors with activations between conditions that are significantly different according to a predefined threshold value (e.g. $p < .001$ according to mass univariate t-tests). Clusters are then identified by grouping adjacent significant sensors and time points, and these clusters are used for subsequent statistical analysis (Groppe et al., 2011).

In the case of more exploratory analyses whereby data reduction is less desirable, there are other approaches available which may be used to control for multiple comparisons whilst still maintaining adequate statistical power to detect potential treatment effects. The first of these approaches, which is considerably less conservative than Bonferroni family-wise error correction, is the method of *false discovery rate* (FDR) (Benjamini & Hochberg, 1995; Benjamini & Yekutieli, 2001). The basic principle behind the FDR approach is that if all the significant $p$-values from a family of tests are considered together, then the false discovery proportion (FDP) is the expected number of significant results which are expected to be type I errors (or incorrect rejections). For example, if 10,000 significant $p$-values are uncovered using mass univariate testing, and the FDP is set at 5%, then the highest 500 $p$-values out of these tests would be subsequently rejected. There are a number of algorithms available to calculate the FDR, and for a more thorough consideration of this technique, the reader is referred to Benjamini and Hochberg (1995), Benjamini and Yekutieli (2001) or Groppe et al. (2011).

Another approach which can be used to address the issue of multiple comparisons in mass univariate testing involves the use of non-parametric data-driven statistics. In contrast to the standard parametric approaches, which utilise the general linear model, non-parametric approaches rely on far fewer assumptions and resample the *actual* (current) data in order to calculate parameter estimates. Two common techniques which can account for dependence in the data, and hence are useful in the context of controlling for multiple comparisons, are the Bootstrap method and random permutation tests (RPTs). Bootstrapping involves continually resampling from the current sample, *with* replacement, in order to generate confidence intervals or *p*-values associated with group means (Efron & Tibshirani, 1986). For example, if there were 20 individuals in our treatment group and we wished to estimate the confidence interval for the group mean using bootstrapping, then we would repeatedly take a random sample of 20 values from our sample in order to establish a sampling distribution. In order for the sample to be different each time, there needs to be an allowance for duplication of values in each random selection of values, which is known as resampling with replacement. After resampling several thousand times, then a 95% confidence interval for the group means can be established.

RPTs involve repeatedly assigning the values in one's sample, *without* replacement, to the various treatment groups on the basis of the null hypothesis of no difference between treatment groups (Nichols & Holmes, 2002). For example, in a sample of 50 participants who were evenly divided between placebo and treatment groups, the RPT would involve randomly assigning 25 participants to placebo and 25 participants to the treatment group and repeating this process several times. After a thousand permutations, a sampling distribution for the difference between the two group means on the outcome measure of interest could be established, and this could be used to determine the probability of obtaining the actual mean difference obtained in one's sample according to the null hypothesis.

In order to use bootstrapping or RPT in order to control for multiple comparisons, the same approach is used as for a single outcome measure, except that *all* topographical and/or temporal values can be considered simultaneously. A common approach is to calculate a $t_{max}$ distribution, whereby for each permutation of the data, the most extreme *t*-value from the family of t-tests is identified. On the basis of a large number of permutation, the distribution of extreme *t*-values, or $t_{max}$, can be compared to the real data that were obtained in the experiment. For any specific data point, the probability of obtaining a value as least as extreme as the one obtained, across the whole family of tests, can then be determined by calculating the proportion of $t_{max}$ values which are greater than or equal to it. Another common approach to using RPT or bootstrapping is to establish a distribution associated with the total number of sites which are found to be significant within a specified time range. The first step to conducting this type of analysis is similar to the

ROI analysis and requires that a value for a statistical threshold is set, whereby differences between groups (e.g. treatment and placebo) are determined to be statistically significant at any individual site. The most basic test statistic to use in this example would be a between-groups t-test, where any difference greater than a critical *t*-value associated with a *p*-value of <0.05 would be labelled as significant. This single threshold test would then be applied to all topographical sites (e.g. 64-channels in a typical EEG recording) and the total number of sites which exceeded the threshold would be tallied. In the second step of the analysis, the bootstrap procedure or RPT procedure would then be used in order to establish a sampling distribution associated with the total number of sites exceeding the threshold. So after several thousand permutations, the number of sites that were found to be significantly greater than threshold in the current sample could be compared to the sampling distribution of this number in order to determine a *p*-value that is corrected for multiple comparisons. For further information on controlling for multiple comparisons in neuroimaging, and the use of more advanced methods such as supra-threshold testing, please refer to the excellent review papers by Nichols and Hayasaka (2003) and Groppe et al. (2011).

## 12.7   CONCLUSIONS AND FUTURE DIRECTIONS

Whilst the study of the neurocognitive effects of nutraceutical interventions is still in its infancy, neuroimaging research over the past 20 years has already begun to uncover some important and valuable insights. By far, the greatest contribution to this field to date has come from electrophysiological research methods, largely due to the favourable cost and availability of this technology. However, NIRS, another highly accessible technology, also promises to provide valuable complementary information on cerebral oxygen metabolism in the coming years. Whilst fMRI remains the superior technology for imaging brain activity in cortical and subcortical structures with a high degree of spatial resolution, the costs associated with this technology are still prohibitive for many psychopharmacology research laboratories. Similarly, PET also has great potential to increase our understanding of cerebral metabolic processes associated with nutraceuticals, yet the costs as well as the problems associated with the use of radioisotopes continue to be a hindrance. Whilst not included in the current review, MEG is another imaging modality which has excellent temporal and spatial resolution. MEG has great potential to elucidate in vivo mechanisms of action of natural substances in the brain, yet the application of this technology to psychopharmacology is yet to eventuate. In future research, it is recommended that a greater effort be made on the part of disparate research labs to arrive at common methods, involving both cognitive activation tasks as well as analysis techniques, so that systematic review and meta-analysis of neuroimaging outcome measures (a necessary next step) can begin to occur. If current trends continue, then the next decade of human psychopharmacology research will enable robust and replicable in vivo neural effects to be established for a greatly augmented range of nutraceutical nootropics.

## TOP 6 SUMMARY POINTS FROM CHAPTER

- A clear justification for the use of neuroimaging in a cognitive intervention study should precede its inclusion in the study. The major benefits of including neuroimaging in an intervention study include (1) to better understand *in vivo* mechanisms of action within the human brain and (2) to capture subtle neurocognitive effects that may be difficult to determine using standard behavioural measures.

- EEG is the imaging modality that has been utilised most frequently in relation to psychopharmacological studies of nutraceutical and nutritional interventions. Power spectral analysis and ERP analysis have a long history of use in cognitive-affective neuroscience and are measures of cortical electrical activity which possess excellent temporal resolution. SST is also a technique with potential, although further research is required.

- NIRS is a cost-effective measure of CBF that has begun to be used in relation to nutritional interventions. Future research using CW systems with optodes spanning an extended range of cortical regions will further improve the applicability of this technique.

- fMRI provides superior spatial resolution in comparison to other techniques and for this reason, is the method of choice for examining the neurocognitive effects of interventions at a subcortical level. However, measurement of the BOLD signal limits temporal precision, and the costs associated with fMRI scans are often prohibitive for smaller laboratories.

- PET, most commonly used in conjunction with the radiotracer fluoro-deoxy-glucose (FDG), enables direct observation of cerebral metabolism, although the costs associated with scanning, together with the use of radioisotopes, mean that the number of nutritional studies to have used this technique are limited.

- A number of considerations should be taken into account when designing and interpreting the results of a neuroimaging study. These include the following: (1) clearly directionalised hypotheses, (2) careful selection of an activation task that has a difficulty level appropriate for the sample under consideration, (3) the timing of neuroimaging data collection which takes into account the pharmacokinetic properties of the intervention under investigation and (4) statistical analysis that is sophisticated enough to take into account the typically large number of outcome variables, with recommended techniques including ROI analysis, FDR, bootstrapping and/or multiple-permutations testing.

## WHERE TO FROM HERE?

- With an increasing number of nutraceutical and nutritional neuroimaging studies appearing in the literature, it is envisaged that a more nuanced use of these technologies will continue to evolve.
- The establishment of standard operating procedures will ensure greater quality control in data collection, whilst the establishment of common outcome metrics across laboratories will enable meta-analysis of effect sizes across different studies.
- The use of more powerful electrophysiological analysis techniques such as temporal principle components analysis (tPCA) and time–frequency analysis will facilitate greater sensitivity in the detection of treatment effects.
- The use of fMRI and PET in a wider range of nutraceutical intervention studies will be of great utility in complementing the existing electrophysiological literature.
- The application of MEG to nutritional studies will enable the temporal precision of *ERP* to be combined with enhanced spatial resolution, resulting in greater understanding of in vivo mechanisms of action in the human brain.

## REFERENCES

Baldeweg, T., Wong, D., & Stephan, K. E. (2006). Nicotinic modulation of human auditory sensory memory: Evidence from mismatch negativity potentials. *International Journal of Psychophysiology, 59*(1), 49–58. doi: 10.1016/j.ijpsycho.2005.07.014

Barry, R. J., Clarke, A. R., Hajos, M., McCarthy, R., Selikowitz, M., & Dupuy, F. E. (2010). Resting-state EEG gamma activity in children with Attention-Deficit/Hyperactivity Disorder. *Clinical Neurophysiology, 121*(11), 1871–1877. doi: 10.1016/j.clinph.2010.04.022

Barry, R. J., Clarke, A. R., & Johnstone, S. J. (2011). Caffeine and opening the eyes have additive effects on resting arousal measures. *Clinical Neurophysiology, 122*(10), 2010–2015. doi: 10.1016/j.clinph.2011.02.036

Barry, R. J., & De Blasio, F. M. (2013). Sequential processing in the equiprobable auditory Go/NoGo task: A temporal PCA study. *International Journal of Psychophysiology, 89*(1), 123–127. doi: 10.1016/j.ijpsycho.2013.06.012

Barry, R. J., De Blasio, F. M., & Borchard, J. P. (2014). Sequential processing in the equiprobable auditory Go/NoGo task: Children vs. adults. *Clinical Neurophysiology.* doi: 10.1016/j.clinph.2014.02.018

Barry, R. J., Johnstone, S. J., Clarke, A. R., Rushby, J. A., Brown, C. R., & McKenzie, D. N. (2007). Caffeine effects on ERPs and performance in an auditory Go/NoGo task. *Clinical Neurophysiology, 118*(12), 2692–2699. doi: 10.1016/j.clinph.2007.08.023

Bayram, A., Bayraktaroglu, Z., Karahan, E., Erdogan, B., Bilgic, B., Özker, M., ... Demiralp, T. (2011). Simultaneous EEG/fMRI analysis of the resonance phenomena in steady-state visual evoked responses. *Clinical EEG and Neuroscience, 42*(2), 98–106.

Bendlin, B. B., Trouard, T. P., & Ryan, L. (2007). Caffeine attenuates practice effects in word stem completion as measured by fMRI BOLD signal. *Human Brain Mapping, 28*(7), 654–662. doi: 10.1002/hbm.20295

Benjamini, Y., & Hochberg, Y. (1995). Controlling the false discovery rate: A practical and powerful approach to multiple testing. *Journal of the Royal Statistical Society, 57*(1), 289–300.

Benjamini, Y., & Yekutieli, D. (2001). The control of the false discovery rate in multiple testing under dependency. *Annals of Statistics, 29*(4), 1165–1188. doi: 10.1214/aos/1013699998

Borgwardt, S., Hammann, F., Scheffler, K., Kreuter, M., Drewe, J., & Beglinger, C. (2012). Neural effects of green tea extract on dorsolateral prefrontal cortex. *European Journal of Clinical Nutrition, 66*(11), 1187–1192. doi: 10.1038/ejcn.2012.105

Brown, L. A., & Riby, L. M. (2013). Glucose enhancement of event-related potentials associated with episodic memory and attention. *Food and Function, 4*(5), 770–776. doi: 10.1039/c3fo30243a

Camfield, D. A., Scholey, A., Pipingas, A., Silberstein, R., Kras, M., Nolidin, K., … Stough, C. (2012). Steady state visually evoked potential (SSVEP) topography changes associated with cocoa flavanol consumption. *Physiology and Behavior, 105*(4), 948–957. doi: 10.1016/j.physbeh.2011.11.013

Camfield, D. A., Scholey, A. B., Pipingas, A., Silberstein, R. B., Kure, C., Zangara, A., … Stough, C. (2013). The neurocognitive effects of *Hypericum perforatum* special extract (Ze 117) during smoking cessation. *Phytotherapy Research, 27*(11), 1605–1613. doi: 10.1002/ptr.4909

Croft, R. J., & Barry, R. J. (2000a). EOG correction of blinks with saccade coefficients: A test and revision of the aligned-artefact average solution. *Clinical Neurophysiology, 111*(3), 444–451. doi: 10.1016/S1388-2457(99)00296-5

Croft, R. J., & Barry, R. J. (2000b). EOG correction of blinks with saccade coefficients: A test and revision of the aligned-artefact average solution. *Clinical Neurophysiology, 111*, 444–451.

Croft, R. J., & Barry, R. J. (2000c). Removal of ocular artifact from the EEG: A review. *Neurophysiologie Clinique, 30*(1), 5–19. doi: 10.1016/S0987-7053(00)00055-1

Croft, R. J., Chandler, J. S., Barry, R. J., Cooper, N. R., & Clarke, A. R. (2005). EOG correction: A comparison of four methods. *Psychophysiology, 42*(1), 16–24. doi: 10.1111/j.1468-8986.2005.00264.x

Cropley, V., Croft, R., Silber, B., Neale, C., Scholey, A., Stough, C., & Schmitt, J. (2012). Does coffee enriched with chlorogenic acids improve mood and cognition after acute administration in healthy elderly? A pilot study. *Psychopharmacology, 219*(3), 737–749. doi: 10.1007/s00213-011-2395-0

Dien, J. (2012). Applying principal components analysis to event-related potentials: A tutorial. *Developmental Neuropsychology, 37*(6), 497–517. doi: 10.1080/87565641.2012.697503

Dimpfel, W., Kler, A., Kriesl, E., Lehnfeld, R., & Keplinger-Dimpfel, I. K. (2006). Neurophysiological characterization of a functionally active drink containing extracts of ginkgo and ginseng by source density analysis of the human EEG. *Nutritional Neuroscience, 9*(5–6), 213–224. doi: 10.1080/10284150601043713

Dimpfel, W., Kler, A., Kriesl, E., Lehnfeld, R., & Keplinger-Dimpfel, I. K. (2007). Source density analysis of the human EEG after ingestion of a drink containing decaffeinated extract of green tea enriched with L-theanine and theogallin. *Nutritional Neuroscience, 10*(3–4), 169–180. doi: 10.1080/03093640701580610

Diukova, A., Ware, J., Smith, J. E., Evans, C. J., Murphy, K., Rogers, P. J., & Wise, R. G. (2012). Separating neural and vascular effects of caffeine using simultaneous EEG-FMRI: Differential effects of caffeine on cognitive and sensorimotor brain responses. *NeuroImage, 62*(1), 239–249. doi: 10.1016/j.neuroimage.2012.04.041

Donchin, E., & Coles, M. G. H. (1988). Is the P300 component a manifestation of context updating? *Behavioural Brain Science, 11*, 357–374.

Efron, B., & Tibshirani, R. (1986). Bootstrap methods for standard errors, confidence intervals, and other measures of statistical accuracy. *Statistical Science, 1*, 54–77.

Fontani, G., Corradeschi, F., Felici, A., Alfatti, F., Migliorini, S., & Lodi, L. (2005). Cognitive and physiological effects of Omega-3 polyunsaturated fatty acid supplementation in healthy subjects. *European Journal of Clinical Investigation, 35*(11), 691–699. doi: 10.1111/j.1365-2362.2005.01570.x

Francis, S. T., Head, K., Morris, P. G., & Macdonald, I. A. (2006). The effect of flavanol-rich cocoa on the fMRI response to a cognitive task in healthy young people. *Journal of Cardiovascular Pharmacology, 47*(Suppl. 2), S215–S220. doi: 10.1097/00005344-200606001-00018

Gagnon, C., Desjardins-Crépeau, L., Tournier, I., Desjardins, M., Lesage, F., Greenwood, C. E., & Bherer, L. (2012). Near-infrared imaging of the effects of glucose ingestion and regulation on prefrontal activation during dual-task execution in healthy fasting older adults. *Behavioural Brain Research, 232*(1), 137–147.

Gevins, A., Smith, M. E., & McEvoy, L. K. (2002). Tracking the cognitive pharmacodynamics of psychoactive substances with combinations of behavioral and neurophysiological measures. *Neuropsychopharmacology, 26*(1), 27–39. doi: 10.1016/S0893-133X(01)00300-1

Gomez-Ramirez, M., Kelly, S. P., Montesi, J. L., & Foxe, J. J. (2009). The effects of L-theanine on alpha-band oscillatory brain activity during a visuo-spatial attention task. *Brain Topography, 22*(1), 44–51. doi: 10.1007/s10548-008-0068-z

Grabner, R. H., Fink, A., Stipacek, A., Neuper, C., & Neubauer, A. C. (2004). Intelligence and working memory systems: Evidence of neural efficiency in alpha band ERD. *Cognitive Brain Research, 20*(2), 212–225. doi: 10.1016/j.cogbrainres.2004.02.010

Griffeth, V. E. M., Perthen, J. E., & Buxton, R. B. (2011). Prospects for quantitative fMRI: Investigating the effects of caffeine on baseline oxygen metabolism and the response to a visual stimulus in humans. *NeuroImage, 57*(3), 809–816. doi: 10.1016/j.neuroimage.2011.04.064

Groppe, D. M., Urbach, T. P., & Kutas, M. (2011). Mass univariate analysis of event-related brain potentials/fields I: A critical tutorial review. *Psychophysiology, 48*(12), 1711–1725. doi: 10.1111/j.1469-8986.2011.01273.x

Haller, S., Rodriguez, C., Moser, D., Toma, S., Hofmeister, J., Sinanaj, I., … Lovblad, K. O. (2013). Acute caffeine administration impact on working memory-related brain activation and functional connectivity in the elderly: A BOLD and perfusion MRI study. *Neuroscience, 250*, 364–371. doi: 10.1016/j.neuroscience.2013.07.021

Herrmann, C. S., Rach, S., Vosskuhl, J., & Strüber, D. (2014). Time-frequency analysis of event-related potentials: A brief tutorial. *Brain Topography, 27*(4), 438–450. doi: 10.1007/s10548-013-0327-5

Itil, T. M., Eralp, E., Tsambis, E., Itil, K. Z., & Stein, U. (1996). Central nervous system effects of *Ginkgo biloba*, a plant extract. *American Journal of Therapeutics, 3*(1), 63–73.

Jackson, P. A., & Kennedy, D. O. (2013). The application of near infrared spectroscopy in nutritional intervention studies. *Frontiers in Human Neuroscience*(AUG). doi: 10.3389/fnhum.2013.00473

Jackson, P. A., Reay, J. L., Scholey, A. B., & Kennedy, D. O. (2012a). DHA-rich oil modulates the cerebral haemodynamic response to cognitive tasks in healthy young adults: A near IR spectroscopy pilot study. *The British Journal of Nutrition, 107*(8), 1093–1098. doi: 10.1017/S0007114511004041

Jackson, P. A., Reay, J. L., Scholey, A. B., & Kennedy, D. O. (2012b). Docosahexaenoic acid-rich fish oil modulates the cerebral hemodynamic response to cognitive tasks in healthy young adults. *Biological Psychology, 89*(1), 183–190. doi: 10.1016/j.biopsycho.2011.10.006

Keane, M. A., & James, J. E. (2008). Effects of dietary caffeine on EEG, performance and mood when rested and sleep restricted. *Human Psychopharmacology, 23*(8), 669–680. doi: 10.1002/hup.987

Keane, M. A., James, J. E., & Hogan, M. J. (2007). Effects of dietary caffeine on topographic EEG after controlling for withdrawal and withdrawal reversal. *Neuropsychobiology, 56*(4), 197–207. doi: 10.1159/000120625

Kenemans, J. L., & Lorist, M. M. (1995). Caffeine and selective visual processing. *Pharmacology Biochemistry and Behavior, 52*(3), 461–471. doi: 10.1016/0091-3057(95)00159-T

Kennedy, D. O., & Haskell, C. F. (2011). Cerebral blood flow and behavioural effects of caffeine in habitual and non-habitual consumers of caffeine: A near infrared spectroscopy study. *Biological Psychology, 86*(3), 298–306. doi: 10.1016/j.biopsycho.2010.12.010

Kennedy, D. O., Scholey, A. B., Drewery, L., Marsh, V. R., Moore, B., & Ashton, H. (2003). Electroencephalograph effects of single doses of *Ginkgo biloba* and *Panax ginseng* in healthy young volunteers. *Pharmacology Biochemistry and Behavior, 75*(3), 701–709. doi: 10.1016/S0091-3057(03)00120-5

Kennedy, D. O., Wightman, E. L., Reay, J. L., Lietz, G., Okello, E. J., Wilde, A., & Haskell, C. F. (2010). Effects of resveratrol on cerebral blood flow variables and cognitive performance in humans: A double-blind, placebo-controlled, crossover investigation. *American Journal of Clinical Nutrition, 91*(6), 1590–1597. doi: 10.3945/ajcn.2009.28641

Kim, S. G., Richter, W., & Ugurbil, K. (1997). Limitations of temporal resolution in functional MRI. *Magnetic Resonance in Medicine, 37*(4), 631–636. doi: 10.1002/mrm.1910370427

Klaassen, E. B., De Groot, R. H. M., Evers, E. A. T., Snel, J., Veerman, E. C. I., Ligtenberg, A. J. M., ... Veltman, D. J. (2013). The effect of caffeine on working memory load-related brain activation in middle-aged males. *Neuropharmacology, 64*, 160–167. doi: 10.1016/j.neuropharm.2012.06.026

Klimesch, W. (1999). EEG alpha and theta oscillations reflect cognitive and memory performance: A review and analysis. *Brain Research Reviews, 29*(2–3), 169–195. doi: 10.1016/S0165-0173(98)00056-3

Klimesch, W., Doppelmayr, M., Schwaiger, J., Auinger, P., & Winkler, T. (1999). 'Paradoxical' alpha synchronization in a memory task. *Cognitive Brain Research, 7*(4), 493–501. doi: 10.1016/s0926-6410(98)00056-1

Klimesch, W., Sauseng, P., & Hanslmayr, S. (2007). EEG alpha oscillations: The inhibition-timing hypothesis. *Brain Research Reviews, 53*(1), 63–88. doi: 10.1016/j.brainresrev.2006.06.003

Koppelstaetter, F., Poeppel, T. D., Siedentopf, C. M., Ischebeck, A., Verius, M., Haala, I., ... Krause, B. J. (2008). Does caffeine modulate verbal working memory processes? An fMRI study. *NeuroImage, 39*(1), 492–499. doi: 10.1016/j.neuroimage.2007.08.037

Li, Y., Ma, Z., Lu, W., & Li, Y. (2006). Automatic removal of the eye blink artifact from EEG using an ICA-based template matching approach. *Physiological Measurement, 27*(4), 425–436. doi: 10.1088/0967-3334/27/4/008

Liau, J., Perthen, J. E., & Liu, T. T. (2008). Caffeine reduces the activation extent and contrast-to-noise ratio of the functional cerebral blood flow response but not the BOLD response. *NeuroImage, 42*(1), 296–305. doi: 10.1016/j.neuroimage.2008.04.177

Macpherson, H., Silberstein, R., & Pipingas, A. (2012). Neurocognitive effects of multivitamin supplementation on the steady state visually evoked potential (SSVEP) measure of brain activity in elderly women. *Physiology and Behavior, 107*(3), 346–354. doi: 10.1016/j.physbeh.2012.08.006

Mattay, V. S., Fera, F., Tessitore, A., Hariri, A. R., Berman, K. F., Das, S., ... Weinberger, D. R. (2006). Neurophysiological correlates of age-related changes in working memory capacity. *Neuroscience Letters, 392*(1–2), 32–37. doi: 10.1016/j.neulet.2005.09.025

Näätänen, R., Paavilainen, P., Rinne, T., & Alho, K. (2007). The mismatch negativity (MMN) in basic research of central auditory processing: A review. *Clinical Neurophysiology, 118*(12), 2544–2590. doi: 10.1016/j.clinph.2007.04.026

Neubauer, A. C., & Fink, A. (2009). Intelligence and neural efficiency. *Neuroscience and Biobehavioral Reviews, 33*(7), 1004–1023. doi: 10.1016/j.neubiorev.2009.04.001

Neubauer, A. C., Fink, A., & Schrausser, D. G. (2002). Intelligence and neural efficiency: The influence of task content and sex on the brain – IQ relationship. *Intelligence, 30*(6), 515–536. doi: 10.1016/S0160–2896(02)00091-0

Neubauer, A. C., Grabner, R. H., Fink, A., and Neuper, C. (2005). Intelligence and neural efficiency: Further evidence of the influence of task content and sex on the brain-IQ relationship. *Cognitive Brain Research, 25*(1), 217–225. doi: 10.1016/j.cogbrainres.2005.05.011

Nichols, T., & Hayasaka, S. (2003). Controlling the familywise error rate in functional neuroimaging: A comparative review. *Statistical Methods in Medical Research, 12*(5), 419–446. doi: 10.1191/0962280203sm341ra

Nichols, T. E., & Holmes, A. P. (2002). Nonparametric permutation tests for functional neuroimaging: A primer with examples. *Human Brain Mapping, 15*(1), 1–25. doi: 10.1002/hbm.1058

Nugent, S., Croteau, E., Pifferi, F., Fortier, M., Tremblay, S., Turcotte, E., & Cunnane, S. C. (2011). Brain and systemic glucose metabolism in the healthy elderly following fish oil supplementation. *Prostaglandins Leukotrienes and Essential Fatty Acids, 85*(5), 287–291. doi: 10.1016/j.plefa.2011.04.008

Oakes, T. R., Pizzagalli, D. A., Hendrick, A. M., Horras, K. A., Larson, C. L., Abercrombie, H. C., … Davidson, R. J. (2004). Functional coupling of simultaneous electrical and metabolic activity in the human brain. *Human Brain Mapping, 21*(4), 257–270. doi: 10.1002/hbm.20004

Parent, M. B., Krebs-Kraft, D. L., Ryan, J. P., Wilson, J. S., Harenski, C., & Hamann, S. (2011). Glucose administration enhances fMRI brain activation and connectivity related to episodic memory encoding for neutral and emotional stimuli. *Neuropsychologia, 49*(5), 1052–1066.

Park, C. A., Kang, C. K., Son, Y. D., Choi, E. J., Kim, S. H., Oh, S. T., … Cho, Z. H. (2014). The effects of caffeine ingestion on cortical areas: Functional imaging study. *Magnetic Resonance Imaging, 32*(4), 366–371. doi: 10.1016/j.mri.2013.12.018

Perthen, J. E., Lansing, A. E., Liau, J., Liu, T. T., & Buxton, R. B. (2008). Caffeine-induced uncoupling of cerebral blood flow and oxygen metabolism: A calibrated BOLD fMRI study. *NeuroImage, 40*(1), 237–247. doi: 10.1016/j.neuroimage.2007.10.049

Pfurtscheller, G. (1992). Event-related synchronization (ERS): An electrophysiological correlate of cortical areas at rest. *Electroencephalography and Clinical Neurophysiology, 83*(1), 62–69.

Pham, T. T. H., Croft, R. J., Cadusch, P. J., & Barry, R. J. (2011). A test of four EOG correction methods using an improved validation technique. *International Journal of Psychophysiology, 79*(2), 203–210. doi: 10.1016/j.ijpsycho.2010.10.008

Poldrack, R. A. (2007). Region of interest analysis for fMRI. *Social Cognitive and Affective Neuroscience, 2*(1), 67–70. doi: 10.1093/scan/nsm006

Portas, C. M., Rees, G., Howseman, A. M., Josephs, O., Turner, R., & Frith, C. D. (1998). A specific role for the thalamus in mediating the interaction of attention and arousal in humans. *Journal of Neuroscience, 18*(21), 8979–8989.

Riby, L. M., Sünram-Lea, S. I., Graham, C., Foster, J. K., Cooper, T., Moodie, C., & Gunn, V. P. (2008). P3b versus P3a: An event-related potential investigation of the glucose facilitation effect. *Journal of Psychopharmacology, 22*(5), 486–492. doi: 10.1177/0269881107081561

Ritter, P., & Villringer, A. (2006). Simultaneous EEG-fMRI. *Neuroscience and Biobehavioral Reviews, 30*(6), 823–838. doi: 10.1016/j.neubiorev.2006.06.008

Royan, J., Tombaugh, T. N., Rees, L., & Francis, M. (2004). The Adjusting-Paced Serial Addition Test (Adjusting-PSAT): Thresholds for speed of information processing as a function of stimulus modality and problem complexity. *Archives of Clinical Neuropsychology, 19*(1), 131–143. doi: 10.1016/S0887-6177(02)00216-0

Rypma, B., Berger, J. S., Genova, H. M., Rebbechi, D., & D'Esposito, M. (2005). Dissociating age-related changes in cognitive strategy and neural efficiency using event-related fMRI. *Cortex, 41*(4), 582–594.

Rypma, B., Eldreth, D. A., & Rebbechi, D. (2007). Age-related differences in activation-performance relations in delayed-response tasks: A multiple component analysis. *Cortex, 43*(1), 65–76. doi: 10.1016/S0010–9452(08)70446-5

Schmidt, A., Hammann, F., Wölnerhanssen, B., Meyer-Gerspach, A. C., Drewe, J., Beglinger, C., & Borgwardt, S. (2014). Green tea extract enhances parieto-frontal connectivity during working memory processing. *Psychopharmacology*. doi: 10.1007/s00213-014-3526-1

Scholey, A., Bauer, I., Neale, C., Savage, K., Camfield, D., White, D., ... Hughes, M. (2013). Acute effects of different multivitamin mineral preparations with and without guaraná on mood, cognitive performance and functional brain activation. *Nutrients, 5*(9), 3589–3604. doi: 10.3390/nu5093589

Scholey, A., Downey, L. A., Ciorciari, J., Pipingas, A., Nolidin, K., Finn, M., ... Stough, C. (2012). Acute neurocognitive effects of epigallocatechin gallate (EGCG). *Appetite, 58*(2), 767–770. doi: 10.1016/j.appet.2011.11.016

Scholey, A. B., Camfield, D. A., Macpherson, H., Owen, L., Nguyen, P., & Riby, L. (2014). Hippocampal involvement in Glucose Facilitation of Recognition Memory: Event-related potential components in a dual-task paradigm. *Nutrition & Ageing*. doi: 10.3233/NUA-140042, online June 2005.

Serra-Grabulosa, J. M., Adan, A., Falcõn, C., & Bargallõ, N. (2010). Glucose and caffeine effects on sustained attention: An exploratory fMRI study. *Human Psychopharmacology, 25*(7–8), 543–552. doi: 10.1002/hup.1150

Silberstein, R. B. (1995). Steady-state visually evoked potentials, brain resonances, and cognitive processes. In P. L. Nunez (Ed.), *Neocortical dynamics and human EEG rhythms* (pp. 272–303). New York: Oxford University Press.

Sizonenko, S. V., Babiloni, C., De Bruin, E. A., Isaacs, E. B., Jönsson, L. S., Kennedy, D. O., ... Sijben, J. W. (2013). Brain imaging and human nutrition: Which measures to use in intervention studies? *British Journal of Nutrition, 110*(Suppl. 1), S1–S30. doi: 10.1017/S0007114513001384

Small, G. W., Silverman, D. H. S., Siddarth, P., Ercoli, L. M., Miller, K. J., Lavretsky, H., ... Phelps, M. E. (2006). Effects of a 14-day healthy longevity lifestyle program on cognition and brain function. *American Journal of Geriatric Psychiatry, 14*(6), 538–545. doi: 10.1097/01.JGP.0000219279.72210.ca

Steinbrink, J., Villringer, A., Kempf, F., Haux, D., Boden, S., & Obrig, H. (2006). Illuminating the BOLD signal: Combined fMRI-fNIRS studies. *Magnetic Resonance Imaging, 24*(4), 495–505. doi: 10.1016/j.mri.2005.12.034

Stone, W. S., Thermenos, H. W., Tarbox, S. I., Poldrack, R. A., & Seidman, L. J. (2005). Medial temporal and prefrontal lobe activation during verbal encoding following glucose ingestion in schizophrenia: A pilot fMRI study. *Neurobiology of Learning and Memory, 83*(1), 54–64.

Stough, C., Silberstein, R. B., Pipingas, A., Song, J., Camfield, D. A., & Nathan, P. J. (2011). Examining brain-cognition effects of *Ginkgo biloba* extract: Brain activation in the left temporal and left prefrontal cortex in an object working memory task. *Evidence-Based Complementary and Alternative Medicine, 2011*, 1–10. Article No. 164139. doi: 10.1155/2011/164139

Stough, C. K., Scholey, A., Kure, C., Tarasuik, J., Kras, M., Zangara, A., & Camfield, D. (2013). An open label study investigating the efficacy of *Hypericum perforatum* special extract (ZE117), nicotine patches and combination (ZE117)/nicotine patches for smoking cessation. *Alternative & Integrative Medicine, 2*(9). Article No. 147. doi: http://dx.doi.org/10.4172/2327-5162.1000147

Strangman, G., Boas, D. A., & Sutton, J. P. (2002). Non-invasive neuroimaging using near-infrared light. *Biological Psychiatry, 52*(7), 679–693. doi: 10.1016/S0006-3223(02)01550-0

Tal, O., Diwakar, M., Wong, C. W., Olafsson, V., Lee, R., Huang, M. X., & Liu, T. T. (2013). Caffeine-induced global reductions in resting-state BOLD connectivity reflect widespread decreases in MEG connectivity. *Frontiers in Human Neuroscience, 7*, 1–10. Article No. 63. doi: 10.3389/fnhum.2013.00063

Thompson, J. C., Tzambazis, K., Stough, C., Nagata, K., & Silberstein, R. B. (2000). The effects of nicotine on the 13 Hz steady-state visually evoked potential. *Clinical Neurophysiology, 111*(9), 1589–1595. doi: 10.1016/S1388-2457(00)00334-5

Tieges, Z., Richard Ridderinkhof, K., Snel, J., & Kok, A. (2004). Caffeine strengthens action monitoring: Evidence from the error-related negativity. *Cognitive Brain Research, 21*(1), 87–93. doi: 10.1016/j.cogbrainres.2004.06.001

Tieges, Z., Snel, J., Kok, A., Plat, N., & Ridderinkhof, R. (2007). Effects of caffeine on anticipatory control processes: Evidence from a cued task-switch paradigm. *Psychophysiology, 44*(4), 561–578. doi: 10.1111/j.1469-8986.2007.00534.x

Tombaugh, T. N., Stormer, P., Rees, L., Irving, S., & Francis, M. (2006). The effects of mild and severe traumatic brain injury on the auditory and visual versions of the Adjusting-Paced Serial Addition Test (Adjusting-PSAT). *Archives of Clinical Neuropsychology, 21*(7), 753–761. doi: 10.1016/j.acn.2006.08.009

Wallstrom, G. L., Kass, R. E., Miller, A., Cohn, J. F., & Fox, N. A. (2004). Automatic correction of ocular artifacts in the EEG: A comparison of regression-based and component-based methods. *International Journal of Psychophysiology, 53*(2), 105–119. doi: 10.1016/j.ijpsycho.2004.03.007

Watanabe, A., Kato, N., & Kato, T. (2002). Effects of creatine on mental fatigue and cerebral hemoglobin oxygenation. *Neuroscience Research, 42*(4), 279–285. doi: 10.1016/S0168-0102(02)00007-X

Wightman, E. L., Haskell, C. F., Forster, J. S., Veasey, R. C., & Kennedy, D. O. (2012). Epigallocatechin gallate, cerebral blood flow parameters, cognitive performance and mood in healthy humans: A double-blind, placebo-controlled, crossover investigation. *Human Psychopharmacology, 27*(2), 177–186. doi: 10.1002/hup.1263

Wong, C. W., Olafsson, V., Tal, O., & Liu, T. T. (2012). Anti-correlated networks, global signal regression, and the effects of caffeine in resting-state functional MRI. *NeuroImage, 63*(1), 356–364. doi: 10.1016/j.neuroimage.2012.06.035

Yimit, D., Hoxur, P., Amat, N., Uchikawa, K., & Yamaguchi, N. (2012). Effects of soybean peptide on immune function, brain function, and neurochemistry in healthy volunteers. *Nutrition, 28*(2), 154–159. doi: 10.1016/j.nut.2011.05.008

# 13 Evidence, Innovations and Implications

*Louise Dye and Talitha Best*

## CONTENTS

## SUMMARY

This volume has considered the evidence for effects of nutrition on cognition and *brain health*. The role of diet both early and later in life and its impact on our mental performance and risk of age-related cognitive impairment or Alzheimer's disease has been explored. Diets and specific nutrients have been discussed which could confer protection against cognitive impairment or facilitate cognitive performance acutely.

## 13.1 EVIDENCE

The promising evidence of protective effects of certain dietary patterns identified by epidemiological studies reviewed by Andreeva and Kesse-Guyot (Chapter 2) demonstrates that the early adoption of a healthy dietary pattern could confer long-term benefits for cognitive function and prevent age-related cognitive impairment. In particular they identify the Mediterranean diet, rich in fruit and vegetables, plant-derived products and seafood as a dietary pattern which seems to confer long-term benefits for health in general and brain health specifically.

It is important to consider what is not eaten as well as what is consumed when evaluating the impact of a dietary pattern on health outcomes. The Mediterranean diet includes only low intakes of meat, alcohol, saturated fats and sugar. A meta-analysis of prospective studies indicated that consumption of fresh red meat and processed red meat as well as total red meat was associated with increased risk of stroke (Kaluza et al., 2012). Stroke more than doubles the risk of dementia (Zhu et al., 1998; Ivan et al., 2004). The recent Cochrane review (Rees et al., 2013) concluded that, despite limited evidence to date, a Mediterranean dietary pattern reduces some cardiovascular risk factors including risk of stroke. Psaltopoulou et al. (2013) estimate the reduced risk of stroke to be 29% with high adherence to the Mediterranean diet along with a 40% reduction in cognitive impairment and 32% reduced risk of depression. Hence, the avoidance of some foods coupled with high intakes of others could account for the beneficial effects conferred by the Mediterranean diet.

In addition to the whole diet approach identified epidemiologically, the chapters in this volume have identified food components such as polyphenols (Lamport and Keane, Chapter 10), herbs and botanicals (Scholey et al., Chapter 9) and omega 3 fatty acids (McNamara and Valentine, Chapter 7) as well as vitamins (de Jager and Ahmed, Chapter 8) which have been shown to confer cognitive benefits in short-term acute studies and longer term interventions across the lifespan and in young, healthy and older adults.

The role of glucose as the main neural fuel of the brain and the potential to influence glucose availability by modulating the glycaemic index of specific foods and food components as described by Sunram-Lea and colleagues (Chapter 6) is fundamental to our understanding of the impact of nutrition on cognition. The glycaemic properties of the whole diet and the modification of this by food choice or even ingenious food technological advances may be a fruitful avenue for public health interventions. The association of poor glucose regulation and the resultant states of ill health, impaired glucose tolerance and type 2 diabetes mellitus with obesity clearly underlines the importance of diet for health. Moreover, the demonstration of cognitive impairment along this trajectory of glucoregulation points to an important and worrying trend for physical and brain health. A number of systematic reviews of prospective studies of people with T2DM have suggested increased risk of dementia and Alzheimer's disease (Cukierman et al., 2005; Biessels, 2006). Recent studies have demonstrated impairment of hippocampal function, which is reflected by impairment in memory (Strachan et al., 1997; Lamport et al., 2014). Some of these impairments are evident in people with impaired glucose tolerance which precedes T2DM often by a period of years (Lamport et al., 2009, 2013, 2014).

Rates of obesity are increasing and are closely related to impaired glucose tolerance and the development of type 2 diabetes. The proportion of the adult English population that were overweight or obese increased from 58% to 65% in men and from 49% to 58% in women between 1993 and 2011 (the Health and Social Care Information Centre, 2013). The proportion of adults that were obese almost doubled in the same period (from 13% to 24% in men and from 16% to 26% in women). Although the United Kingdom has one of the highest rates of obesity in the Europe, Australia has recently overtaken the United States in incidence (WHO, 2014). Obesity, particularly in midlife, is associated with increased risk of cognitive impairment and the development of vascular dementia and Alzheimer's disease. This relationship has been found independently of age and co-morbidities such as T2DM, which is also associated with cognitive impairment (Profenno et al., 2010). Cross-sectional and longitudinal studies which compare obese and non-obese individuals generally show poorer performance in the obese across a range of cognitive domains (Elias et al., 2003, 2005; Gunstad et al., 2011). Specific decrements in memory (Gunstad et al., 2010, 2011, 2006), executive function (Gunstad et al., 2007; Fergenbaum et al., 2009) and complex attention and psychomotor processing speed (Cournot et al., 2006) have been reported, and it has been hypothesised that these may be due to pathophysiological mechanisms directly related to adiposity (Stanek and Gunstad, 2013). Whilst midlife adiposity is clearly critically related to the risk of dementia and Alzheimer's disease, recent evidence suggests that obese children and adolescents show cognitive and brain abnormalities (see Stanek and Gunstad, 2013 for a review) which could indicate a developmental trajectory, and hence research and early intervention in young people will be an important future priority. There is a clear and direct link between food intake and body weight, but the consequences of excessive body weight for cognitive function are only just beginning to be understood, and interventions which reduce obesity may well have beneficial effects on cognitive function.

The genomic tools described by Jose Ordovas (Chapter 3) have allowed us to identify genes involved in the regulation of glucose and lipid metabolism that are also associated with obesity and type 2 diabetes and cognitive impairment/Alzheimer's disease. Specifically, the allele *APOE4* is currently the most interesting candidate gene. GWAS has not led to the identification of many more alleles, but linking this genomic technology to brain imaging studies (discussed by Camfield and Scholey, Chapter 12) will provide a more integrated picture of genetic-behaviour links and allow us to test the impact of dietary interventions on cognition mediated by effects of these interventions on gene expression. For example, the BDNF gene is associated with cognitive function. Interventions with flavonoids increase the expression of BDNF in the hippocampus and induce changes in neuronal morphology detectable using MRI, with observable increases in cognitive function measured by suitable tests in the domain of memory.

We have considered existing methodologies (Ahmed and de Jager, Chapter 4) and new technologies (Camfield and Scholey, Ordovas in Chapters 12 and 3) and explored the potential for brain-level interventions which when combined with dietary interventions might confer even greater benefits for mental performance and psychological brain health in terms of effects on depression and mood (Teo, Chapter 11). These new methods help to elucidate mechanisms of action of nutrients on the brain and cognitive function and to confirm the validity of existing methods.

## 13.2 METHODOLOGICAL INNOVATIONS AND RECOMMENDATIONS FOR RESEARCHING THE NUTRITION–COGNITION RELATIONSHIP

The critical appraisal of the available evidence for specific nutrients, diets or approaches presented in this volume highlights the importance of the design and analysis of studies in this area. There is huge scope for innovation in the field of nutrition and cognition, building on some of the advances outlined in this volume and the adaptation of existing methods to enable us to develop our understanding of the mechanism by which nutrition can influence our cognitive and brain health. Such advances require sophistication in the measurement of cognitive function, the determination of mechanisms of action of the ingested nutrients, consideration of genetic predisposition and gene expression modulated by both diet and lifestyle. In addition, we can improve our study design and analysis strategies, our sharing of data and the added value that is conferred by systematic reviews and meta-analyses.

### 13.2.1 Measuring Cognitive Function

Uncovering the effects of nutrition on cognitive function and brain health requires the employment of sensitive tests to assess performance on a number of cognitive domains. The process and recommendations for this was described by Ahmed and de Jager (Chapter 4) in this volume. Cognitive tests which may be useful for screening dementia or for the measurement of stable traits are inappropriate for evaluating nutritional interventions. For example, the Mini–Mental State Examination (MMSE) is primarily a tool for identifying and diagnosing dementia (Folstein et al., 1975), unlikely to change in response to a nutritional intervention and not recommended as an outcome measure, especially in cognitively healthy populations, likely to show ceiling effects (de Jager et al., 2014). As discussed in Chapter 4, cognitive tests should be chosen on the basis of the hypothesised effect on a specific cognitive domain underpinned by plausible mechanism of action of the intervention.

The increased registration of nutritional trials on clinical trial databases (e.g. www.clinicaltrials.gov) and the growing insistence on open access and data sharing of studies funded by public bodies may present a valuable opportunity to inspect and verify data collection in such studies and to advance the methodology for the administration and analysis of cognitive test data. For example, norms based on age, gender and IQ of the samples tested on a wide variety of cognitive tests in nutritional interventions can be determined or improved, version equivalence of parallel forms of well used tests verified and more sophisticated analyses of existing datasets performed including systematic reviews and meta-analyses.

### 13.2.2 Measuring Mood

It is important to also consider the impact of diet or nutritional intervention on mood elucidated in the chapter by Polak and colleagues (Chapter 5). Mood may interact with objective performance (Hoyland et al., 2008) and be critical for engagement and motivation of participants in studies, particularly children (Hoyland et al., 2009). It is a valuable outcome measure in its own right. However, although often measured in studies of nutrient effects on cognitive function, few authors have linked this dependent variable directly with objective performance outcomes, probably due to a lack of statistical sophistication. There have been some exciting developments in the measurement of mood, for example, ecological momentary assessment and experience sampling (see Chapter 5 by Polak and colleagues and http://www.saa2009.org). These real-time data capture methodologies offer the capability to measure physiological processes concurrently with psychological functions and experiences such as hunger, mood and alertness in free-living situations. A future innovation will be to harness these techniques to aid our understanding and capacity to intervene effectively to promote mental and cognitive health, well-being and physical state.

### 13.2.3 Assessment of Dietary Intake

Valid and reliable measures of dietary intake and methods to characterise dietary patterns accurately and consistently are required. Several techniques are available for measuring habitual diet (e.g. food frequency questionnaires [FFQs], food diaries, dietary interviews, 24 h recall and doubly labelled water). A discussion of these approaches has been provided by Andreeva and Kesse-Guyot (Chapter 2) and future innovations in the area include apps which use mobile phone technology such as myfood24 and commercial food intake apps. Of course these technologies do not reduce the reactive effect of recording food intake but they do improve on the capture of intake data.

### 13.2.4 Sampling and Sample Selection

Volunteers for psychological research have been shown to differ from the general population in many ways (Rosenthal and Rosnow, 1975). Volunteers for dietary intervention studies are typically from populations who have a high degree of interest and knowledge regarding diet and health. They are more likely than the general population to consume high levels of specific nutrients, for example, flavonoids, or be regular breakfast or supplement consumers depending on the nature of the study and the way this is advertised. Consequently, they may be least likely to benefit from the intervention and samples should be screened and well characterised on the basis of their habitual diet. Other important participant characteristics which should be reported to allow accuracy between study comparisons and appropriate interpretation of findings include age, IQ, education, socio-economic status, mental health problems such as depression, smoking and type 2 diabetes (mentioned in Chapter 1). These characteristics can exert an influence on response to intervention, and failure to take this into account in the analysis may reduce the likelihood of observing the subtle effects that dietary interventions may have on cognitive outcomes.

Differences in samples' genetic profile could be one reason for variable effects in the studies reviewed. Ordovas has explained that the beneficial effects of some nutrients (in this case omega 3 fatty acids) on cognitive function are conferred only in those individuals who do not possess the *APOE4* allele. Given that those with *APOE4* are at greatest risk of cognitive decline, targeting this intervention at those with this genetic predisposition is unlikely to be beneficial. Certainly genotyping samples included in dietary studies would help to unravel more of the gene–diet interactions in the development of and diet-mediated prevention of cognitive decline. As yet unidentified genetic predispositions both to cognitive impairment and to nutrient responsivity may explain some failures to reject the null hypothesis.

### 13.2.5 Statistical Analysis

There are a number of areas where those examining nutrition–cognition relationships could improve their sensitivity to explain variance in the analyses which they perform. Most studies adopt the Neyman–Pearson approach testing the null hypothesis that there is no effect of a nutrient on the primary cognitive outcome. Many studies, however, do not identify a primary cognitive outcome, and cognitive measures may be added to a range of other, usually physical outcomes, for example, blood pressure and cholesterol. This means that the study may not have sufficient power to detect a change in a cognitive outcome resulting in a failure to reject the null hypothesis.

Detecting no effect on a measure of cognition following a nutritional intervention could mean that the intervention really does not influence the cognitive parameter measured. Alternatively, it could reflect a lack of sensitivity of that measure to small or subtle changes in performance. An effect may also fail to be detected because of inadequate power which is also related to the magnitude of the experimental effect or individual differences in the use of a scale which increase variability and decrease sensitivity of the measure. Null or inconsistent effects may also be attributable to the use of insensitive experimental designs (e.g. between subjects) or inappropriate selection of baseline measures and the failure to include these in the statistical analysis.

A null result may be due to a lack of sensitivity of the selected measure rather than a true absence of an effect. Two psychological tests of cognitive performance may claim to measure the same function, but it may be that only one is sufficiently sensitive to detect effects of a nutritional manipulation. It is feasible that commonly employed measures may be inadequate measures of cognitive function in relation to nutrient intervention and mask real effects. A lack of effect on some measures could be due to a subtle effect of a nutrient on only one component of the task, for example, reaction time which when computed into a composite score is no longer detected. Many studies have simply administered *off-the-shelf* tests and report the factor scores or summed components based on previous validation studies or factor analyses which are not based on the same populations in the same state, for example, following a nutritional intervention.

Appropriate analysis of data from studies where cognitive function is the outcome variable poses some unique problems. Even where participants can be randomised to nutrient or placebo interventions, it cannot be assumed that baseline measures will not differ and hence change from baseline or inclusion of baseline as a covariate is the recommended statistical approach. In these randomised studies, both ANOVA on change from baseline and ANCOVA with baseline as a covariate will be unbiased (van Breukelen, 2006). In nonrandomised studies where baseline differences may pre-exist, both methods may contradict each other since neither can be unbiased. Moreover, the overuse and over-interpretation of subgroup analyses poses further problems in this field (Pocock et al., 2002), as does the splitting of samples using median splits (Scott and Delaney, 1993).

The importance of controlling for lifestyle factors and other residual confounders to establish causal effects of nutrition on cognitive health cannot be underestimated. Many epidemiologically studied dietary patterns could reflect healthy lifestyle. For example, Devore et al. (2012) analysed data from the Nurses' Health Study and reported that higher polyphenol intake was associated with less cognitive decline than seen in nurses whose polyphenol intake was low. However, those consuming high levels of polyphenols were also more affluent and engaged in more physical activity. Similarly, despite finding a positive relationship between breakfast and academic outcomes, Adolphus et al. (2013) report presence of residual confounding which links breakfast consumption to other potentially beneficial behaviours linked to better academic performance.

## 13.3  THE FUTURE

It is clear from the range of nutritional interventions and dietary patterns considered in this volume that there is great potential for these to influence physical and psychological health. The field, however, is complex, and the consumer needs protection from unsubstantiated claims which purport and promise beneficial, sometimes even life-saving, effect of certain dietary supplements or practices, for which there is little evidence.

The European Food Safety Authority (EFSA) in Europe, the Food and Drug Administration in the United States and the Food Standards Australia New Zealand (FSANZ) all regulate and approve claims on foods. Key to claim approval is the establishment of a cause and effect relationship between consumption of a sufficiently characterised ingredient or food and a specified outcome and based on evidence from human randomised controlled trials and observational studies performed in the appropriate target population under specified conditions of use. Claims relating to nutrition and cognition are reviewed by the EFSA Panel on Dietetic Products, Nutrition and Allergies (NDA). EFSA issues guidance documents and publishes opinions, positive and negative, in the EFSA journal on the EFSA website http://ec.europa.eu/nuhclaims which has a search facility to view current authorised and rejected claims. Function claims are based on evidence which demonstrates that the intake of a food/constituent contributes to maintaining a physiological function or to improving a physiological function, for example, maintaining normal cognitive function with age. To date, about one in five claims submitted have been adopted. Claims for nutrients that have been approved in relation to cognition are summarised in the Table 13.1.

More than 30 claims relating to specific cognitive functions such as learning or memory have been rejected to date. Thus, one future development will be increased

## TABLE 13.1
## Summary of Approved Health Claims for Cognition

| Claim Term: Contributes to (Maintenance of) | | | | |
|---|---|---|---|---|
| Normal Nervous System Function | Normal Brain Function | Normal Cognitive Function | Brain/Cognitive Development | Mental Performance |
| Biotin | Carbohydrate | Iodine | DHA | Pantothenic acid |
| Riboflavin B2 | DHA | Iron | Folic acid | |
| B6 | | Water | | |
| B12 | | Zinc | | |
| Copper | | | | |
| Vitamin C | | | | |
| Iodine | | | | |
| Magnesium | | | | |
| Niacin | | | | |
| Potassium | | | | |
| Thiamine | | | | |

scientific activity which establishes the evidence for appropriate claims on food and food constituents. Another aspect will be the development of novel foods which confer health benefits on which such claims might be made. Such product innovation will require research to demonstrate the efficacy of new formulations or ingredients for physical and cognitive health.

As we learn more about the role of diet early and later in life in shaping and maintaining our cognitive functions as we age, it becomes apparent that there is much which is still unknown. Nutrition and other behaviours, such as physical activity, are modifiable lifestyle factors making them key public health targets for behaviour change interventions. An important challenge will be determining how best to implement such interventions to improve and maintain cognitive and brain health. This is critical in the light of the ageing population in the Western world, and how to achieve the prolongation of an active, healthy and independent life for the elderly represents a major challenge for society. A greater understanding and careful application of nutrition–cognition research could increase healthy life years and reduce costly disability life years associated with poor cognitive function, age-related memory impairment, dementia and Alzheimer's disease and the enormous social and psychological burden which they portend.

There is much about impact of diet on health and longevity which we do not yet understand and many unanswered questions. This volume has suggested new avenues to propel this field forward from new ways of evaluating, researching and recommending nutrition for brain health to the potential of genomic-based personalised nutrition. Nevertheless, there are many areas that a book of this type and length cannot consider but that is not to say that these are unimportant or do not play a role in *brain health*. Some of these potentially fruitful avenues of investigation are suggested in this book and others considered here in terms of future directions which the advancing techniques and technologies outlined in the book may enable us to soon explore.

## REFERENCES

Adolphus, K., Lawton, C.L., and Dye, L. (2013). The effects of breakfast on behaviour and academic performance in children and adolescents. *Frontiers in Human Neuroscience*: http://www.frontiersin.org/Human_Neuroscience/10.3389/fnhum.2013.00425/full#h1.

Biessels, G.J., Staekenborg, S., Brunner, E., Brayne, C., and Scheltens, P. (2006). Risk of dementia in diabetes mellitus: A systematic review. *Lancet Neurology*, 5(1):64–74.

Cournot, M., Marquié, J.C., Ansiau, D., Martinaud, C., Fonds, H., Ferrières, J. et al. (2006). Relation between body mass index and cognitive function in healthy middle-aged men and women. *Neurology*, 67:1208–1214.

Cukierman, T., Gerstein, H.C., and Williamson, J.D. (2005). Cognitive decline and dementia in diabetes – Systematic overview of prospective observational studies. *Diabetologia*, 48(12):2460–2469.

De Jager, C., de Bruin, E., Butler, L., Dye, L., Fletcher, J., Lamport, D. et al. (2014). Markers of cognitive function: Criteria for validation and considerations for investigating the effects of foods and nutrients. *Nutrition Reviews*, 72(3):162–179.

Devore, E.E., Kang, J.H., Breteler, M.M., and Grodstein, F. (2012). Dietary intakes of berries and flavonoids in relation to cognitive decline. *Annals of Neurology*, 72(1):135–143.

Elias, M.F., Elias, P.K., Sullivan, L.M., Wolf, P.A., and D'Agostino, R.B. (2003). Lower cognitive function in the presence of obesity and hypertension: The Framingham heart study. *International Journal of Obesity and Related Metabolic Disorders*, 7:260–268.

Elias, M.F., Elias, P.K., Sullivan, L.M., Wolf, P.A., and D'Agostino, R.B. (2005). Obesity, diabetes and cognitive deficit: The Framingham Heart Study. *Neurobiol Aging*, 26(Suppl. 1):11–16.

Fergenbaum, J.H., Bruce, S., Lou, W., Hanley, A.J., Greenwood, C., and Young, T.K. (2009). Obesity and lowered cognitive performance in a Canadian first nations population. *Obesity*, 17:1957–1963.

Folstein, M.F., Folstein, S.E., and McHugh, P.R. (1975). Mini-mental state. A practical method for grading the cognitive state of patients for the clinician. *Journal of Psychiatric Research*, 12(3):189–198.

Gunstad, J., Lhotsky, A., Wendell, C.R., Ferrucci, L., and Zonderman, A.B. (2010). Longitudinal examination of obesity and cognitive function: Results from the Baltimore longitudinal study of aging. *Neuroepidemiology*, 34:222–229.

Gunstad, J., Paul, R.H., Cohen, R.A., Tate, D.F., and Gordon, E. (2006). Obesity is associated with memory deficits in young and middle-aged adults. *Eating and Weight Disorders*, 11:15–19.

Gunstad, J., Paul, R.H., Cohen, R.A., Tate, D.F., Spitznagel, M.B., and Gordon, E. (2007). Elevated body mass index is associated with executive dysfunction in otherwise healthy adults. *Comprehensive Psychiatry*, 48:57–61.

Gunstad, J., Strain, G., Devlin, M., Wing, R., Cohen, R., Paul, R. et al. (2011). Improved memory function 12 weeks after bariatric surgery. *Surgery for Obesity and Related Diseases*, 7(4):465–472.

Hoyland, A., Dye, L., and Lawton, C.L. (2009). A systematic review of the effect of breakfast on the cognitive performance of children and adolescents. *Nutrition Research Reviews*, 22(2):220–243.

Hoyland, A., Lawton, C., and Dye, L. (2008). Acute effects of macronutrient manipulations on cognitive test performance in healthy young adults: A systematic research review. *Neuroscience & Biobehavioral Reviews*, 32:72–85.

Ivan, C.S., Seshadi, S., Beiser, A., Au, R., Kase, C.S., Kelly-Hayes, M., and Wolf, P.A. (2004). Dementia after stroke: The Framingham study. *Stroke*, 35: 1264–1268.

Kaluza, J., Wolk, A., and Larsson, S.C. (2012). Red meat consumption and risk of stroke: A meta-analysis of prospective studies. *Stroke*, 43(10):2556–2560.

Lamport, D.J., Dye, L., Mansfield, M.W., and Lawton, C.L. (2013). Acute glycaemic load breakfast manipulations do not attenuate cognitive impairments in adults with type 2 diabetes. *Clinical Nutrition*, 32(2), 265–272.

Lamport, D.J., Lawton, C.L., Mansfield, M.W., and Dye, L. (2009). Impairments in glucose tolerance can have a negative impact on cognitive function: A systematic research review. *Neuroscience & Biobehavioral Reviews*, 33(3):394–413.

Lamport, D.J., Lawton, C.L., Mansfield, M.W., Moulin, C.A., and Dye, L. (2014). Type 2 diabetes and impaired glucose tolerance are associated with word memory source monitoring recollection deficits but not simple recognition familiarity deficits following water, low glycaemic load, and high glycaemic load breakfasts. *Physiology & Behavior*, 124:54–60.

Pocock, S.J., Assmann, S.E., Enos, L.E., and Kasten, L.E. (2002). Subgroup analysis, covariate adjustment and baseline comparisons in clinical trial reporting: Current practice and problems. *Statistics in Medicine*, 21:2917–2930.

Profenno, L.A., Porsteinsson, A.P., and Faraone, S.V. (2010). Meta-analysis of Alzheimer's disease risk with obesity, diabetes, and related disorders. *Biological Psychiatry*, 67:505–512.

Psaltopoulou, T., Sergentanis, T.N., Panagiotakos, D.B., Sergentanis, I.N., Kosti, R., and Scarmeas, N. (2013). Mediterranean diet, stroke, cognitive impairment, and depression: A meta-analysis. *Annuals of Neurology*, 74(4):580–591.

Rees, K., Hartley, L., Flowers, N., Clarke, A., Hooper, L., Thorogood, M., and Stranges, S. (2013). 'Mediterranean' dietary pattern for the primary prevention of cardiovascular disease. *Cochrane Database of Systematic Reviews 2013*, Issue 8. Art. No.: CD009825.

Rosenthal, R. and Rosnow, R.L. (1975). *The Volunteer Subject*. John Wiley & Sons, New York.

Scott, M.E. and Delaney, H.D. (1993). Bivariate median splits and spurious statistical significance. *Psychological Bulletin*, 113(1):181–190.

Stanek, K.M. and Gunstad, J. (2013). Can bariatric surgery reduce risk of Alzheimer's disease? *Progress in Neuro-Psychopharmacology & Biological Psychiatry*, 47:135–139.

Strachan, M.W., Deary, I.J., Ewing, F.M., and Frier, B.M. (1997). Is type II diabetes associated with an increased risk of cognitive dysfunction? A critical review of published studies. *Diabetes Care*, 20(3):438–445.

The Health and Social Care Information Centre. (2013). *Statistics on Obesity, Physical Activity and Diet: England*. London, U.K. February 20, 2013, http://www.hscic.gov.uk/catalogue/PUB10364.

van Breukelen, G.J. (2006). ANCOVA versus change from baseline had more power in randomized studies and more bias in nonrandomized studies. *Journal of Clinical. Epidemiology*, 59:920–925.

World Health Organisation. (2014). *Overweight and Obesity Factsheet 311*. WHO, Geneva, Switzerland.

Zhu, L., Fratiglioni, L., Guo, Z., Agüero-Torres, H., Winblad, B., and Viitanen, M. (1998). Association of stroke with dementia, cognitive impairment, and functional disability in the very old: A population-based study. *Stroke*, 29: 2094–2099.

# Index

Printed in the United States
by Baker & Taylor Publisher Services